CAPD Update
Continuous Ambulatory Peritoneal Dialysis

CAPD Update

Continuous Ambulatory Peritoneal Dialysis

edited by

Jack W. Moncrief, M.D.
Austin Diagnostic Clinic
Austin, Texas

and

Robert P. Popovich, Ph.D.
Department of Chemical & Biomedical Engineering
The University of Texas at Austin
Austin, Texas

MODERN PROBLEMS IN KIDNEY DISEASE:
A SERIES SPONSORED BY THE NATIONAL KIDNEY
FOUNDATION

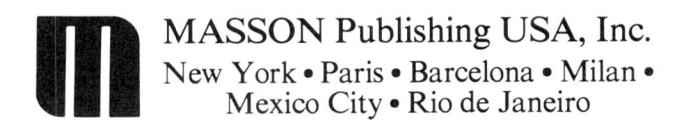

MASSON Publishing USA, Inc.
New York • Paris • Barcelona • Milan •
Mexico City • Rio de Janeiro

Library of Congress Cataloging in Publication Data
Main entry under title:

CAPD update.

   (Modern problems in kidney disease ; 1)
   "Proceedings of the CAPD International Symposium
II, May 9–10, 1980, Austin, Texas"—T.p. verso.
   Includes index.
   1. Peritoneal dialysis—Congresses. 2. Ambulatory
medical care—Congresses. I. Moncrief, Jack W.
II. Popovich, Robert P. III. CAPD International
Symposium (2nd : 1980 : Austin, Tex.) IV. Series.
   [DNLM: 1. Peritoneal dialysis. 2. Ambulatory care.
WJ 378 C236]
   RC901.7.P47C37   617'.461059   81-8260

ISBN 0-89352-134-5   AACR2

Proceedings of the CAPD International Symposium II, May 9–10, 1980, Austin, Texas

This publication was made possible by a grant from Travenol Laboratories, Inc., Deerfield, Illinois

Copyright © 1981 by Masson Publishing USA, Inc.

All rights reserved. No part of this book may be reproduced in any form,
by photostat, microform, retrieval system, or any other means, without the
prior written permission of the publisher.

ISBN 0-89352-134-5

Library of Congress Catalogue Card Number: 81-8260

Printed in the United States of America

FOREWORD

Continuous Ambulatory Peritoneal Dialysis is now four years old. Dialysis facilities around the world are engaged in the training and management of patients with End-Stage Renal Disease using this new modality. This is the 2nd International Symposium relating to CAPD; the first was held in Paris in November 1979. This symposium is designed as a discussion by physicians and nurses who have had various experiences and areas of interest relating to CAPD. It is organized to promote, up-date, and stimulate research. We appreciate the support of the following sponsors:

>Austin Diagnostic Clinic Foundation
>
>Department of Chemical Engineering
>The University of Texas at Austin
>
>National Kidney Foundation
>
>United Dialysis Services, Inc.
>
>Artificial Organs Division/Baxter
>Travenol Laboratories, Inc.
>
>American Kidney Fund

This book is published through the courtesies of the National Kidney Foundation. The editors are grateful to all the participants and special thanks must go to Betty Moncrief who did the real work.

CONTRIBUTORS

STEVEN R. ALEXANDER, M.D., *Assistant Professor in Pediatric Nephrology, Department of Pediatrics and Medical Director, CAPD Training Program, University of Oregon Health Sciences Center, Portland, Oregon.*

H. V. BAEYER, *Department of Nephrology, Freie Universität Berlin, Klinikum Charlottenburg, West Germany.*

JOHN WILLIAMSON BALFE, M.D., F.R.C.P.(C), *Associate Professor of Pediatrics, University of Toronto, Director of CAPD Program, The Hospital for Sick Children, Toronto, Canada.*

SHERRY BARLOW-SNEAD, R.D., *Renal Dietician, The Methodist Hospital, Community Dialysis Unit, Houston, Texas.*

H. BECKER, *Department of Nephrology, Freie Universität Berlin, Klinikum Charlottenburg, West Germany.*

JONAS BERGSTROM, M.D., *St. Erik's Hospital, Stockholm, Sweden.*

MICHAEL J. BLUMENKRANTZ, M.D., *Coordinator, Veterans Cooperative Dialysis Study and Associate Professor, UCLA School of Medicine, Los Angeles, California.*

B. BOROWZAK, *Department of Nephrology, Freie Universität Berlin, Klinikum Charlottenburg, West Germany.*

D. BRANA, M.D., *Military Central Hospital, Buenos Aires (1426), Argentina.*

LIDIA BRANDES, B.SC., *Research Assistant, Peritoneal Dialysis Unit, Toronto Western Hospital, Canada.*

HOWARD J. BURTON, M.SC., M.S.W., *Associate Director, The Health Care Research Unit, University of Western Ontario, London, Canada.*

VINCENZO CALDERARO, M.D., *Research Fellow, Peritoneal Dialysis Unit, Toronto Western Hopsital, Canada.*

ROBERT A. CAMPBELL, M.D., *Professor of Pediatrics and Chief, Section of Pediatric Nephrology, Department of Pediatrics, University of Oregon Health Sciences Center, Portland, Oregon.*

F. CANTAROVICH, M.D., *Military Central Hospital, Buenos Aires (1426), Argentina.*

DON CARMICHAEL, M.SC., *Department of Preventative Medicine-Biostatistic, University of Toronto, Canada.*

L. CASTRO, M.D., *Military Central Hospital, Buenos Aires (1426), Argentina.*

C. CHENA, M.D., *Military Central Hospital, Buenos Aires (1426), Argentina.*

JEAN NOEL COLLIN, PH.D., *Assistant, Department of Pharmacology, Groupe Hospitalier Pitié-Salpêtrière, Paris, France.*

JOHN A. CONLEY, B.SC., B.P.E., M.S.C. PH.D., *Project Director, The Health Care Research Unit, University of Western Ontario, London, Canada.*

C. CORREA, M.D., *Military Central Hospital, Buenos Aires (1426), Argentina.*

PETER O. CRASSWELLER, M.D., F.R.C.S., *Division of Urology, Toronto Western Hospital, Canada.*

MARY CUPIT, R.N., *Nursing Coordinator, CAPD Program, Lankenau Hospital, Philadelphia, Pennyslvania.*

JUAN FERNANDEZ DE CASTRO, M.D., *Head of Nephrology Department, Hospital "Valentin Gomez Farias," Guadalajara, Jal., Mexico.*

ALFIO DE MARTIN, M.D., *Assistant, Department of Nephrology, Groupe Hospitalier Pitié-Salpêtrière, Paris, France.*

HEWETT A. ELLIS, M.D., PH.D., F.R.C., PATH., *Reader in Pathology, University of Newcastle upon Tyne, England.*

PETER C. FARRELL, B.E. (Sydney), S.M. (MIT), PH.D. (Wash.), D.SC. (UNSW), *Director, Centre for Biomedical Engineering, University of New South Wales, Kensington, N.S.W. 2033.*

G. M. GAHL, *Department of Nephrology, Freie Universität Berlin, Klinikum Charlottenburg, West Germany.*

RAMAN GOKAL, M.B. CH.B., M.R.C.P., M.D., *Lecturer in Medicine, University of Newcastle upon Tyne, England.*

ENF. MARTHA GONZÁLEZ, *Nurse of the Dialysis Unit, Nephrology Department, Hospital de Especialidades, La Raza, Medical Center, I.M.S.S., Mexico 15, D.F.*

GUSTAVO GORDILLO PANIAGUA, M.D., *Head of Nephrology Department, Hospital Infantil de Mexico, Mexico D.F.*

LAZARO GOTLOIB, M.D., *Visiting Scientist, Division of Nephrology, Toronto Western Hospital, Canada.*

AGNES C. HAFF, M.S., *Division of Research, Lankenau Hospital, Philadelphia, Pennsylvania.*

HARRY HUSDAN, PH.D., *Director, Metabolic Renal Laboratory, Toronto Western Hospital, Canada.*

MARGARET-ANN IRWIN, R.N., R.M.N., B.SC., C.D.P., *Head Nurse, Dialysis Unit, The Hospital for Sick Children, Toronto, Canada.*

BRIGID JAYNES, R.N., *Staff Development Coordinator, The Methodist Hospital, Community Dialysis Unit, Houston, Texas.*

V. JULIANELLI, M.D., *Military Central Hospital, Buenos Aires (1426), Argentina.*

DAVID N.S. KERR, M.SC., F.R.C.P.(L), F.R.C.P.(E), *Professor of Medicine, University of Newcastle upon Tyne, England.*

M. KESSEL, *Department of Nephrology, Freie Universität Berlin, Klinikum Charlottenburg, West Germany.*

RAMESH KHANNA, M.D., *Renal Fellow, Division of Nephrology, Toronto Western Hospital, Canada.*

THOMAS F. KNIGHT, M.D., *Assistant Chief, Renal Metabolic Research Laboratory, Veterans Administration Medical Center and Assistant Professor of Medicine, Baylor College of Medicine, Houston, Texas 77211.*

EDWARD C. KOHAUT, M.D., *Associate Professor of Pediatrics, University of Alabama in Birmingham, Alabama.*

SOPHIA M. KOZAK, R.N., *Nursing Service, Veterans Administration Medical Center, Houston, Texas 77211.*

VICKI JO KRUGER, R.M.A., *Chief Technician CAPD, Acorn Research Laboratory and Austin Diagnostic Clinic, 3410 Owen, Austin, Texas 78705.*

CHRISTINE E. LACKE, P.A.-C, *Renal Section, Department of Internal Medicine, Veterans Administration Medical Center, Houston, Texas 77211.*

MARCEL LEGRAIN, M.D., *Professeur, Head of the Department of Nephrology, Groupe Hospitalier Pitié-Salpétrière, Paris, France.*

ROBERT M. LINDSAY, M.D., F.R.C.P.(E)., F.R.C.P.(C)., F.A.C.P., *Associate Professor of Medicine, University of Western Ontario, Director, Renal Unit, Victoria Hospital, London, Ontario, Canada.*

ALBERTO J. LOCATELLI, M.D., *Auxiliary Professor of Medicine U.N.B.A., Chief of Nephrology Division, Policlinico Metalurgico Central, Buenos Aires, Argentina.*

J. PÉREZ LOREDO, M.D., *Military Central Hospital, Buenos Aires (1426), Argentina.*

JEANNE LOVELL, R.N., *Supervisor, Peritoneal Dialysis, The Methodist Hospital, Community Dialysis Unit, Houston, Texas.*

JOHN F. MAHER, M.D., *Professor of Medicine, Uniformed Services University of the Health Sciences, Bethesda, Maryland.*

KRISTINE A. MAKSYM, R.N., B.S.N., *Nurse-Specialist in Pediatric Nephrology and Head Nurse, Continuous Ambulatory Peritoneal Dialysis Program, University of Oregon Health Sciences Center, Portland, Oregon.*

JAMES A. MAY, *Arizona/New Mexico Community Hemodialysis Services, Inc., 7351 East Osborn Road, Suite 200, Scottsdale, Arizona 85251.*

WILLIAM G. MCCREADY, M.B., M.R.C.P., *Renal Fellow, Peritoneal Dialysis Unit, Toronto Western Hospital, Canada.*

ERIC H. MEEMA, M.D., F.R.C.P.(C), *Professor of Radiology, Toronto Western Hospital, Canada.*

JACK W. MONCRIEF, M.D., *Acorn Research Laboratory and Austin Diagnostic Clinic, 3410 Owen, Austin, Texas 78705.*

FRANCISCO JAVIER MONTEÓNA RAMAS, M.D., *Nephrologist of the Dialysis Unit, Nephrology Department, Hospital de Especialidades, La Raza, Medical Center, I.M.S.S., Mexico 15, D.F.*

CAROL VIRGINIA MULLINS-BLACKSON, R.N., *Assistant Head Nurse CAPD, Acorn Research Laboratory and Austin Diagnostic Clinic, 3410 Owen, Austin, Texas 78705.*

KARL D. NOLPH, M.D., *Professor of Medicine and Director of Nephrology, University of Missouri Health Sciences Center and V.A. Hospital, Columbia, Missouri.*

RAYMOND OGILVIE, PH.D., *Director, Department of Biochemistry, Toronto Western Hospital, Canada.*

D.G. OREOPOULOS, M.D., PH.D., F.R.C.P.(C)., F.A.C.P., *Professor of Medicine, University of Toronto and Director, Peritoneal Dialysis Unit, Toronto Western Hospital, Canada.*

STEPHEN PERRY, M.S., *Assistant Administrator, The Children's Hospital, Birmingham, Alabama.*

R. P. POPOVICH, PH.D., *Biomedical Engineering Program, Chemical Engineering Department, The University of Texas at Austin, Austin, Texas.*

CRAIG G. PRICE, P.A., *The Methodist Hospital, Community Dialysis Unit, Houston, Texas.*

W. K. PYLE, PH.D., *Biomedical Engineering Program, Chemical Engineering Department, The University of Texas at Austin, Austin, Texas.*

CHARLOTTE QUINTON, R.N., *Home Peritoneal Dialysis Unit, Toronto Western Hospital, Canada.*

D. H. RANDERSON, B.E. (**Monash**), M.SC. PH.D. (**UNSW**), *Postdoctoral Fellow at Medical Klinikum Grosshardern, Munich, Federal Republic of Germany.*

GEORGE A. REICHARD, PH.D., *Director, Division of Biochemistry and Physiology, Division of Research, Lankenau Hospital, Philadelphia, Pennsylvania.*

M. REICHART, M.D., *Military Central Hospital, Buenos Aires (1426), Argentina.*

R. RIEDINGER, *Department of Nephrology, Freie Universität Berlin, Klinikum Charlottenburg, West Germany.*

HELEN RODELLA, B.SC., *Research Assistant, Peritoneal Dialysis Unit, Toronto Western Hospital, Canada.*

MARIA LUISA ROJAS CASTAÑEDA, *Biochemist of the Dialysis Laboratory, Nephrology Department, Hospital De Especialidades, La Raza, Medical Center, I.M.S.S., Mexico 15, D.F.*

D. ROSENTHAL, M.S., *Biomedical Engineering Program, Chemical Engineering Department, The University of Texas at Austin, Austin, Texas.*

JACQUES ROTTEMBOUR, M.D., *Chef de Clinque, Assistant Department of Nephrology, Groupe Hospitalier Pitié-Salpétrière, Paris, France.*

R. SCHURIG, *Department of Nephrology, Freie Universität Berlin, Klinikum Charlottenburg, West Germany.*

CHARLES R. SCHLEIFER, M.D., *Director, CAPD Program, Lankenau Hospital, Philadelphia, Pennsylvania.*

HARRY O. SENEKJIAN, M.D., *Assistant Chief, Dialysis Unit, Veterans Administration Medical Center, and Assistant Professor of Medicine, Baylor College of Medicine, Houston, Texas 77221.*

JAMES SHMERLING, M.S., *Administrative Assistant, The Children's Hospital, Birmingham, Alabama.*

MILES H. SIGLER, M.D., *F.A.C.P., Director, Division of Nephrology, Lankenau Hospital, Philadelphia, Pennsylvania.*

PAMELA SIMON, R.N., *Acorn Research Laboratory and Austin Diagnostic Clinic, 3410 Owen, Austin, Texas 78705.*

ERIC SINGLAS, PH.D., *Assistant, Department of Pharmacology, Groupe Hospitalier Pitié-Salpêtrière, Paris, France.*

MICHAEL I. SORKIN, M.D., *Assistant Professor of Medicine, University of Missouri Health Sciences Center, Columbia, Missouri.*

"P" ALICE JANE SORRELS, R.N., *Research Coordinator, Head Nurse CAPD, Acorn Research Laboratory and Austin Diagnostic Clinic, 3410 Owen, Austin, Texas 78705.*

WADI N. SUKI, M.D., *Professor of Medicine, Chief, Renal Section, Baylor College of Medicine and The Methodist Hospital, Houston, Texas.*

YESHAWANT B. TALWALKAR, M.D., *Associate Professor in Pediatric Nephrology, Department of Pediatrics, University of Oregon Health Sciences Center, Portland, Oregon.*

DISA K. TAUNTON, R.N., B.S.N., *Unit Director, Renal Unit, Oschsner Foundation Hospital, New Orleans, Louisiana.*

BRENDAN P. TEEHAN, M.D., F.A.C.P., *Director, Haverford Dialysis Unit, Lankenau Hospital, Philadelphia, Pennsylvania.*

J. TIZADO, B.CH., *Military Central Hospital, Buenos Aires (1426), Argentina.*

ALEJANDRO TREVIÑO BECERRA, M.D., *Chief of the Neprology Department, Hospital de Especialidades, La Raza, Medical Center, I.M.S.S., Mexico 15, D.F.*

CLEVERT H. TSENG, M.D., *Clinical Instructor in Pediatric Nephrology, Department of Pediatrics, University of Oregon Health Sciences Center, Portland, Oregon.*

STEPHEN VAS, M.D., PH.D., F.R.C.P.(C), *Chief, Department of Medical Microbiology, and Professor of Medicine, Toronto Western Hospital, Canada.*

MARIA DEL PILAR VELÁZQUEZ, *Nurse of the Dialysis Unit, Nephrology Department, Hospital de Especialidades, La Raza, Medical Center, I.M.S.S., Mexico 15, D.F.*

J. VERNETTI, M.D., *Military Central Hospital, Buenos Aires (1426), Argentina.*

FERNANDO VILLARROEL, PH.D., *Division Director, Bureau of Medical Devices, Food and drug Administration, Silver Spring, Maryland 20910.*

MICHAEL K. WARD, M.B., CH.B., M.R.C.P., *Consultant Physician, Royal Victoria Infirmary, Newcastle upon Tyne, England.*

EDWARD J. WEINMAN, M.D., *Chief, Renal Section, Veterans Administration Medical Center and Professor of Medicine, Baylor College of Medicine, Houston, Texas 77211.*

GEORGE WELLS, M.SC., *Health Care Research Unit, University of Western Ontario, London, Canada.*

R. WILBERG, M.D., *Military Central Hospital, Buenos Aires (1426), Argentina.*

ROBERT J. WINEMAN, PH.D., *Program Director, Chronic Renal Disease Program, National Institute of Arthritis, Metabolism and Digestive Diseases, National Institutes of Health, Bethesda, Maryland 20205.*

GABOR G. ZELLERMAN, M.S.B.I.D., ENG., *President, Accurate Surgical Instrument Co., Toronto, Canada.*

CONTENTS

Foreword		v
Contributors		vii

Peritoneal Dialysis International Resurgence

1	**Peritoneal Dialysis and The National Institutes of Health** F. Villarroel, R. J. Wineman	1
2	**CAPD International Symposium, Paris 1979** M. Legrain	7
3	**Early CAPD Experiences in Patients Originally Treated with Intermittent Peritoneal Dialysis** A. Treviño, F. J. Monteóná, M. L. Rojas, M. P. Velazquez, M. González	11
4	**The Future of Chronic Ambulatory Peritoneal Dialysis in Guadalajara, Jalisco, Mexico** J. F. de Castro, G. G. Paniagua	19
5	**Factors Affecting a Continuous Ambulatory Peritoneal Dialysis (CAPD) Program** A. J. Locatelli	23
6	**ESRD: An Unclear Future in the USA** J. A. May	27

Kinetics of Peritoneal Dialysis—Adults and Children

7	**Peritoneal Transport Evaluation in CAPD** W. K. Pyle, J. W. Moncrief, R. P. Popovich	35
8	**Blood Flow to the Peritoneum: Physiological and Pharmacological Influences** J. F. Maher	53
9	**Pharmacokinetics of Co-Trimoxazole Using the Peritoneal Route: Consequence for the Treatment of Peritonitis in Patients Maintained on Peritoneal Dialysis** E. Singlas, J. Rottembourg, A. de Martin, J. N. Collin, M. Legrain	63

xiv Contents

| 10 | **Peritoneal Dialysis Limitations and Continuous Ambulatory Peritoneal Dialysis**
K. D. Nolph, M. I. Sorkin | 67 |
| 11 | **Metabolite Generation and Clearance Variation in Long-Term CAPD**
D. H. Randerson, P. C. Farrell | 75 |

Nutrition

12	**CAPD: Nutritional Concerns—Have We Learned from the Experiences in the 1960s and 1970s?** M. J. Blumenkrantz	83
13	**Caloric Intake and Nitrogen Balance in Patients Undergoing CAPD** G. M. Gahl, H. v. Baeyer, R. Riedinger, B. Borowzak, R. Schurig, H. Becker, M. Kessel	87
14	**Acid-Base Studies in Continuous Ambulatory Peritoneal Dialysis** B. P. Teehan, G. A. Reichard, M. H. Sigler, C. R. Schleifer, M. C. Cupit, A. C. Haff	95
15	**Finding the Uremic Molecule(s)** J. Bergström	103

Solutions

16	**Further Experience with the Use of Amino Acid Containing Dialysate (Amino-Dianeal) in Peritoneal Dialysis** D. G. Oreopoulos, J. W. Balfe, R. Khanna, P. Crassweller, L. Gotloib, H. Rodella, G. Zellerman, L. Brandes, W. McCready, R. Ogilvie, H. Husdan	109
17	**Additives in CAPD** F. Cantarovich, J. Pérez Loredo, C. Chena, M. Reichart, J. Tizado, L. Castro, K. Brana, V. Julianelli	117
18	**CAPD: Three Daily Exchanges** F. Cantarovich, J. Pérez Loredo, C. Chena, R. Wilberg, J. Vernetti, C. Correa, J. Tizado	125

Clinical Application

| 19 | **The Initiation of a CAPD Program**
D. K. Taunton | 133 |
| 20 | **The Quality of Life of the CAPD Patient**
"P" A. J. Sorrels, C. Mullins-Blackson, J. W. Moncrief, R. P. Popovich | 135 |

Contents xv

21	Peritoneal Catheter Complications in CAPD Patients C. Lacke, S. M. Kozak, H. O. Senekjian, T. F. Knight, E. J. Weinman	139
22	Hypertriglyceridemia, Diabetes Mellitus, and Insulin Administration in Patients Undergoing Continuous Ambulatory Peritoneal Dialysis J. W. Moncrief, W. K. Pyle, P. Simon, R. P. Popovich	143
23	New Materials "P" A. J. Sorrels, V. Kruger, J. W. Moncrief, R. P. Popovich	167
24	A Comparison of CAPD and Hemodialysis in Adaptation to Home Dialysis R. M. Lindsay, D. G. Oreopoulos, H. Burton, J. Conley, G. Wells	171
25	Chronic Intermittent and Continuous Ambulatory Peritoneal Dialysis: A Comparison W. N. Suki, S. Barlow-Snead, C. G. Price, B. Jaynes, J. Lovell	181

CAPD in Children

26	Cost and Social Benefits of CAPD in a Pediatric Population J. Shmerling, E. Kohaut, S. Perry	189
27	Clinical Parameters in Continuous Ambulatory Peritoneal Dialysis for Infants and Children S. R. Alexander, C. H. Tseng, K. A. Maksym, R. A. Campbell, Y. B. Talwalkar, E. C. Kohaut	195
28.	An Assessment of Continuous Ambulatory Peritoneal Dialysis (CAPD) in Children J. W. Balfe, M.-A. Irwin, D. G. Oreopoulos	211
29	Ultrafiltration in the Young Patient on CAPD E. C. Kohaut, S. R. Alexander	221
30	Kinetics of Peritoneal Dialysis in Children R. P. Popovich, W. K. Pyle, D. A. Rosenthal, S. R. Alexander, J. W. Balfe, J. W. Moncrief	227

Bone Disease

31	Renal Osteodystrophy in Patients on Continuous Ambulatory Peritoneal Dialysis (CAPD): A Biochemical and Radiological Study V. Calderaro, D. G. Oreopoulos, E. H. Meema, R. Khanna, S. Quinton, D. Carmichael	243
32	Histological Renal Bone Disease in Patients on Continuous Ambulatory Peritoneal Dialysis R. Gokal, H. A. Ellis, M. K. Ward, D. N. S. Kerr	249

Peritonitis

33	**Treatment of *Candida* Peritonitis with Peritoneal Lavage** M. J. Blumenkrantz	253
34	**Treatment of Peritonitis (in Patients on CAPD)** D. G. Oreopoulos, S. Vas, R. Khanna	259
35	**Diagnosis and Treatment of Peritonitis** K. D. Nolph, M. I. Sorkin	265
	Index	273

CHAPTER ONE

Peritoneal Dialysis and The National Institutes of Health

FERNANDO VILLARROEL, Ph.D.

ROBERT J. WINEMAN, Ph.D.

THE MILESTONES IN THE DEVELOPMENT OF PERITONEAL DIALYSIS as maintenance therapy for chronic uremic patients occurred almost simultaneously with other achievements that permitted the development of modern hemodialysis. Extracorporeal technology, however, lent itself more readily to engineering improvements that permitted higher solute and fluid removal rates. These latter made hemodialysis a more attractive mode of treatment and diminished the implementation of peritoneal dialysis.

Recent developments have created the potential for a broader application of peritoneal dialysis to a degree not anticipated a few years ago. Contemporary peritoneal dialysis with its innovations holds a potential for becoming a more widespread and important mode of therapy for the maintenance of chronic renal disease patients. Nevertheless, well-controlled clinical trials are necessary for adequate assessment of its benefits and risks. Further research is needed to resolve a number of technical and scientific aspects of peritoneal dialysis. Among such unresolved issues are: incidence and cause of complications; immunological status of patients; nutritional status, including effects upon glucose and lipid metabolism; effects on the pediatric age group, especially upon growth and maturation; parathormone and calcium and homeostasis; acid/base balance; development of alternative osmotic agents, and long-term effects on peritoneal transport.

The National Institutes of Health (NIH) has supported research and development in the field of peritoneal dialysis for more than 15 years. NIH's support contributed to many of the important developments in this field, from

---

Bureau of Medical Devices, Food and Drug Administration, U.S. Department of Health and Human Services, Silver Spring, Maryland
National Institute of Arthritis, Metabolism, and Digestive Diseases, National Institutes of Health, Bethesda, Maryland

2   CAPD Update

the reverse osmosis dialysate delivery equipment begun in 1970 to continuous ambulatory peritoneal dialysis (CAPD) started in 1976. Studies sponsored by NIH also include the development of a sorbent-type peritoneal dialysis machine, which is undergoing clinical trials currently; theoretical studies of physiological transport parameters and mathematical modeling; comparisons between hemodialysis and peritoneal dialysis; application of drugs for the enhancement of peritoneal mass transfer; microcirculation studies related to peritoneal mass transfer mechanisms; and manipulation of peritoneal dialysis regimens in order to augment its efficiency.

Most of NIH's support has been funded by the National Institute of Arthritis, Metabolism, and Digestive Diseases (NIAMDD). A modest, but significant, amount of funding for studies of peritoneal dialysis has been provided by the NIH Division of Research Resources through the General Clinical Research Centers (GCRC). The impact of NIH support on peritoneal dialysis research and development could be evaluated by reviewing the results obtained from NIH supported projects, but it is evident in the reports submitted for presentation at scientific meetings and in the literature. The relationship of NIH's funding to the over-all peritoneal dialysis research activity of the scientific community will be presented here.

METHODOLOGY

A comparison of consecutive annual funding levels with the annual number of publications in this field, during the period 1971 through 1979, has been

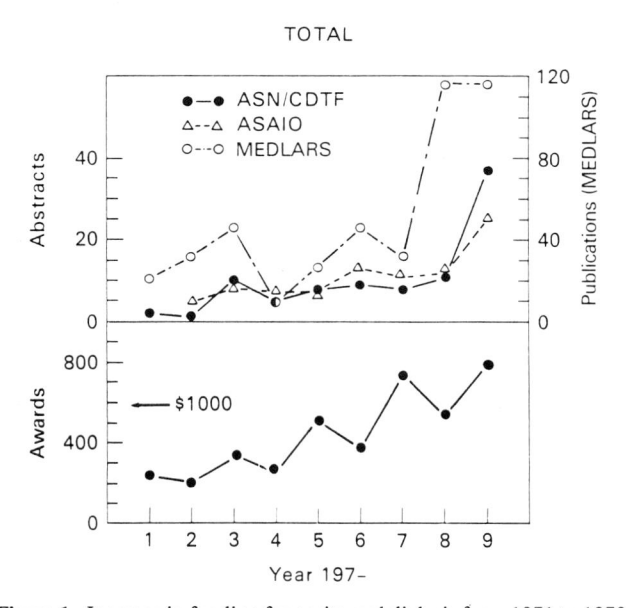

Figure 1. Increase in funding for peritoneal dialysis from 1971 to 1979.

made as an assessment of NIH's impact on peritoneal dialysis research. Three groups of publications were selected as indices of research productivity: (1) abstracts submitted to the American Society of Nephrology and to the Clinical Dialysis and Transplant Forum (ASN/CDTF), (2) abstracts submitted to the American Society of Artificial Internal Organs (ASAIO), and (3) a computerized literature search from the National Library of Medicine (MEDLARS). The authors felt that the two sources of abstracts would provide a general indication of the level of activity in this area. The MEDLARS literature search, on the other hand, would be somewhat affected by the evaluation of peer reviewers.

The peritoneal dialysis research field was subdivided arbitrarily into four categories: Group I—Solute Kinetics and Mathematical Modeling; Group II—Dialysate, Equipment and Access; Group III—Patient Response and Complications; and Group IV—Metabolism and Balance Studies. Publications, as well as the NIH level of funding, were analyzed in total, as well as for each individual group.

RESULTS

The funding and publications data are presented in Figures 1–4. Awards were distributed mostly among Groups I, II, and III; practically no funds were allocated directly to Group IV. The majority of the publications and abstracts covered in this analysis were from authors who received no NIH support.

Figure 1 shows a steady increase in funding for peritoneal dialysis from

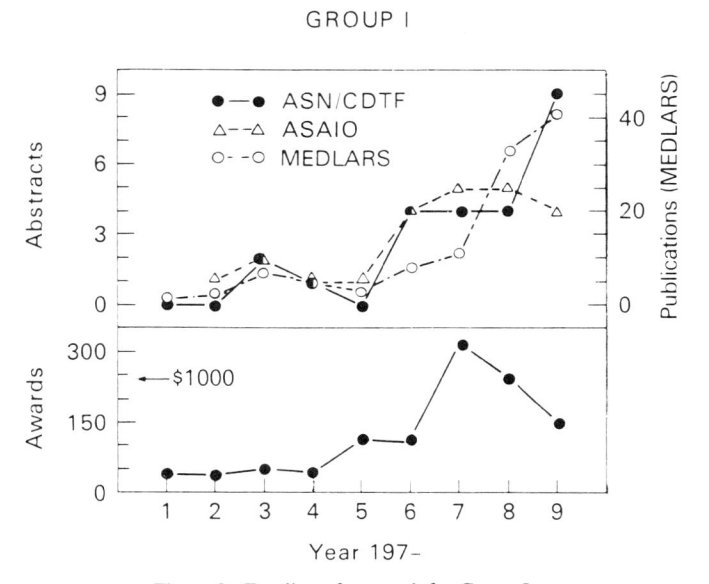

Figure 2. Funding of research for Group I.

1971 to 1979, with funding increasing approximately fourfold during this period. The number of abstracts and publications experienced a twofold increase from 1971 through 1977. However, within the last 3 years, there has been a fourfold increase in publications about peritoneal dialysis. In 1976, as a result of a request for proposal, NIAMDD issued several awards in the area of peritoneal dialysis.

Funding of research for Group I, shown in Figure 2, doubled in 1975, and again in 1977. The number of publications increased in consonance with this increase in research support. Since 1977, funding of this area of peritoneal dialysis research has declined steadily through 1979.

Funding of research for Group II, shown in Figure 3, has remained fairly constant over several years. Within the last 2 years of the analysis period, it has diminished markedly. Publications in this area have remained relatively constant, except for a slight increase in the number of abstracts in 1978 and 1979.

Group III, shown in Figure 4, received the largest allocation of research funds. The response observed in the publications curve appears to reflect well the funding activity.

Very few publications were found in the area covered by Group IV, an area lacking significant NIH support during the period of observation. For these reasons, no graphic representation of Group IV is included.

An important element in increasing publication activity was the advent of CAPD in 1976. Since 1976, CAPD has received continuous support from NIH, with special emphasis in 1978 and 1979. Abstracts related to CAPD have increased steadily, numbering almost 50% of the peritoneal dialysis

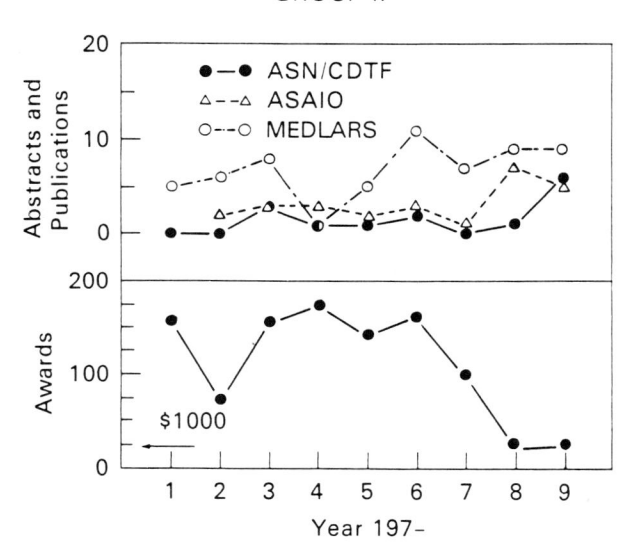

Figure 3. Funding of research for Group II.

Peritoneal Dialysis 5

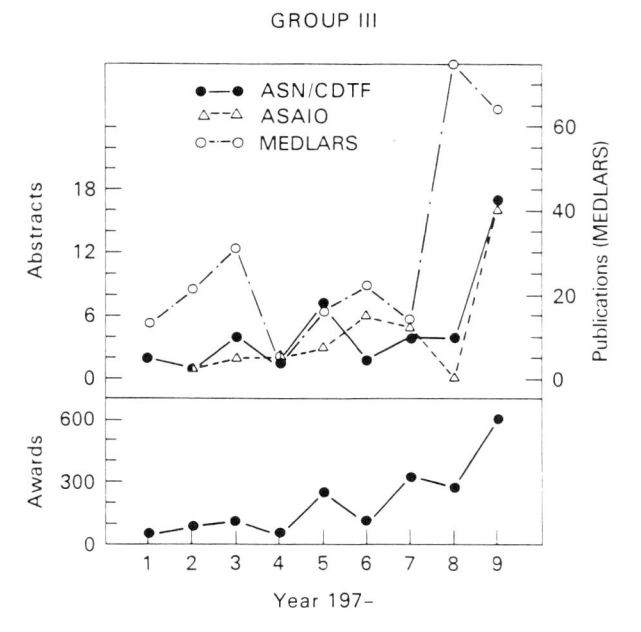

Figure 4. Funding of research for Group IV.

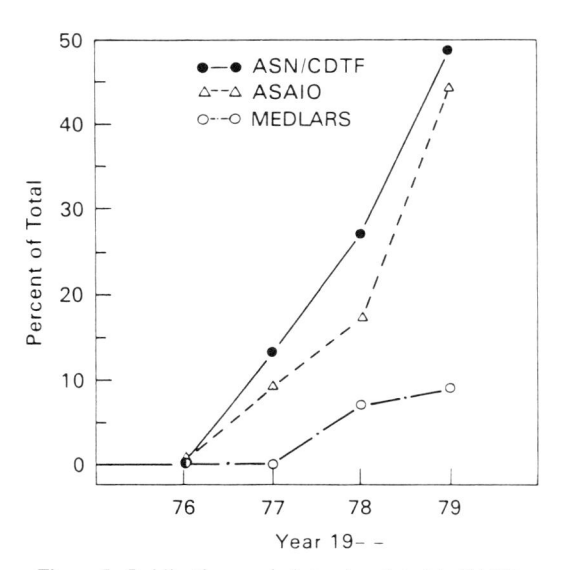

Figure 5. Publications and abstracts related to CAPD.

abstracts published in 1979, as shown in Figure 5. The MEDLARS publication search shows a more modest but significant increase in 1979.

CONCLUSIONS

Based on this analysis, one may conclude that NIH funding of research in peritoneal dialysis has had a significant impact within the time period of observation. It is apparent that this impact on research activity has extended beyond the boundary encompassing the research directly supported by NIH.

It is interesting to note that the area of Metabolism and Balance Studies (Group IV) has received little encouragement from NIH and has been neglected by the scientific community in general. It appears logical to assume that this area will become more important now than CAPD is assuming importance as a maintenance therapy for chronic uremic patients. The future support of this area of research by NIH will be primarily by investigator-initiated research grants.

ACKNOWLEDGMENT

The views expressed here are the authors' own. No official support or endorsement by the Department of Health and Human Services is intended nor should be inferred.

CHAPTER TWO

CAPD International Symposium, Paris 1979

MARCEL LEGRAIN, M.D.

SINCE 1976, CONTINUOUS AMBULATORY PERITONEAL DIALYSIS (CAPD) has opened up a new era in the treatment of chronic renal insufficiency. At the end of 1979 about 1,000 patients with end-stage renal failure had been treated with CAPD mainly in Canada, the United States, and Western Europe. The purpose of the Symposium was to present to a highly qualified audience a critical appraisal of CAPD based upon experimental work and clinical results concerning quality of life, morbidity and mortality rates, real costs, etc. Such information is indeed required in order to offer to physicians and patients the guidelines on which to base a free and well-informed treatment of choice to the benefit of each individual case.

As Chairman of the first CAPD International Symposium[1] initiated and sponsored by Travenol Laboratories, it was a real pleasure and honor to welcome in Paris on November 2 and 3, 1979, the pioneers of CAPD: J. Moncrief, R. Popovich, K. Nolph, and D. Oreopoulos as well as the world's experts involved in the development of this technique. All authors and participants in the discussions must be congratulated on the originality and quality of the data presented dealing with all aspects of a stimulating topic: life with plastic bags.

The first session chaired by K. Nolph was entirely devoted to *anatomy, physiology, and kinetics of peritoneal transport* during peritoneal dialysis. A better understanding of the physiology of the peritoneum and of the mesenteric microcirculation is expected to be reached in the coming years. K. Nolph summarizes the characteristics of the peritoneal resistances to solute movement as follows:

> "Peritoneal capillary walls offer some resistance to movement of larger solutes, such as protein.
> Capillaries are still more permeable than standard cellulosic membranes.

Service de Néphrologie, Groupe Hospitalier Pitié-Salpêtrière, 75013 Paris, France

The peritoneal interstitium may be a major site for all solute movements. Intraperitoneal fluid films also contribute to resistance.

There is probably no major capillary blood flow limitation. Total pore area may be relatively small because of low number of capillaries."

Dr. Wayland from the California Institute of Technology underlined through his elegant studies, including three-dimensional computer reconstruction of the peritoneum wall, the possibly important role played by the state of hydration of the tissue lining the peritoneal cavity and stressed the importance of a better knowledge of factors controlling the permeability both of the mesothelium and of the microvascular walls. Augmentation of peritoneal clearances by drugs was discussed by Dr. Maher. With intermittent peritoneal dialysis, many drugs have proved to be effective using either the intraperitoneal or the intravenous route. Data on patients on CAPD are lacking but, as stated by Nolph during the discussion, if an augmentating agent acting in the low molecular weight range is used, large solute clearances and protein losses will also increase. To reduce protein leak the idea of adding a vasoconstrictor to the solutions has been considered.

Technical requirements dealing with fluids, bags, lines, and connectors were discussed during the session chaired by F. Boen. New and safer designs are expected in the near future. "Connectology" is already an active research field, everyone being aware that appropriate material is critical if the risk of peritoneal infection is to be kept to a minimum. Different types of catheters and connectors were presented at the Symposium. Definitely, a longer follow-up and well-controlled clinical studies are required to allow conclusions on what is best for a given patient.

The conditions of a good training program have been carefully reviewed during the session chaired by J.W. Moncrief. Organizational aspects, medical and nurse staffing, and costs were discussed according to the large experience of that pioneer group. As for any dialysis technique, the role of the Head Nurse is essential. The reports of Barbara Prowant, Sheila Clayton, and "Poppy" Sorrels received a warm reception. The data presented illustrated different training approaches and the necessary flexibility of any CAPD home training program in relation to each case. Hospitalization is not compulsory and outpatient training is routinely performed in Austin and other centers. A two-bed unit allows a training capacity of 30 patients per year.

Medical management of patients on CAPD looks simple. Nevertheless, as stated by C.M. Gahl, Chairman of the session devoted to this topic, careful follow-up is required to avoid infections and vascular and metabolic complications in relation with the technique. Well-trained and dedicated staff are a requisite to a successful CAPD program.

Prevention of *peritonitis* is the cornerstone for an extension of CAPD as the treatment of first choice for a large number of patients. Appropriate technology and careful selection and training of patients are the main factors in mastering this delicate problem. Some technical improvements are expected. A bacteriological filter in the dialysate infusion line has been presented by C. Mion and co-workers. Routine use of this equipment seems to reduce the incidence of peritonitis, which should, according to over-all agreement, be less than one per patient-year. Cause of peritonitis is mainly bacterial infection but may be also the consequence of fungal and opportunistic contamination of the fluid. Adequate diagnosis may require a thorough bacteriological examination, including broth culture and concentrative procedure. A small number of bacteria are, in some cases, present in the peritoneal fluid. The proportion of sterile peritonitis varies greatly from one group to another, being not more than 4.3% in Oreopoulos' group in Toronto, whereas it is about 50% in Australia. Various causes have been emphasized. The possible role of acetate solution and providone-iodine contamination has been considered.

Early detection and emergency treatment should provide a rapid cure of peritonitis and reduce the duration of hospitalization. Home treatment of mild forms is performed by Nolph. Continuous lavage is advocated by most investigators as the first procedure of treatment in association with administration of antibiotics, using the systemic and/or intraperitoneal route. Successful use of co-trimoxazole added to the dialysate followed by oral complementary therapy has been reported by J. Rottembourg. Reduction of peritoneal clearance after a few episodes of peritonitis was considered as unlikely by all participants but has been reported in relation with subacute peritoneal infection.

Besides peritonitis, *various complications* have been reported, including occlusive episodes, severe hypotension, hernia, and abdominal and lumbar pain.

Potential metabolic problems were carefully investigated and discussed during the session chaired by J. Bergström. It should be pointed out that the length of follow-up and the number of patients treated with CAPD for more than a year do not permit, as yet, a definitive evaluation of the long-term metabolic consequences of CAPD.

Poor nutritional status can be encountered if food intake is inadequate for various reasons. Peritonitis can lead some patients to a critical situation aggravated by high protein losses in the dialysate. Surprisingly, a daily protein loss of around 10 g through the dialysate does not induce a nephrotic syndrome and all groups are reporting serum albumin levels in the low normal range. P. Fürst has reported normal plasma-free amino acid concentration in spite of losses of protein and amino acid by the peritoneal route.

The continuous glucose supply represents a unique situation. Although advantageous from a nutritional point of view in some undernourished patients, it may also be harmful. Obesity, plasma lipid abnormalities with high levels of triglycerides, low concentration of high density lipoproteins, and high concentration of very low density lipoproteins have been reported. Prevention of such disorders by adequate regimen and use of amino acids in the dialysate as an osmotic agent instead of glucose has been discussed. Dialysate with amino acids raises many still unsolved questions from a technical, metabolic, and financial point of view.

The hemoglobin level commonly rises even in bilateraly nephrectomized patients, during the first 3 months of treatment with CAPD, and levels off thereafter over the next 7 months. A decline of hemoglobin level has been reported by Oreopoulos after the 10th month of treatment.

As far as *indications* are concerned, various opinions were given. A small group believed, with Oreopoulos, that CAPD could be the treatment of first choice except if contraindications, such as uncooperative patients, various hernias, preexisting lumbar disc, and congenital hypertriglyceridemias, are present. In most units the selection criteria for CAPD remains essentially negative. Most of the patients treated with this method belong to the older age group or represent cases in whom other methods, either dialysis or transplantation, have either failed or are partly or totally contraindicated. Comparative studies performed in Ontario by Lindsay and collaborators have shown that among young patients "young males holding down a demanding job may be best treated by hemodialysis while the young female with a family may prefer CAPD." *Diabetics* can be excellent candidates and an improved control of diabetes has been reported by different groups. Insulin can be given through the peritoneal route. As outlined by C.T. Flynn, CAPD offers to dialysed diabetics a unique possibility of both self-care and home care. The rate of peritonitis does not seem to be more frequent in these patients than in those without diabetes mellitus.

Early experience of some groups treating *children,* including very young ones, has been encouraging. Definite effect of CAPD on growth is not yet available. Transplantation can be performed without particular problems even in patients who have presented with peritonitis. Peritoneal dialysis has been used when necessary after transplantation.

Survival data at 1 and 2 years involving large series of patients are not yet available. The death and drop-out rates remain high, around 30% at 1 year in many series. Such figures are not surprising if one considers the mean age and the negative selection of patients treated with CAPD in most centers. Nevertheless the first results presented before and during the Symposium raised a "cynical critique" of CAPD by Shaldon who stated that data currently available do not justify widespread use of the technique.

Major discrepancies in the proportions in which different methods including CAPD are used to treat terminal renal failure are observed in different countries. Prospective evaluation of various types of treatment is always difficult and hazardous. In any case the expected extension of the CAPD program should not preclude the development of other therapeutic facilities, since the total number of uremic patients requiring treatment will increase in the coming years.

Data presented during the Symposium have convinced all participants, if necessary, that CAPD is "here to stay," but more time is required to define clearly the shortcomings and advantages of the method when compared to other standard dialysis techniques. We personally believe that patient compliance will remain the major limiting factor to a large extension of CAPD. Whatever the future may be, the nephrologist is already amazed and happy that "life with plastic bags" has already offered to many patients with end-stage renal failure an unexpected feeling of well-being and freedom.

Reference

1. Legrain, M., Ed.: *CAPD: Proceedings of an International Symposium.* Excerpta Medica, Amsterdam, 1980.

CHAPTER THREE

Early CAPD Experiences in Patients Originally Treated with Intermittent Peritoneal Dialysis

ALEJANDRO TREVIÑO, M.D.

FRANCISCO JAVIER MONTEÓNÁ, M.D.

MARÍA LUISA ROJAS

MARÍA DEL PILAR VELÁZQUEZ

MARTHA GONZÁLEZ

INTRODUCTION

RECENT RESEARCH AND DEVELOPMENT OF PERITONEAL DIALYSIS have brought new interest into the traditional uremic treatments. Extracorporeal dialysis and renal transplant have certain limitations and in some places their use is not as widespread as in the developed countries. Because of this fact, we are greatly interested in the progress of continuous ambulatory peritoneal dialysis (CAPD).[1-5] Our dialytic peritoneal program had been changed in the last 12 months; first, becasue of the availability of soft catheters and second, because of the semiautomatic peritoneal dialysis machine. But even with these new developments our peritoneal treatment had been quite short and limited to hospital patients.[6] Our results obtained with intermittent peritoneal dialysis had been as good as those obtained in other places but limited to a few selected patients.

At the beginning of this year and with great confidence and expectations, we started a CAPD program on patients who had been subjected previously to intermittent dialytic treatment. It is necessary to say that the population group that attends our hospital does not have good living conditions because of low income. So patients that we are dealing with are not the same as those in other countries that have started CAPD.[7]

Departamento de Nefrología, Hospital de Especialidades, Centro Médico La Raza, I.M.S.S., México

MATERIALS AND METHODS

Our hospital's dialysis unit was started a year ago with six patients on hemodialysis and later on peritoneal dialysis with indwelling Tenckhoff catheters. Data of patients of this study are shown in Table 1. We included eight patients, four from each sex, ages ranging from 20 to 53 years, average 38.5. Causes for chronic renal failure were: four cases of glomerulonephritis, two cases of pyelonephritis, one case each of gout nephropathy and polycystic disease (Table 1). The Silastic, 2 band Dacron Tenckhoff catheter is inserted by microlaparotomy making a 4-cm infroumbilical incision dissecting to the peritoneum that is incised to introduce the catheter, pulling out the distal end through a contralateral opening. Once the catheter is in place and functional in the abdominal wall, the patient is referred from the operating theater to the dialysis unit to start treatment using a semiautomatic machine. Dialysate volume was 2,000 ml of standard solution for the first 72 hours, rechanging every 8 hours adding 2,000 of heparin and 250 mg of cephalosporin each exchange. Initially patients received intermittent peritoneal dialysis, from 3 to 8 months three times a week, with a total of 30 exchanges of 2 liters per week. They received a diet of 80 g of protein, 1,500 ml of fluid, 3 g of calcium chloride, and only occasionally vitamins.

With the availability of 2-liter peritoneal dialysis plastic bags, since January 1980, we started training patients for CAPD. Once the patients finished the 2-week training course, treatment was continued at home and patients came to the outpatient department every 2 weeks to be checked and for their material supply. Then monthly appointments were made. Our CAPD schedule consists of four exchanges in 24 hours, at 7, 12, 17, and 22 hours. The last exchange of 1 liter is left in the abdominal cavity overnight.

TABLE 1.

Patients in Treatment with Intermitent Peritoneal Dialysis and Continuous Ambulatory Peritoneal Dialysis

Name	Sex	Age	Number of IPD Procedures	Antiquity in CAPD (Weeks)
1. P.E.L.	M	49	1,008[b]	14
2. E.G.J.	F	53	73	16
3. T.Z.E.	M	32	47	16
4. T.M.M.	F	42	42	15
5. P.R.M.	M	20	10	16
6. Z.M.C.	F	50	15	8
7. R.D.M.	F	30	10	8
8. P.C.A.	M	33	10	8
9. H.G.M.L.[a]	F	36	42	5
10. P.V.J.[a]	M	21	45	2

[a] Catheter removed.
[b] Dialysis at home.

Patients are dialyzed 6 days a week. A comparative study was made of serum values of urea, creatinine, sodium, potassium, calcium, phosphorus, and albumin on samples obtained every 2 weeks, also before starting treatment with peritoneal dialysis, with intermittent peritoneal dialysis, and on CAPD. Weight and blood pressure were also recorded. For statistical studies of mean values Student's t-test was used.

RESULTS

The Tenckhoff catheter was left in place from 2 to 12 months, average 6.25 months. In patients 9 and 10 the catheter had to be removed because of peritonitis after 9 and 6 months of treatment. This gives a total of 1,400 days/catheter, 1,215 intermittent peritoneal dialysis procedures, and 107 patient-weeks on CAPD. We had seven cases of peritonitis; two patients on intermittent peritoneal dialysis and five patients on continuous ambulatory peritoneal dialysis. That represents 0.9% days/per dialysis. In four cases the etiological agent was *Staphylococcus epidermidis,* in two cases, *Staphylococcus aureus,* and in one case there was no bacterial growth. In those two cases in which the catheter had to be removed, the causal agent was enterobacter and *Proteus* and the patients did not respond to treatment. Five peritonitis episodes were observed in four patients. Case 4 has been free of infection for 8 months.[4,8]

Improvement in the biochemical conditions of these patients was observed and the following values were obtained: urea in the first dialysis was 306 ± 68.2, in intermittent peritoneal dialysis, 235.9 ± 56.4, and with CAPD, a reduction to 134.75 ± 53.9 mg% ($p < 0.01$). Creatinine in the first dialysis was 21.05 ± 2.7, decreasing on intermittent peritoneal dialysis to 16.9 ± 3.64

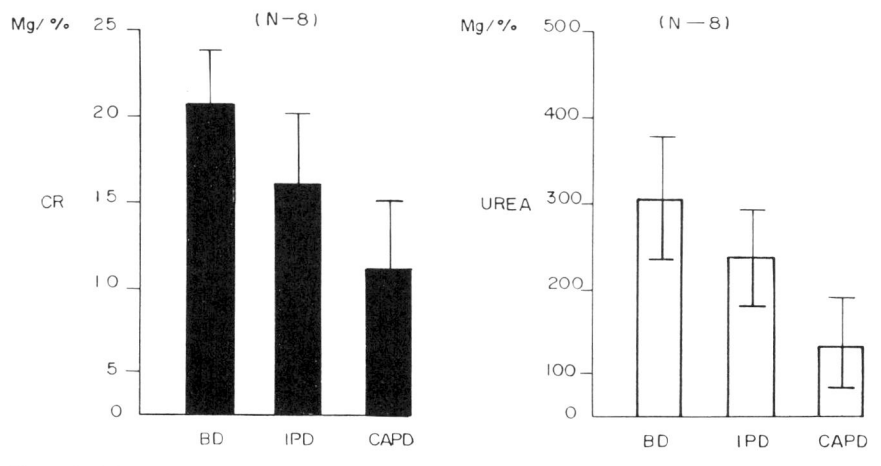

Figure 1. Mean serum values of creatinine and urea on patients before dialysis (BD), intermittent peritoneal dialysis (IPD), and continuous ambulatory peritoneal dialysis (CAPD).

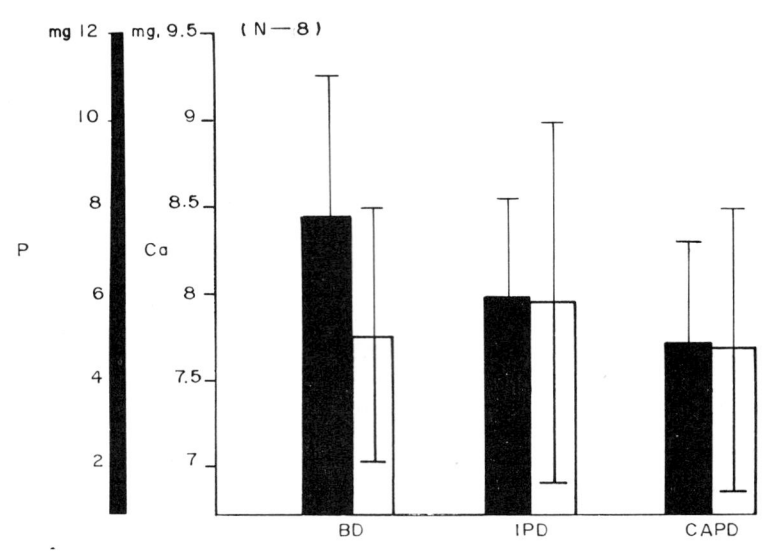

Figure 2. Mean serum values of phosphorus and calcium on patients before dialysis (BD), intermittent peritoneal dialysis (IPD), and continuous ambulatory peritoneal dialysis (CAPD).

and even more on CAPD, to 11.1 ± 3.87 mg% ($p < 0.001$) (Fig. 1). Phosphorus showed a significant decrease, from first dialysis, 7.78 ± 3.25, to intermittent peritoneal dialysis, 5.95 ± 2.35, and in CAPD, 4.94 ± 2.45 mg% ($p < 0.001$). Calcium levels did not show statistically significant changes. First dialysis was 7.75 ± 0.77, on intermittent peritoneal dialysis, 7.88 ± 1.19, and in CAPD, 7.7 ± 0.82 mg% (Fig. 2). Sodium levels showed significant increase within normal ranges, due to a better control of extracellular fluid. Average in the first dialysis was 138.6 ± 3.5 mEq/liter, in intermittent peritoneal dialysis, 135 ± 6.74, and in CAPD, 140.5 ± 3.02, keeping it steadier ($p < 0.05$). Potassium values did not show statistically significant

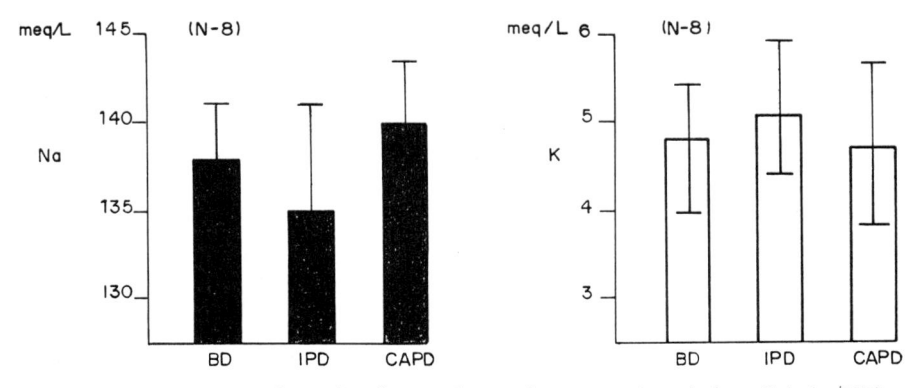

Figure 3. Mean serum values of sodium and potassium on patients before dialysis (BD), intermittent peritoneal dialysis (IPD), and continuous ambulatory peritoneal dialysis (CAPD).

variance, as can be seen in Figure 3, in spite of the fact that there was an increase in potassium intake from 50 to 60 mEq/day. Serum potassium levels remained in normal range from 3.7 to 5.7 mEq/liter (Fig. 3).

Serum albumin showed a significant decrease in patients on CAPD, 2.75 ± 0.86, as compared to values obtained in the first dialysis of 3.6 ± 0.7 mg% ($p < 0.02$) (Fig. 4). No statistically significant changes were observed in body weight and blood pressure levels in spite of edema reduction, except that there was an increase in lean tissue (Fig. 5). We noticed better patient hematocrit with mean values of 30 mg%. Patients did not require blood transfusion. Control of blood pressure was improved, therefore requiring less hypotensive agents, and the hypotensive drugs were discontinued in four patients.

DISCUSSION

As soon as we had the necessary equipment (plastic bags) ready 4 months ago, we started a CAPD program. Our data shown here show primarily that it is possible to maintain patients with CAPD in our environment. Patients were easily transferred from intermittent peritoneal dialysis when biochemical and hemodynamic stabilization had been obtained to treatment with CAPD.

Our results showed that patients improved from one treatment to the other, obtaining a reduction on urea levels, from 235.9 ± 56.4 to 134.75 ± 53.9

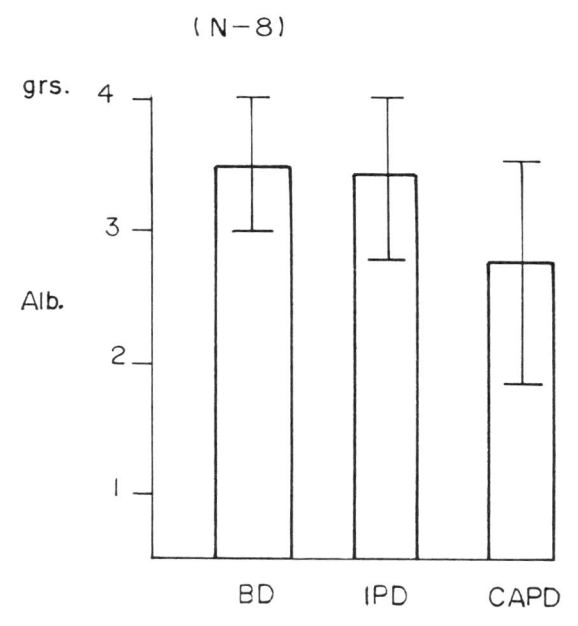

Figure 4. Mean serum values of albumin in patients before dialysis (BD), intermittent peritoneal dialysis (IPD), and continuous ambulatory peritoneal dialysis (CAPD).

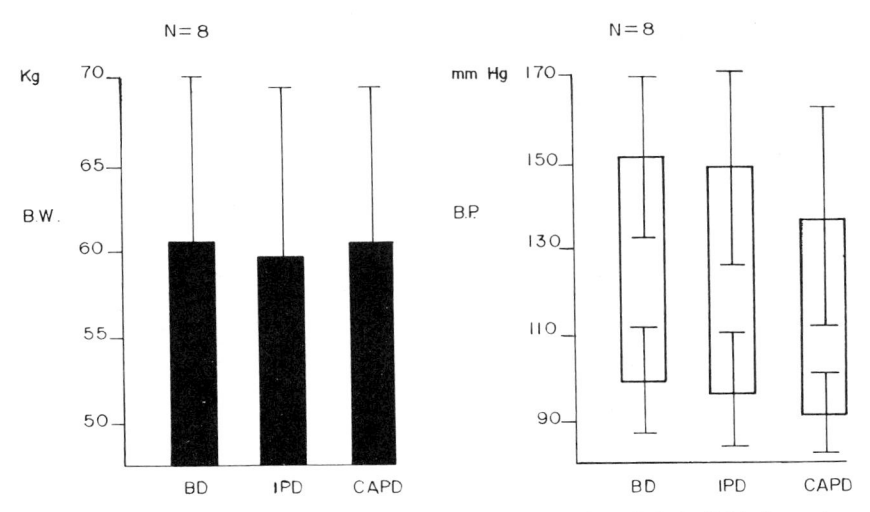

Figure 5. Mean body weight and blood pressure of patients before dialysis (BD), intermittent peritoneal dialysis (IPD), and continuous ambulatory peritoneal dialysis (CAPD).

mg%, and creatinine levels were reduced from 16.9 ± 3.64 to 11.1 ± 3.87 mg% ($p < 0.001$). Sodium was stabilized in average values of 140.5 mEq/liter with a better regulation of sodium chloride and fluid balance preventing water retention, which resulted in a better blood pressure control. Other biochemical parameters that show the correction of alterations observed in the uremic syndrome are values of phosphorus, 4.94 ± 1.45 mg%; calcium, 7.7 ± 0.82 mg%; potassium, 4.75 ± 0.97 mEq/liter. Nutritional behavior in these patients showed that a stable lean body weight was obtained. Albumin levels decreased to adequate figures, 2.75 ± 0.86 g% and hematocrit was stable at 30 mg%. No transfusions were required.

This analysis shows that CAPD is useful to control uremia in patients in end-stage chronic renal failure, allowing a better correction of urea, creatinine, and phosphorus levels; likewise, there is better control of blood pressure, body weight, hematocrit, sodium, and calcium.

Among complications, albumin loss is easily controlled by an adequate intake of protein that, as a matter of fact, is practically a normal diet. Peritonitis episodes have been few and transient, though quite severe in patients 4 and 10, making catheter removal necessary. Those two patients died even though they were put on hemodialysis treatment.

These results are obtained with greater simplicity, less cost, and more acquiescence from the patient because of the feeling of welfare and freedom experienced.

Finally, we feel that the possibility of treatment of patients by means of CAPD will decrease the great hospital load that chronic uremic patients represent, at the same time giving them a therapeutic regimen that will maintain them in better condition than with any other type of dialysis regimen.[9-11]

ACKNOWLEDGMENTS

We are indebted to Ramón Paniagua, M.D., for his technical assistance.

References

1. Boen, S. T.: Overview and history of peritoneal dialysis. *Dial Transplant* **6:** 12–18, 1977.
2. Popovich, R. P., Moncrief, J. W., Decherd, J. F., Pyle, W. K., Morris, S., and Lindley, J.D.: Clinical development of the low dialysis clearance hypothesis via equilibrium peritoneal dialysis. *Proc Annu Contractor's Conf Artif Kidney-Chronic Uremia Prog (NIAMDD)* **10:** 123–125, 1977.
3. Burton, B. T.: End-stage renal disease: Better treatment at lower cost. *Ann Intern Med* **88:** 567–568, 1978.
4. Oreopoulos, D. G.: Maintenance peritoneal dialysis. In *Strategy in Renal Failure*, E. A. Friedman, Ed. John Wiley & Sons, New York, 1978, pp. 393–414.
5. Popovich, R. P., Moncrief, J. W., Nolph, K. D., Ghods, A. J., Twardowski, Z. P., and Pyle, M. K.: Continuous ambulatory peritoneal dialysis. *Ann Intern Med* **88:** 444–56, 1978.
6. Erbessd, L. M., Treviño, B. A., Zúñiga, V., Almeida M., González, L., and Velázquez, J.: Aspectos biopsicosociales de pacientes con insuficiencia renal crónica en la zona norte del valle de México (in press).
7. Tenckhoff, H.: Home peritoneal dialysis. In *Clinical Aspects of Uremia and Dialysis*, S. G. Massry and A. L. Sellers, Eds. Charles C Thomas, Springfield, Ill., 1976, pp. 583–615.
8. Rubin, J., Rogers, W. A., Taylor, H. M., Everett, E. D., Prowant, B. F. Fruto, L. V., and Nolph, K. D.: Peritonitis during continuous ambulatory peritoneal dialysis. *Ann Intern Med* **92:** 7–12, 1980.
9. Friedman, E. A., Deland, B. G., and Butt, K. M. H.: Pragmatic realities in uremia therapy. *N Engl J Med* **298:** 368–371, 1978.
10. Oreopoulos, D. G.: Letter to editor. *N Engl J Med* **302:** 755, 1980.
11. Treviño, B. A.: Does extracorporeal dialysis dissapear?. *J Dial*, 1978.

CHAPTER FOUR

The Future of Chronic Ambulatory Peritoneal Dialysis in Guadalajara, Jalisco, Mexico

JUAN FERNANDEZ DE CASTRO, M.D.

GUSTAVO GORDILLO PANIAGUA, M.D.

CHRONIC RENAL FAILURE, which is the terminal stage of progressive renal failure, is present mainly in the young adults at the time they are in the most productive stage of their lives (Table 1).[1]

There is a variable period of time between the onset of chronic renal failure and its terminal phase. The dietary regimens and symptomatic therapeutics (antihypertensives, diuretics) for some years might control the situation until the progressive loss of nephrones cannot be compensated for and the use of dialysis becomes necessary to maintain homeostasis. During this period, the patient usually declines in physical activity until he becomes an invalid with mental depression, anorexia, and chronic malnutrition.

Regardless of the definite rehabilitation program chosen, these patients require the use of dialysis to prevent progressive physical damage and keep them in good condition in order to be prepared for renal transplantation and to be able to continue with their normal activities, which will consequently help restore their emotional stability. Chronic hemodialysis (HD) programs have tried to resolve this problem, and in countries where the government is in charge of supplying this service to all uremic patients, the success rate for these programs has been higher. However, the same result is not observed in those countries where there is no match between the technological development available and the social and cultural level of the patients.

In Guadalajara there are 30 artificial kidneys available, but only 35 patients are now in the chronic HD program. This is a very small percentage

---

Hospital Regional Dr. Valentin Gomez Farias, Guadalajara, Jalisco, Mexico
Hospital Infantil de Mexico, Mexico

19

TABLE 1.

Causes of Chronic Renal Failure in Adults

Glomerulonephritis	43.4%
Pyelonephritis	19.8%
Cystic kidney disease	8.4%
Renal vascular disease	4.9%
Drug-induced nephropathy	3.2%

(Reprinted with permission from Gurland et al.: Combined report on regular dialysis and transplantation in Europe, Proc Euro Dial Transplant Assoc **13:** 3, 1975.)

of patients when considering that for the 2,000,000 inhabitants in Guadalajara, approximately 100–150 uremic patients[2] die annually (Table 2). This reveals mainly that only a few uremic patients are able to afford hemodialysis and shows the economic and cultural inability in Guadalajara to supply this therapeutic measure to all uremic patients needing it.

The advent of chronic peritoneal dialysis with its intermittent modalities and, even better, continuous ambulatory peritoneal dialysis (CAPD) might radically change this situation. It is convenient to discuss briefly some advantages of CAPD in relation to chronic HD so that we can further establish which procedure is the more indicated for an economically limited system with few possiblities for resolving the clinical problem with renal transplantation.

ECONOMIC ASPECTS

In the Regional Hospital for Government Employees (ISSSTE) HD has a monthly net cost of $700 per patient and CAPD has less than $400. Of course, the possibilities of realizing both procedures are equally feasible but in this circumstance there is greater freedom for those patients on CAPD for attending school and work than for those on HD.

MEDICAL ASPECTS

Patients under CAPD have more dietary alternatives than with HD. As we have observed, the former are able to stabilize their blood pressure within normal limits which indicates the absence of hypervolemia. Thus, these patients are more assured of maintaining a good state of nutrition. Also their

TABLE 2.

Use of Hemodialysis in Guadalajara

Population	Uremic Patients/Year	On Chronic Dialysis	Kidney Machines
>2,000,000	100–150	35	30

anemia improves, since there are no losses through vascular access, not even during the procedure. Furthermore, with CAPD we can maintain their serum metabolites closer to normal levels.

Although the side effects are greater with HD than with CAPD, we must point out the risk of peritonitis, which becomes more likely with the number of connections and with the resting periods of CAPD. However, the use of collapsible plastic bags and of the titanium adaptor for the catheter has decreased the risk of infection. The tube that connects the bags with the catheter can remain unchanged for a month. The patient only needs to touch the bags when he changes them in order to be connected to the tube. Under the circumstances, it can be assured that in a place like Guadalajara and with the cultural background of Mexican uremic patients CAPD is the proper selection that requires less training time, is less expensive, and gives better possibilities of performance, with less risk for the patients.

References

1. Gurland, H. J., Brunner, F. P., Chantler, C., Jacobs, C, Schrarer, K., Selwood, N. H., Spies, G., and Wing, A. J.: Combined report on regular dialysis and transplantation in Europe. *Proc Eur Dial Transplant Assoc* **13**: 3, 1975.
2. Delano, B. G.: Realities of home hemodialysis. *Urology* **1**: 620, 1973.

CHAPTER FIVE

Factors Affecting a Continuous Ambulatory Peritoneal Dialysis (CAPD) Program

ALBERTO J. LOCATELLI, M.D.

CAPD IS A NEW MODALITY of peritoneal dialysis developed by Popovich and Moncrief[1] in Austin, which began a new era[2] in the treatment of ESRD. It utilizes the capacity of the peritoneal membrane to purify middle and large molecules with low dialysate flow rate, avoiding humoral fluctuations, without machines, and without any dietetic restrictions. In September 1978, a program of CAPD was begun at the Policlínico Metalúgico Central in Buenos Aires.[3]

This experience was obtained on 12 patients with an average of 207 patient-weeks. This first period showed a high rate of peritonitis: one episode every 9 patient-weeks. This incidence is similar to the one obtained by Popovich and Moncrief,[4] who used glass containers. We have used semirigid plastic bags of 1 liter each, with tubings of difficult handling.

When empty, the bags were lying on the abdominal wall fastened by a cloth belt. In general the patients showed a similar evolution to that of Moncrief[5] and Oreopoulos[6] with reference to urea and creatinine values, decrease of oral aluminum hydroxide, and antihypertensive drugs; the most common complication was orthostatic hypotension.

Obviously our main problem was the high incidence of peritonitis, especially gram-negative bacteria (11 of 23 episodes). This was why seven patients were transferred to hemodialysis. The development of CAPD in the last 2 years in the United States[7] and Canada[8] has shown an important decrease in the number of episodes of peritonitis up to one each 10 patient-months. This was possible with a new technology by means of 2-liter plastic bags, exchanges of dialysate four times a day, and simpler and safer tubings. In accordance with the experience obtained all over the world in CAPD, some

---

Policlínico Metalúrgico Central, Buenos Aires, Argentina

factors should be taken into account to start a program of CAPD, above all in developing countries.

TECHNICAL ASPECTS

Due to technological improvement, new bags and tubings are available nowadays. Moreover it will be of high risk to start a program without these systems for connection and disconnection.

PHYSICAL AND PERSONNEL REQUIREMENTS

This matter has been well described by Moncrief[7] and Oreopoulos.[9] I would like to make some comments. It is important that members of the staff who will start patient training believe in CAPD and transmit their feeling to the patients. They should discuss all technical problems according to standardizing the technique. In view of the social situation in developing countries the social worker is an essential member of the staff, reporting about the family environment and prospective patients' habitat.

PATIENT SELECTION CRITERION

It is more important to take into account patients' cooperation and carefulness instead of their intelligence. A social worker's report is also valuable in the selection process.

CONCLUSIONS

We agree with the idea that CAPD will probably be the treatment of choice for most patients suffering from ESRD. With new technology, high incidence of peritonitis has been reduced and in the near future it would be comparable to the level attained with intermittent peritoneal dialysis. In order to include new patients in the plan, it is important to keep one's mind on the previously mentioned factors.

CAPD allows an almost endless variety of tactics to improve efficiency and interest.

References

1. Popovich, R. P., Moncrief, J. W., Decherd, J. F., Bomar, J. B., and Pyle, W. K.: The definition of a novel portable/wearable equilibrium peritoneal dialysis technique. *Abstr Trans Am Soc Artif Intern Organs* **5**: 64, 1976.
2. Robson, M. D., and Oreopoulos, D. G.: Continuous ambulatory peritoneal dialysis. A revolution in the treatment of chronic renal failure. *Dial Transplant* **7**: 999, 1978.
3. Locatelli, A., de Benedetti, L., Chena, C., Montero, J. M., and Ryba, J.: Continuous

ambulatory peritoneal dialysis. Fourth Latin American Congress of Nephrology, May 20–24, 1979.
4. Popovich, R. P., Moncrief, J. W., Nolph, K. D., *et al*.: Continuous ambulatory peritoneal dialysis. *Ann Intern Med* **88**: 449, 1978.
5. Moncrief, J. W.: Continuous ambulatory peritoneal dialysis. *Dial Transplant* **7**: 809, 1978.
6. Oreopoulos, D. G., Robson, M., Izatts, et al.: A simple and safe technique for continuous ambulatory peritoneal dialysis (CAPD). *Trans Am Soc Artif Intern Organs* **24**: 484, 1978.
7. Moncrief, J. W.: Continuous ambulatory peritoneal dialysis. *Dial Transplant* **8**: 1077, 1979.
8. Oreopoulos, D. G.: Peritoneal dialysis is here to stay. *Nephron* **24** (1): 7–9, 1979.
9. Oreopoulos, D. G.: Requirements for the organization of a continuous ambulatory peritoneal dialysis program. *Nephron* **24**(6): 261–263, 1979.

CHAPTER SIX

ESRD: An Unclear Future in the USA

JAMES A. MAY, B.S.

AS I TRAVEL THE NATION consulting with the owners and executives of dialysis facilities and centers, their primary concerns seem to be:

1. What is happening in Baltimore and why can't we get any answers?
2. Are they really going to reduce the reimbursement rate?
3. Don't they understand that the way costs are rising there will soon be no margin left and facilities may well be forced out of business?
4. Don't they care what happens to the patient?

Perhaps I can shed some light on these queries.

First, it is doubtful that anyone in the bureaucracy in Baltimore or Washington understands what is really happening financially in the end-stage renal disease (ESRD) arena. The United States government is groping for solutions to the financial problems.

Even though some of the bureaucrats deny it, others have openly suggested that the current ESRD program is the pilot project for national health care. If this is so, then the bureaucracy must also control and contain the costs of the program if the movement toward national health care is to gain momentum. Even so, the office of ESRD in Baltimore has been in chaos for some time now. Let me illustrate:

In November 1978, Eugene Rubel announced at the American Society of Nephrology (ASN) meeting in New Orleans that a new reimbursement for self-care dialysis was to take place immediately. Facilities would be paid 75% of their current screen, receiving, of course, only 80% of that reduced amount from the Health Care Financing Administration (HCFA). Apparently, someone in the bureaucracy erroneously felt that self-dialysis was significantly less costly than staff-assisted dialysis. The Renal Physicians Association, the Network Forum, and many individuals and organizations enlightened Mr. Rubel and his associates, and the order was rescinded. However, it was replaced by a self-dialysis reimbursement methodology that, although not economically disastrous to the facilities, was ill advised.

Arizona/New Mexico Community Hemodialysis Services, Inc., Scottsdale, Arizona

During that same month, I met with Mr. Rubel in his Washington office. We discussed the concept of a national flat rate for all outpatient maintenance dialysis and whether the ESRD Branch in Baltimore should be strengthened and become somewhat autonomous, or simply be absorbed into the other bureaus. I suspect that my recommendations did not differ from others made to him and we witnessed the organization of the new Office of End Stage Renal Disease with Phil Jos returning to become the Director and reporting directly to Gene Rubel, now Director of the Office of Special Programs.

During this time period, the decision was made to establish one national reimbursement rate for both centers and facilities, to introduce a significant reduction in the screen. In mid-June 1979 I met with several ESRD officials and was informed that the new screen would probably be $123, but it could be as high as $129. I encouraged them to resist pressures from the higher echelons of the Department of Health, Education and Welfare (HEW) for a significant reduction of the screen.

On June 25, 1979, approximately 15 individuals, representing various organizations involved in ESRD, attended a special meeting in Baltimore. At that time, Mr. Rubel announced the new screen of $129, which, according to the statement of officials present, was derived as the mean reported cost for dialysis facilities: The higher costs of centers were not considered in the study. Since facilities represented about 50% of the total, that meant that only 25% of the centers and facilities reported that they could operate at a cost of $129 or less.

We are all aware of the chaos that was apparently precipitated by this announcement:

1. Many reacted swiftly to reverse this new screen.
2. Mr. Rubel announced his resignation.
3. He was replaced a few months later by his Deputy Director, who lasted only a few weeks in that position.
4. Lela Carp resigned.
5. Stanley Weintraub and Michael McMullen were reassigned.
6. Mr. Edmund Kelly, Deputy Director of Health Standards and Quality Bureau (HSQB), became the acting director of the Office of Special Programs.
7. "A large well-established facility" in the east was audited by the Inspector General's office, which then questioned the accuracy of the cost reports submitted by that facility on a voluntary basis.
8. The office of Inspector General audited several more facilities.
9. A new, but lower screen was proposed by high-level HEW officials.
10. The office of ESRD seemingly was relieved of more and more authority and the officers therein were apparently used as input resources rather than in decision making.
11. Phil Jos resigned.
12. A highly secretive document proposing new "incentive rates," including methodology and possible dollar amounts, was prepared and submitted to the Secretary of HEW for approval and publication in the Federal Register.

Now what are the developments of the past few weeks?

1. Ray Brown has resigned.
2. Cor Denian has been reassigned and the Division of Network Administration has been abolished. This responsibility now belongs to the Professional Standards Review Organization project officers at each regional office.
3. Various ESRD functions have been reassigned to other existing agencies within HCFA bureaus.
4. What is left of the office of ESRD is to remain under the Director of the Office of Special Programs.
5. Mr. Kelly expects to return to his primary duties as Deputy Director of HSQB early in 1981.

Now what about the proposed "incentive reimbursement" package?

Surely, we are all aware of the enormous controversy resultant from the various attempts by the bureaucracy to implement a reimbursement plan based on this provision of PL 95-292, which states:

> "Such regulations shall provide for the implementation of appropriate incentives for encouraging more efficient and effective delivery of services (consistent with quality care), and shall include, to the extent determined feasible by the Secretary, a system for classifying comparable providers and facilities, and prospectively set rates or target rates with arrangements for sharing such reductions in costs as may be attributable to more efficient and effective delivery of services.
>
> "Such regulations, in the case of services furnished by proprietary providers and facilities may include, if the Secretary finds it feasible and appropriate, provision for recognition of a reasonable rate of return on equity capital...."

The current plan, which has been selected from several alternatives, proposes that four national base rates be established: 1) urban hospitals, 2) urban independents, 3) rural hospitals, and 4) rural independents.

The rate for each facility is to be calculated by adjusting its base rate by an area wage index similar to the one used in setting hospital cost limits. The rate for each group is to be set as follows: Facility costs will be divided into the labor component and the nonlabor component; the mean for each component will then be calculated, after weighing each facility's cost component by the number of treatments; the base rate for each group equals the sum of the two medians. The base rate for a specific facility is to be determined by adjusting the labor component of the base rate by the area wage index applicable to the facility.

Two exceptions to the national rates are proposed. One is for facilities that have an unusual patient care mix or other circumstances that make higher costs unavoidable. The other is a 1-year transition period during the first year of implementation, to permit facilities that currently have costs above the rate to bring their costs into line. The transition exception is to reimburse the facility at a rate based on its actual cost, or on the 75th percentile of its group; whichever is lower.

Facilities will be required to report their costs and these reports will be used to monitor the program and to establish future rate methodologies and future rates.

If a facility can furnish treatments more efficiently than the rate, it will be allowed to retain the difference between its actual cost and its national rate.

A large number of auditors are currently being trained and 112 facilities are to be audited in the next few weeks. Pending the findings of these audits the current suggested incentive rate package is given in Table 1.

Please keep in mind that Medicare will pay only 80% of this new screen.

Simply stated, the officials in Baltimore and Washington believe that dialysis centers and facilities are earning greater profits than they are reporting. They seemingly are unconcerned about the rate of inflation and its current and future cost impact upon dialysis facilities, nor do they seem to realize that with a profit margin, many facilities have been both willing and able to dialyze the patient who had no financial resource for payment, as well as those who had no means of paying the 20% that Medicare fails to cover. The new rate will make it virtually impossible to continue to extend these life-saving gifts to dialysis patients.

Will some facilities be unable to survive these "economic sanctions" by well-meaning but ill-advised bureaucrats and be forced to close their doors? Many believe the answer is an unquestionable Yes! The results to the patient if two or three facilities in large urban areas or even one facility in rural and some urban areas are forced to shut their doors is obvious.

Perhaps three questions are pertinent at this time.

1. Since the bureaucrats are determined to place all facilities and centers on a cost reimbursement basis, why does HCFA not pay 100% of the costs incurred by facilities and centers rather than only 80%?
2. If the reduced screen is implemented and costs continue to rise, will the screen be raised and, if so, rapidly enough to prevent the demise of facilities?
3. If facilities and centers are somehow able to reduce costs below the new screen, will HCFA on the basis of such cost reports reduce the screen again?

TABLE 1.

Suggested Incentive Rate Package

	Urban ($)	Rural ($)
Nonlabor Component per Treatment		
Independent	95.00	94.00
Hospital	104.00	108.00
Labor Component per Treatment[a]		
Independent	28.00	29.00
Hospital	41.00	39.00
Basic Incentive Rates		
(Nonlabor component plus labor component)		
Independent	123.00	123.00
Hospital	145.00	147.00

[a] Labor component to be adjusted for each facility by the appropriate area wage index to determine the basic incentive reimbursement rate.

May I suggest that one disadvantage of the cost basis is that there is no incentive to hold down costs. This is evident in the experience with the hospital cost reimbursement program.

One disadvantage of the charge basis is that some operators will reduce the quality of care in order to maximize profits.

However, if the reimbursement is reduced and all facilities are placed on a cost basis as proposed, then sooner or later operators will be compelled to lower the quality of care in order to survive.

Although our friends in the bureaucracy have only good intentions and the pressures upon them to lower the federal expenditures are enormous, wisdom clearly indicates that the current course they are pursuing is unsound.

But for us, time is rapidly running out. The entire ESRD community, including patients, had best get involved now if we expect to preserve the ESRD program and be able to offer a responsible quality of patient care.

The federal authorities appear to be solely concerned with the areas of cost and profit. They do not appear to express any major interest in the matter of quality of care or the value received for the dollars expended. Apparently, there has been no questioning as to whether the value received for centers and facilities that have received exceptions to the screen is any greater in terms of the quality of patient care than that delivered by facilities that have not received exceptions to the screen. Rather than auditing dollars, it would be far more important for authorities to audit quality.

It is vital that we, as leaders in ESRD, motivate ourselves, other physicians, executives or organizations, and patients to get involved in an effort to change the thinking of the governmental authorities to understand that it is not profit but poor quality of care that is evil.

APPENDIX: SUMMARY OF MEDICARE COVERAGE FOR CONTINUOUS AMBULATORY PERITONEAL DIALYSIS

CAPD patient training

1. Certification is required by HSQB Regional Office.
2. Covered Training:
   a. Up to 15 training sessions of up to 8 hours each (only one session per day is allowed).
   b. Normally completed within a 2-week period.
   c. 6–8 exchanges can be performed each session.
   d. Up to three supplemental dialyses if medically justified.
   e. CAPD training can be covered when furnished to an inpatient, however, such training itself does not justify inpatient status and is reimbursed at the same rate as the facility's outpatient CAPD training rate. (Coverage determination for inpatient expenses such as hospital room and board would be based on the reason for the patient's hospitalization.)
3. Covered Laboratory Services During Training:
   a. Routine laboratory tests covered for each training session are BUN,

albumin, potassium, SGOT, magnesium, dialysate protein, total protein, sodium, LDH, calcium, Hgb, creatinine, alk. phosphatase, CO_2, Hct, and phosphate.
  b. During home CAPD the above tests are covered on a one time per month basis.
4. Facility Reimbursement Per Training Session:
  a. $150 including routine lab and $145 excluding routine lab if physicians are on alternative method.
  b. $162 including routine lab and $157 excluding routine lab if physicians are on initial method.
  c. Routine lab tests will be reimbursed only to the facility.
  d. Nonroutine lab tests are reimbursed when medically justified to the nonprovider facility, the independent lab or patient on a fee-for-service basis or to the provider facility on a cost basis.
5. Physician Reimbursement:
  a. Under alternate methods the rate is the same as for in facility hemodialysis, prorated for the duration of the training method (usually 2 weeks).
  b. Under the initial method charges are billed through the facility with direct patient care services on a fee-for-service basis.
  c. The flat $500.00 training fee is also applicable for CAPD training.

Covered home CAPD support services, supplies and laboratory

1. Full expense for CAPD support services as specified in the regulations pertaining to PL 95-292 including but not limited to:
  a. Changing administration set (connecting tube).
  b. Visual observation of patient performance of CAPD and reinstruction of techniques omitted by patient.
  c. Inspection of catheter site.
  d. Determination and documentation of evidence of present or past peritonitis.
  e. Instruction in new CAPD techniques and/or modification in apparatus.
2. Frequency of Support Services:
  a. May be furnished monthly, however;
  b. Must be furnished not less than every 90 days.
  c. May be furnished either in the facility or home.
  d. May be performed at time of changing connecting tube.
3. Covered Supplies:
  a. All required to perform CAPD effectively, including consumable and disposable supplies, i.e., dialyzing fluids, tubing and gauge pads.
  b. Weight scales, sphygmomanometer, I.V. stand, dialyzing fluid heaters.
4. Covered Drugs and Biologicals:
  Drugs and biologicals such as blood are covered in the home only if a physician is present and when they are administrated.
5. Routinely Covered Laboratory Test:

If furnished in a certified setting to a CAPD patient at the frequencies specified:
a. Every month: BUN, creatinine, sodium, potassium, CO_2, calcium, magnesium, phosphate, total protein, albumin, alk. phosphatase, LDH, SGOT, Hct, Hgb, and dialysate protein.
b. Every three months: WBC, RBC, and platelet count.
c. Every six months: Residual renal function, 24-hour urine volume, chest x-ray, MNCV, EKG, bone mineral density.

CHAPTER SEVEN

Peritoneal Transport Evaluation in CAPD

W. KEITH PYLE, Ph.D.

JACK W. MONCRIEF, M.D.

ROBERT P. POPOVICH, Ph.D.

THE DEVELOPMENT AND APPLICATION of the continuous ambulatory peritoneal dialysis (CAPD) technique has resulted in renewed interest in peritoneal dialysis as a means of managing chronic uremia.[1-4] Although clinical experience to date has shown that CAPD is indeed an effective treatment,[4-7] many questions about the transport processes in peritoneal dialysis have been generated, which are difficult to answer strictly on the basis of experiential evidence. For example, to determine the volume of dialysate in the peritoneal cavity as a function of dwell time, hundreds of drained volumes from exchanges of varying lengths must be measured.[8] This type of evaluation can be quite involved and still not yield accurate results, since it is dependent upon the degree of drainage, which is variable.

Mathematical modeling, a tool that has been widely used in science and engineering in the evaluation of physical processes, is infrequently available to the clinician. Yet, application of modeling techniques to a process such as peritoneal dialysis can yield a great deal of detailed information about the system in general or in a specific patient. Such information can be of great aid to the physician in understanding and manipulating the peritoneal dialysis process. For example, a thorough evaluation of solute transport can yield correlations that may be used to simulate special dialysis conditions without the need for lengthy clinical trials. Similarly, the results of otherwise expensive studies can be approximated quickly and inexpensively through a verified mathematical model.

Biomedical Engineering Program, Chemical Engineering Department, University of Texas at Austin in conjunction with the Acorn Research Laboratory, Austin Diagnostic Clinic, Austin, Texas

PATIENT-PERITONEAL DIALYSIS MODEL

The most desirable mathematical model is one that closely duplicates natural events through an acceptable compromise of utility and theoretical accuracy of the model. For the patient-peritoneal dialysis system, the model must account for fluid transport and hence variable dialysate volume, diffusive and convective solute transport, intrabody net production or metabolism of a solute, and renal clearance. A schematic of the model that fits these conditions is presented in Figure 1. This model consists of two fluid compartments, dialysate and body, separated by a membrane through which fluid and solute transfer occurs. The dialysate pool is assumed to be well mixed with concentration and volume represented by C_D and V_D, respectively. The body pool is also of uniform concentration, C_B, with volume, V_B. Solute generation is included at the constant rate, G. Removal by remaining renal function is at the constant clearance, K_R. Fluid transfer, ultrafiltration, occurs between the pools at the variable rate, Q_U. The peritoneal membrane is characterized by two parameters: the mass transfer-area coefficient (MTAC) for diffusive transport and the reflection coefficient (RC) for convective transport.

The MTAC and RC are chosen to characterize the peritoneal membrane, since they are dependent primarily on membrane properties and can be assumed to be constant during an exchange in a given patient. Physically, the MTAC is the product of the over-all mass transfer coefficient and the area of the peritoneal membrane available for solute transport. The MTAC may be thought of as the diffusive clearance at infinite dialysate flow rates. Since the MTAC does not vary as does the clearance, comparison of MTACs does not require that measurements be made at the same dwell time with the same volumes.

The rate of metabolite transport across the peritoneum by the process of diffusion will not be equal to the total measured removal rate if any significant convective transport occurs. Hence, a second parameter, the RC, is required to characterize transport completely. The RC describes the relationship between the solute and the membrane pore sizes and may be thought of as the fraction of a solute convected, through ultrafiltration, to the membrane, which does not pass through the membrane.

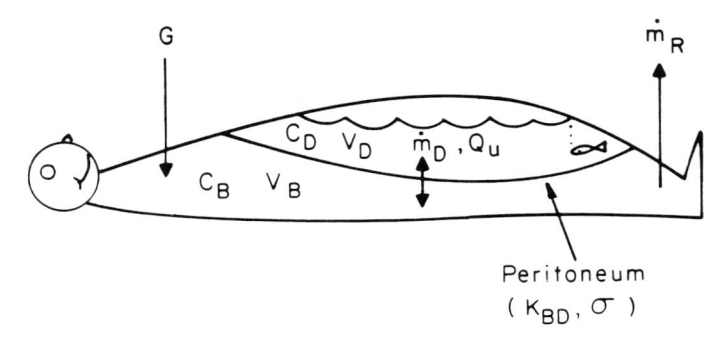

Figure 1. Schematic diagram of the patient-peritoneal dialysis system.

Mathematically, the model encompassing these parameters and effects can be represented by three equations for solute transfer and one for fluid transfer: 1) the peritoneal accumulation rate equation, 2) the membrane transport equation, 3) the over-all mass balance equation, and 4) the ultrafiltration equation. The rate of accumulation of a solute within the peritoneal compartment is given by

$$m = \frac{d(V_D C_D)}{dt}, \qquad (1)$$

where m is the transperitoneal solute transfer rate. From either homogeneous membranes theory[9] or pore theory,[10,11] it may be shown that membrane transport is specified by

$$m = K_{BD}(C_B - C_D) + (1 - \sigma)Q_U \overline{C}, \qquad (2)$$

where

$$\overline{C} = C_B - f(C_B - C_D), \qquad (3)$$

K_{BD} is the mass transfer-area coefficient, σ is the reflection coefficient, Q_U is the ultrafiltration rate,

$$f = \frac{1}{\beta} - \frac{1}{e^\beta - 1}, \qquad (4)$$

$$\beta = \frac{Q_U(1 - \sigma)}{K_{BD}}. \qquad (5)$$

Equation (2) illustrates that solute transfer is the result of two parallel transport mechanisms: diffusion and convection. The rate of diffusion is simply the product of the MTAC, K_{BD}, and the transmembrane solute concentration difference. The convective component is mathematically more complex but is equal to the product of the complement of the RC, the ultrafiltration rate, and the weighted average transmembrane concentration. The weight factor, f, is a function of the ratio of convective to diffusive transport, characterized by the Peclet number, β.[12] An over-all mass balance for the system is

$$C_B V_B + C_D V_D = C_B^0 V_B + C_D^0 V_D^0 + Gt - K_R \int C_B dt. \qquad (6)$$

As will be shown subsequently, the empirical equation,

$$Q_U = a_1 \exp(a_2 t) + a_3, \qquad (7)$$

provides adequate characterization of the ultrafiltration or fluid transfer rates.

Equations (1)–(7) may be combined and solved using Euler's first-order finite difference method[13] to yield characteristic expressions for the dialysate and blood concentrations as functions of the model parameters and time. Equation (7) may be integrated to yield an expression for the dialysate volume:

$$V_D = \frac{a_1}{a_2}[\exp(a_2 t) - 1] + a_3 t + V_D^0. \qquad (8)$$

These characteristic solutions may be fit to clinical data to yield the mass transfer parameters or may be used with prescribed parameter values to simulate desired conditions.

EXPERIMENTAL PROCEDURE AND ANALYSIS

An experimental protocol was designed that allowed collection of data for concurrent evaluation of fluid and solute transport on peritoneal dialysis. Fluid transport data were generated by infusion of a known quantity of sterile, pyrogen-free radioisotopically tagged dextran (mean M.W., 70,000) into a container of fresh dialysis solution. In order to achieve a wide range of osmotic effects, Ringer's lactate, 1.5 and 4.25 g/dl Dianeal® (244, 332, and 477 mOsm/liter, respectively) were chosen for use in the studies.

Following infusion of the prepared solution, dialysate samples were obtained at 0, 20, 40, 60, 90, 120, 180, 240, ... minutes. Since some dextran will transfer despite its large molecular size, blood samples were obtained immediately postinfusion and at the mid and end points of the dwell period to quantitate the transfer. By using the dilution principle corrected for such transfer, intraperitoneal dialysate volumes were calculated at each sample time. Equation (8) was then fit to the calculated volumes using Gauss' nonlinear least squares algorithm.[13,14] The resulting coefficients also specify the ultrafiltration rate curve through Equation (7).

Solute transport data were generated by appropriate analyses on selected samples obtained in the fluid transfer study described. Once the ultrafiltration profile was determined for an exchange, the solutions of the mass transfer Equations (1)–(6) were least squares fit to the concentration–time data for each solute of interest. The resulting mass transfer parameters were then correlated to solute physical properties.

RESULTS

Fluid transfer studies

Nineteen exchanges have been studied in seven CAPD patients. Four studies were performed with Ringer's lactate, eight with 1.5 g/dl Dianeal®, and seven with 4.25 g/dl Dianeal®. Figures 2–4 show typical intraperitoneal volume curves in each of these three solutions. The least squares coefficients are given in Table 1. Since Ringer's lactate is initially somewhat hypotonic, but gradually approaches the serum osmolality, the curve in Figure 2 shows an initial rapid decrease in volume, which asymptomatically approaches a constant rate of decline. That is, ultrafiltration is high from dialysate to blood (negative ultrafiltration) initially, decreasing to the small negative value. Figure 3 illustrates the effects of the moderately hypertonic 1.5-g/dl solution on fluid transfer. In this case, fluid is ultrafiltered from the body increasing

Peritoneal Transport Evaluation in CAPD 39

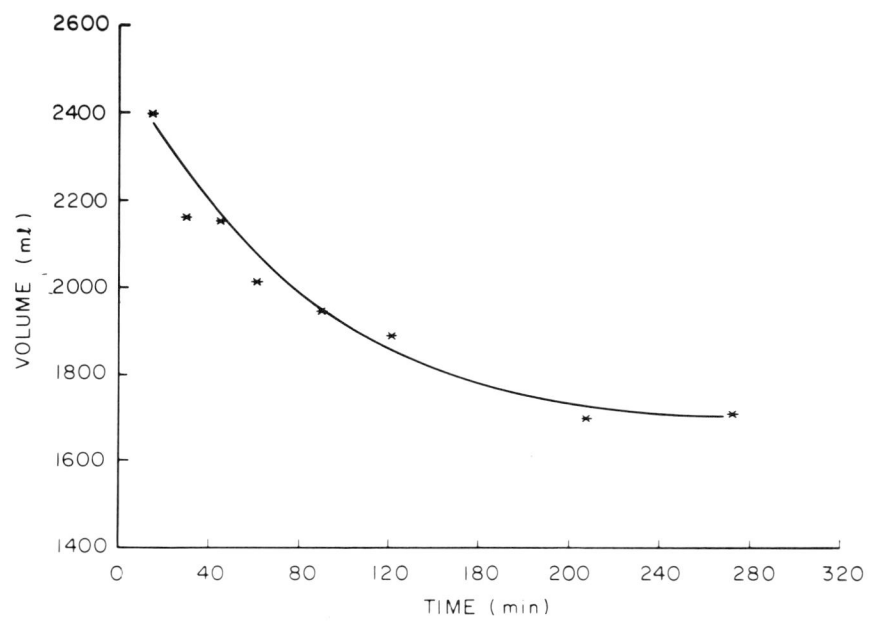

Figure 2. Volume profile resulting from the infusion of Ringer's lactate in patient 1.

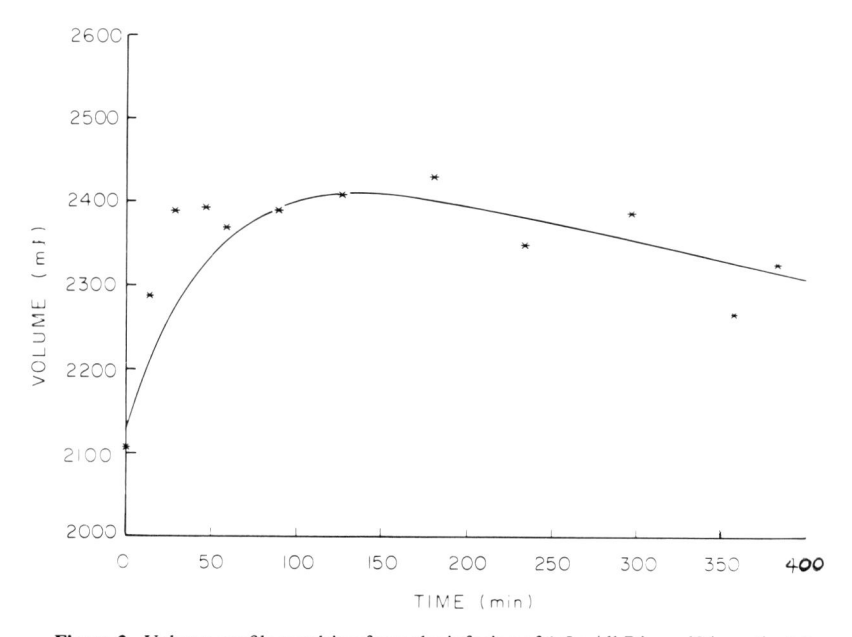

Figure 3. Volume profile resulting from the infusion of 1.5 g/dl Dianeal® in patient 2.

TABLE 1.
Volume Profile Equation Coefficients

Solution	V_D at $t = 0$	a_1	a_2	a_3
Isotonic	2841.	−21.4	−0.0195	−0.231
1.5%	2130.	7.48	−0.0207	−0.452
4.25%	1988.	28.4	−0.0170	−1.40

the intraperitoneal volume to a maximum of approximately 2,408 ml at 136 minutes. Thus, the maximum ultrafiltered volume that could be obtained is 278 ml over the volume at the end of infusion of 2,130 ml. The volume subsequently begins to decrease and approaches a constant rate of reabsorption. Figure 4 shows the fluid transfer characteristics of a 4.25-g/dl solution due to the larger osmotic gradient. The volume increases much more rapidly that it does with the 1.5 solution. The peak volume, at approximately 177 minutes, was 3,325 ml compared to the initial volume of 1,988 ml. In this case approximately 1,337 ml was ultrafiltered. Again, fluid reabsorption begins to occur and approaches a constant rate.

The rate of ultrafiltration can be shown by evaluating the slope or first derivative of the volume curve as a function of time. Figure 5 illustrates the ultrafiltration profile resulting from the 1.5-g/dl volume curve shown in Figure 3. It can be seen that the ultrafiltration rate is about 7 ml/minute

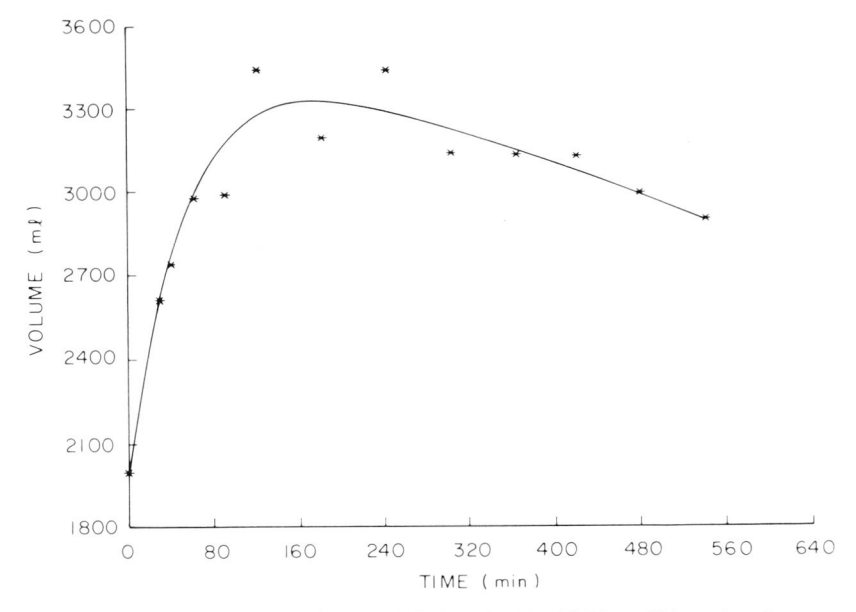

Figure 4. Volume profile from the infusion of 4.25 g/dl Dianeal® in patient 2.

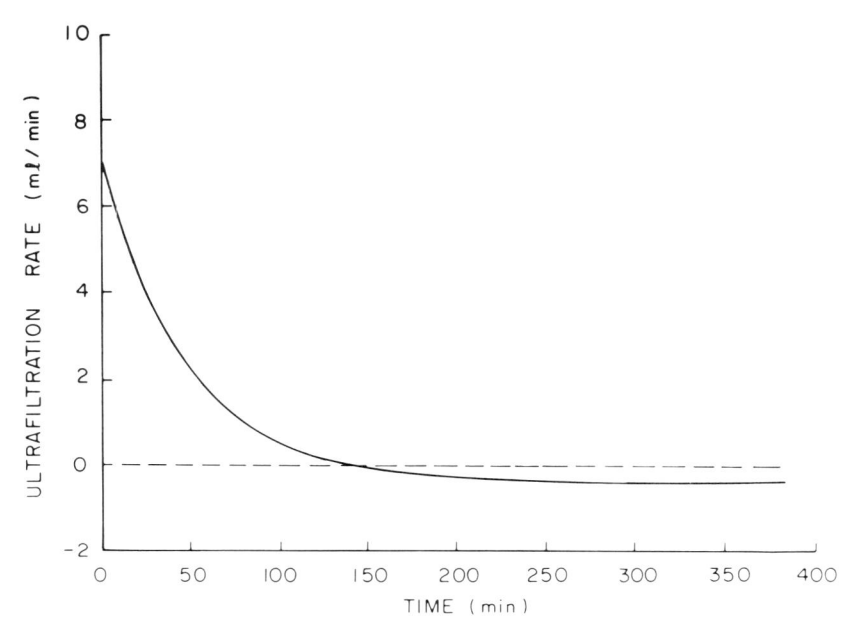

Figure 5. Ultrafiltration profile resulting from the infusion of 1.5 g/dl Dianeal® in patient 2.

immediately postinfusion ($t = 0$), is zero at 136 minutes, and approaches the value of -0.45 ml/minute.* Figure 6 presents the profile derived from the 4.25-g/dl volume curve of Figure 4. Here, the initial ultrafiltration rate exceeds 26 ml/minute and drops to -1.4 ml/minute. Average fluid transfer results are shown in Table 2.

Solute transfer studies

Solute transport was evaluated for urea (M.W., 60), creatinine (M.W., 113), uric acid (M.W., 158), glucose (M.W., 180), inulin (M.W., 5,500), dextran (M.W., 70,000 mean), and total protein (M.W., 340,000 weighted mean). Average MTAC for five CAPD patients are given in Table 3. Mean RCs are shown as a function of molecular size in Figure 7, along with an empirical correlation function.

Figures 8–11 show representative concentration–time profiles for blood urea nitrogen, creatinine, inulin, and total protein, respectively. The dialysate urea level rises rapidly due to its relatively large MTAC of 15.31 ml/minute and low RC of 0.126. The theoretical prediction of the concentration profile for this MTAC value is shown by the solid line in Figure 8. The theoretical

---

*Negative ultrafiltration rates indicate net fluid transfer from dialysate to blood; positive rates indicate transfer from blood to dialysate.

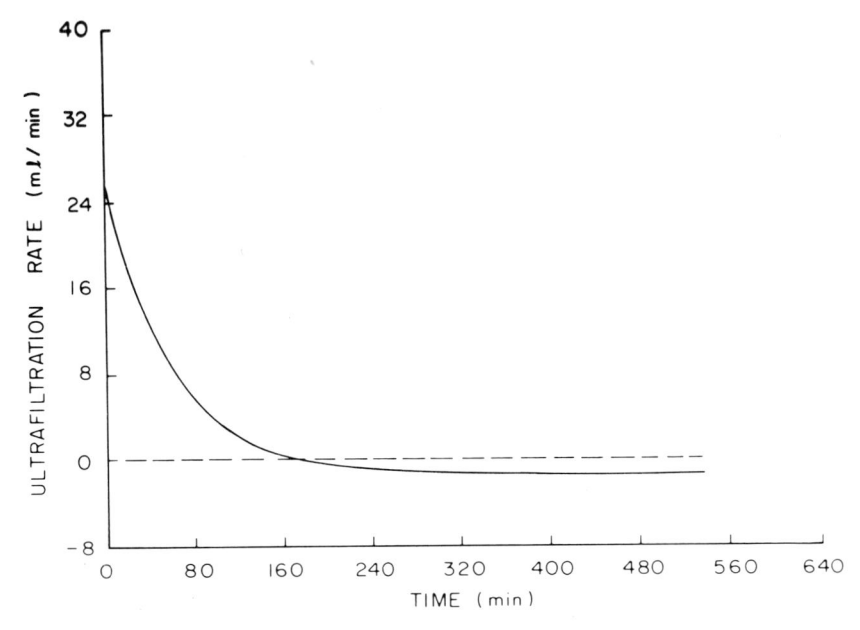

Figure 6. Ultrafiltration profile resulting from the infusion of 4.25 g/dl Dianeal® in patient 2.

plasma concentration, shown by the dashed line, drops slightly during the first 90 minutes of the exchange, then rises back to near the initial level. The dialysate to plasma ratio reaches 0.95, 95% of equilibration in 420 minutes.

Creatinine transfers at a slightly lower rate than does urea due to its larger molecular size. The lower transfer rate is reflected in the lower degree of equilibration, 81% at 360 minutes as illustrated in Figure 9. In this case, the theoretical prediction gives an MTAC of 9.04 ml/minute and a RC of 0.200. As molecular size increases, these effects, that is, lower degree of equilibration, lower MTAC, and higher RC, become even more pronounced. The transfer of inulin from the dialysate into the blood is illustrated in Figure 10.

TABLE 2.
Average Fluid Transfer Results[a]

	1.5 Dianeal®	4.25 Dianeal®
Maximum ultrafiltered volume (ml)	331 ± 187	1,028 ± 258
Maximum volume at (minute)	140 ± 48	247 ± 61
Maximum ultrafiltration rate (ml/minute)	11.7 ± 13.0	16.6 ± 7.7
Reabsorption rate (ml/minute)	−0.68 ± 0.61	−0.87 ± 0.55

[a] Mean ± S.D. ($n = 4$).

TABLE 3.
Average Mass Transfer-Area Coefficients (MTAC)[a]

Patient	Urea	Creatinine	Uric Acid	Glucose	Inulin	Dextran	Total Protein
1	16.2 ± 2.1 (5)	9.0 ± 2.6 (5)	6.3 ± 0.9 (5)	7.2 ± 1.0 (5)	4.1 ± 1.5 (5)	1.46 ± 0.57 (5)	0.041 ± 0.005 (5)
2	20.1 ± 3.8 (7)	11.3 ± 1.7 (7)	9.1 ± 1.4 (7)	9.3 ± 1.7 (7)	8.0 ± 2.4 (7)	1.79 ± 0.33 (7)	0.047 ± 0.025 (7)
3	20.6 (1)	16.9 (1)	14.6 (1)	14.3 (1)	5.2 (1)	3.1 (1)	0.061 (1)
4	21.1 ± 3.7 (2)	13.5 ± 2.4 (2)	12.6 ± 4.8 (2)	9.3 (1)	7.8 ± 5.1 (2)	2.46 ± 0.00 (2)	0.054 (1)
5	16.6 (1)	8.5 (1)	7.3 (1)	9.0 (1)	—	—	—

[a] Mean ± S.D. (n), ml/minute.

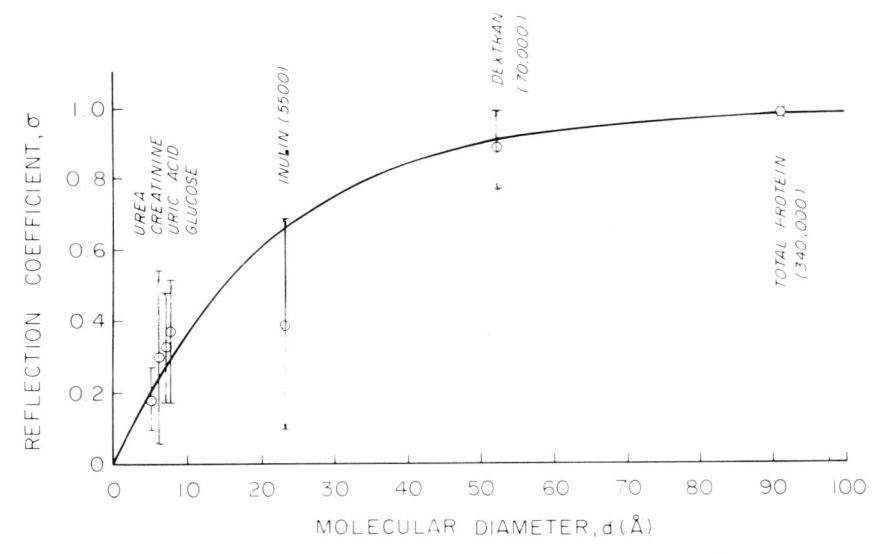

Figure 7. Peritoneal membrane reflection coefficients as a function of solute diameter. $\sigma = 1 - \exp(-.0461d) = 1 - \exp(-.0609 \sqrt[3]{mw})$.

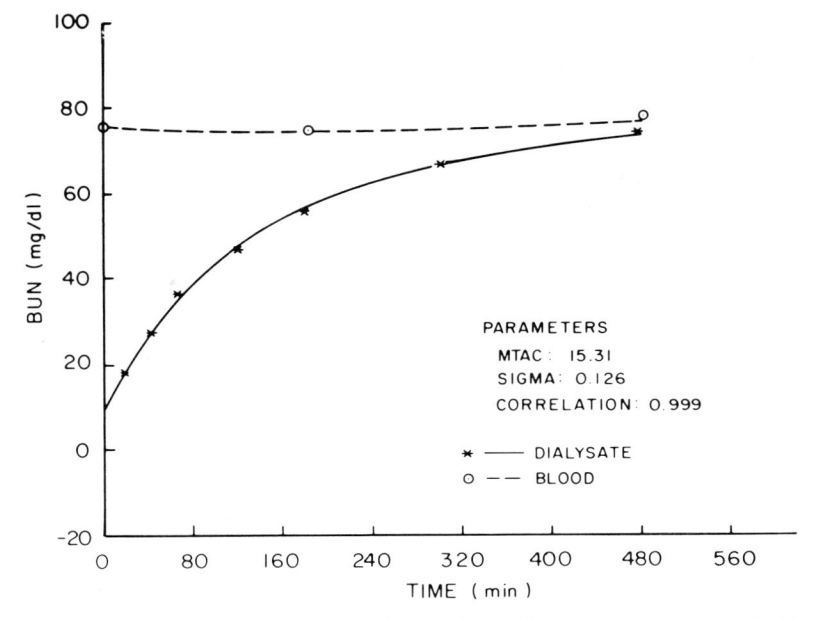

Figure 8. Blood and dialysate concentration profiles for blood urea nitrogen in patient 1.

The dialysate level drops from 15,000 to 7,000 dpm/ml, whereas the blood increases from 0 to 1,300 dpm/ml in 360 minutes. Even though direct comparison of influx and efflux concentration profiles is difficult, it is obvious that the relative blood and dialysate differences shown here are greater at any given time than in either of the two previous cases. For total protein, the serum level of 7.9 g/dl is so high relative to the dialysate that it is not practical to show it in Figure 11, the dialysate concentration profile.

DISCUSSION OF RESULTS

The intraperitoneal volume profiles, Figures 2–4, and the data in Table 2 show the substantial differences in fluid transfer resulting from the use of Ringer's lactate and 1.5 and 4.25 Dianeal® as dialysis solutions. As would be expected, the rate of fluid transfer is dependent on the difference in tonicity between the solution and the blood. The Ringer's solution, initially somewhat hypotonic, shows a consistent absorption of the solution into the body; mildly hypertonic 1.5 Dianeal® results in a modest increase of an average 331 ml in intraperitoneal volume before reabsorption begins; 4.25 Dianeal® provides almost three times the fluid removal capability of 1.5. On the average, 1,028 ml was ultrafiltered with the 4.25 solution. As shown in Table 2, 4.25 Dianeal® results in an initial (maximum) ultrafiltration rate of 16.6 ml/minute, more than 40% greater than that from 1.5, 11.7 ml/minute. Since the decay constants of the ultrafiltration rate profiles for these solutions, coefficients a_2 of Table 1, are nearly equal, the higher initial rate results in positive ultrafiltration for a longer period. On the average, positive ultrafiltration

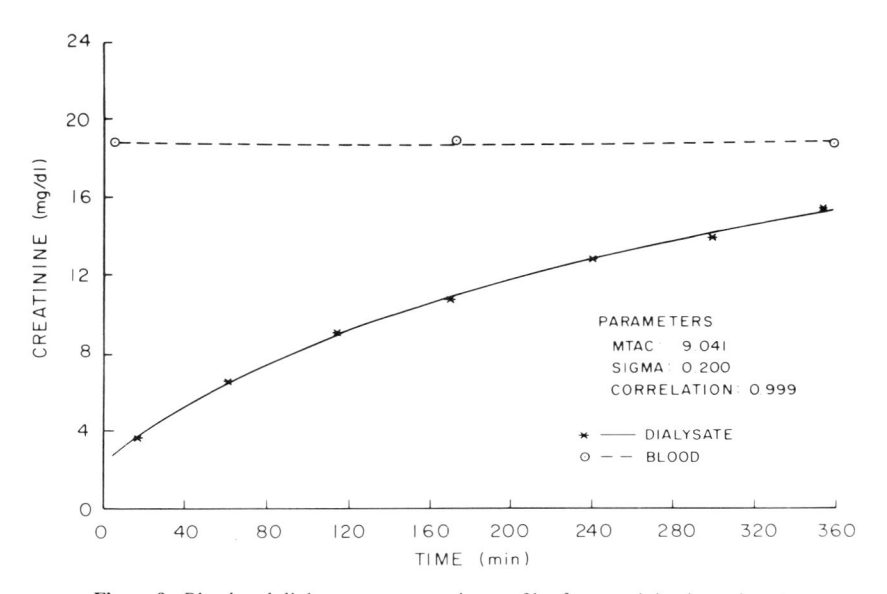

Figure 9. Blood and dialysate concentration profiles for creatinine in patient 1.

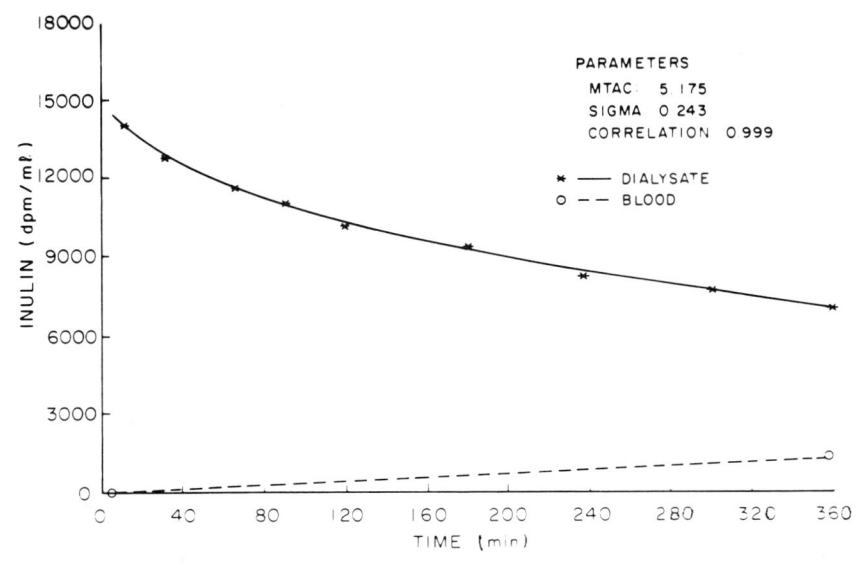

Figure 10. Blood and dialysate concentration profiles for inulin (C-14 tagged) in patient 3.

occurs for the first 140 and 247 minutes in the 1.5 and 4.25 solutions, respectively.

The hypertonicity of dialysis solutions results from the high glucose concentrations used. The blood osmolality, or tonicity, is maintained by the

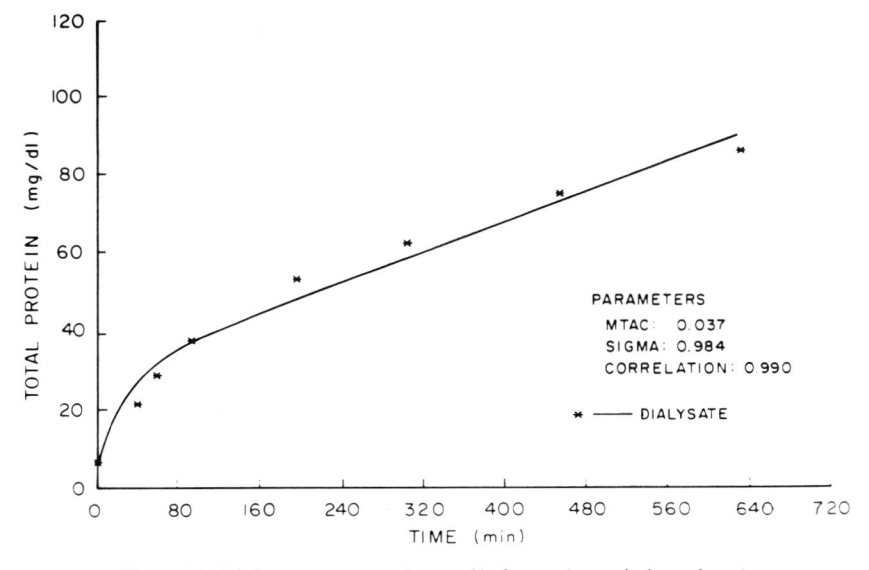

Figure 11. Dialysate concentration profile for total protein in patient 1.

presence of various metabolites, including glucose. However, the blood concentration of glucose is quite low compared to the dialysate. Thus, glucose transfers into the blood and is metabolized. As transfer proceeds, the osmotic driving force is diminished and the ultrafiltration rate declines. At low dialysate glucose levels, the rate asymptotically approaches a constant reabsorption rate. The average reabsorption rates for 1.5 and 4.25 Dianeal® were -0.68 and -0.87 ml/minute. Both values were subject to relatively large variations and may represent a single value ($p > 0.65$). If this is correct, then any changes induced in the peritoneum by the different hypertonicities are not apparent in the reabsorption rate.

The large variations in the reabsorption rate were representative of the patient-to-patient variations in the fluid transfer data. Figure 12 shows the intraperitoneal volume curves resulting from the use of 4.25 Dianeal® in five CAPD patients. From this illustration, it is apparent that the assumption of "average" fluid transfer data could produce significant errors in the analysis of mass transfer data. Thus, results based on such assumed values should be considered general estimates only, unless data supporting the assumption are available.

The ability to dialyze a metabolite across the peritoneum seems primarily dependent on the size of the molecule in question. The size can be expressed as either molecular weight or average molecular radius. The average MTACs in Table 3 show a general decreasing trend with increasing molecular weight,

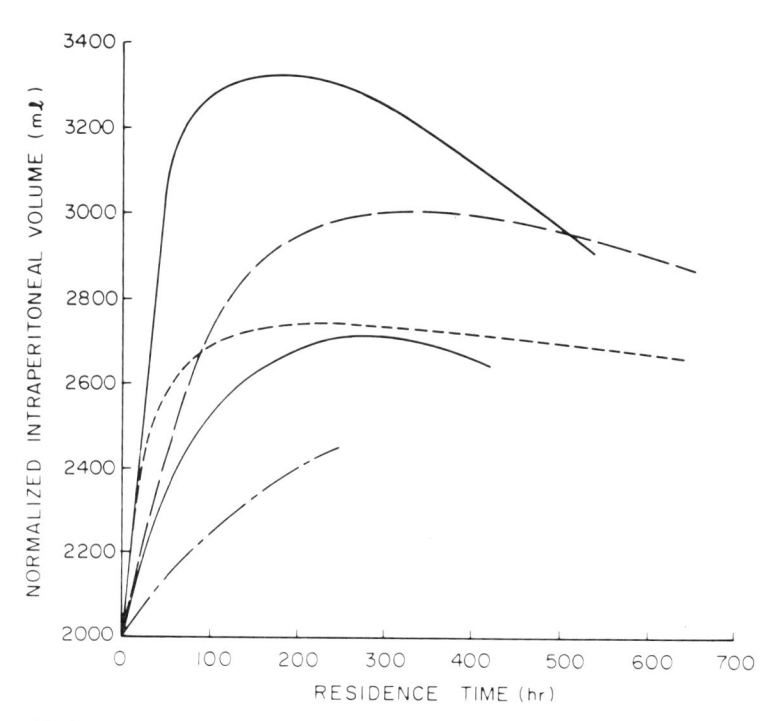

Figure 12. Volume profiles in five CAPD patients normalized to an initial volume of 2,000 ml.

TABLE 4.
Patient Parameters

Patient	Weight (kg)	Surface Area (m^2)
1	64.9	1.76
2	60.8	1.69
3	65.5	1.86
4	83.9	2.11
5	70.1	1.85

ranging from a high of 21.1 ml/minute for urea to a low of 0.041 for mean total protein. Since MTACs contain a measure of the peritoneal transport area, differences in physical size between patients could affect the calculated results. In order to remove such individual variations from the over-all results, two obvious bases for normalization, weight and external body surface area, were chosen. These patient parameters are given in Table 4. The results of the raw and normalized averages, Table 5, suggest that there is little reduction in variation in either of the normalized averages over the raw averages. Results in a larger patient population will be needed to determine the most appropriate basis for normalization. Similar MTACs have been previously reported; however, these have been based on simplifying assumptions, such as constant[15-18] or nonexistent ultrafiltration[19] and constant convective coefficients (analogous to the RC) derived from the literature. From the fluid transfer data presented, it is evident that these assumptions could lead to substantial errors.

The most frequently mentioned work on convective transport coefficients indicates that both urea and inulin have "sieving coefficients" of approximately 0.8.[20] This corresponds to RC of about 0.2. Although these measurements fall within the error range for the corresponding RCs shown in Figure 7, the mistaken conclusion that sieving is equivalent for all solutes could be drawn from the earlier data. In fact, the peritoneal RCs, as determined in this study, range from 0.18 for urea to 0.992 for the proteins and can be predicted

TABLE 5.
Raw and Normalized Average MTACs[a]

Solute	Raw	Weight Norm[b]	S. A. Norm.[c]
Urea	18.9 ± 2.3 (5)	19.4 ± 3.0 (5)	17.7 ± 2.2 (5)
Creatinine	11.8 ± 3.5 (5)	12.1 ± 3.7 (5)	11.0 ± 3.0 (5)
Uric acid	10.0 ± 3.5 (5)	10.1 ± 3.5 (5)	9.3 ± 3.0 (5)
Glucose	9.8 ± 2.7 (5)	10.1 ± 3.1 (5)	9.2 ± 2.5 (5)
Inulin	6.3 ± 1.9 (4)	6.4 ± 2.0 (4)	5.9 ± 1.8 (5)
Dextran	2.2 ± 0.7 (4)	2.3 ± 0.7 (4)	2.0 ± 0.6 (4)
Total protein	0.051 ± 0.009 (4)	0.052 ± 0.010 (4)	0.047 ± 0.007 (4)

[a] Mean + S.D. (*n*), ml/min.
[b] Per 70 kg norm.
[c] Per 1.73 m^2 norm.

with good agreement by the empirical expressions shown in Figure 7. These RCs indicate that the majority of the smaller solutes in the ultrafiltrate are convected through the membrane. Conversely, less than 1% of the protein in the same ultrafiltrate penetrates the peritoneum due to higher RCs. In order to obtain appreciable convective protein transfer, it is necessary to have relatively high ultrafiltration rates to overcome the limit imposed by the high RC.

The concentration–time profiles, Figures 8–11, illustrate the effects quantitated by the parameters discussed above. Low resistance to transport (high MTAC and low RC) allow metabolites, such as urea and creatinine, to nearly equilibrate with the blood in 7–8 hours. Larger solutes, characterized by inulin, dextran, and total protein, may never equilibrate due to higher transport resistances (low MTAC, high RC).

Figure 11, which shows the total protein concentration–time profile, also illustrates the effect of high fluid transport rates in an evaluation of 4.25 Dianeal®. During the first 80 minutes of the residence phase, the ultrafiltration rate was positive and relatively high, similar to the case shown in Figure 6. This caused protein to be convected across the peritoneum at a substantial rate, resulting in the rapid initial rise in protein concentration of about 30 mg/dl. As the ultrafiltration rate stabilizes at the reabsorption rate, the protein transport rate becomes virtually constant, leading to the linear rise in concentration. To rise an additional 30 mg/dl requires about 320 minutes. Thus, even a small degree of convective transport can be quite important in the dialysis of large solutes.

The amount of a given solute removed in an exchange is a complex function of the parameters already described: intraperitoneal volume, ultrafiltration rate, MTAC, and RC. Figure 13 displays the urea dialyzed as a function of the residence time and type of solution used for the parameters of patient 2. It can be seen that the higher tonicity solution is capable of removing about 40% more urea due to the higher intraperitoneal volume. The maximum urea dialysis occurs at about 5.5 and 7 hours for the 1.5 and 4.25 solutions, respectively. It is interesting to note that the mass of urea continues to rise slightly for some time after the volume reaches its maximum. Figure 14 shows similar results for a hypothetical solute (M.W., 5,500) in the same patient. Since solute transfer rates are substantially lower for a molecule of this size, maximum dialysis occurs at significantly greater residence times. For 1.5 and 4.25 Dianeal®, the maxima are approximately 8.5 and 12 hours, respectively. In this case, solute transfer is still appreciable after the fluid maximum is reached; for the 4.25, the mass rises by 62% after this point. Such factors can be of substantial importance in planning treatments for removal of specific solutes.

SUMMARY AND CONCLUSIONS

Fluid transfer is an extremely important factor in peritoneal dialysis, both in clinical treatment and in modeling of the patient-peritoneal dialysis system. Ultrafiltration rates have been shown to vary in an exponential manner with

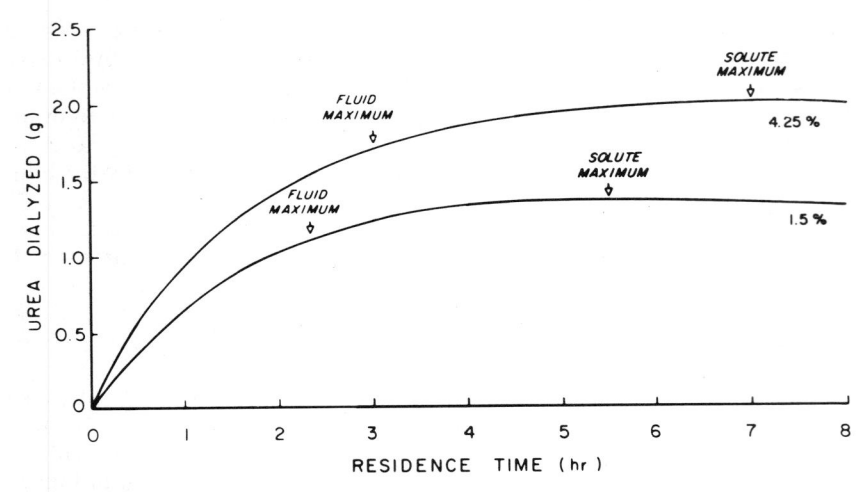

Figure 13. Urea dialyzed (in grams) as a function of residence time in patient 2.

time. Mean fluid transfer results from 19 patient studies were presented. However, patients can often deviate considerably from the average case and mean transport data should be used for initial estimates only. From the similarities of the fluid reabsorption results for 1.5 and 4.25 Dianeal®, it is probable that any changes induced in the peritoneum by the different solutions are of short term and do not greatly affect transport in subsequent exchanges in normal clinical treatment.

The peritoneal membrane MTACs and RCs have been determined for

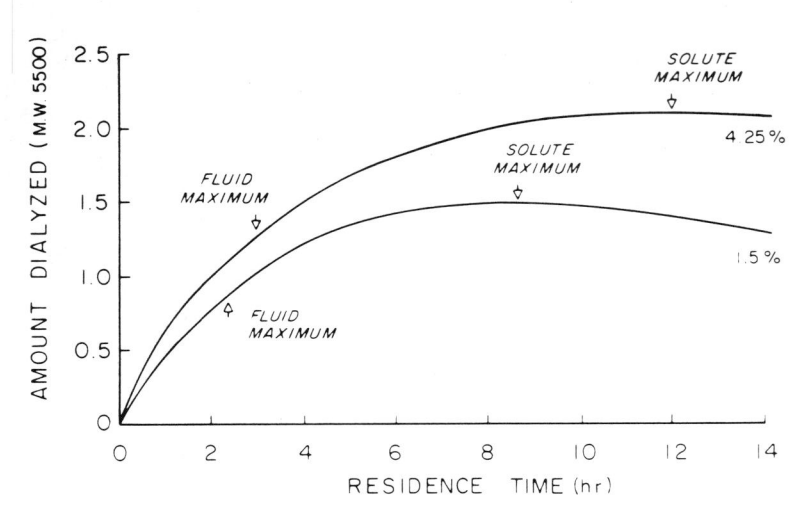

Figure 14. Dialysis of a hypothetical solute (MW, 5,500) as a function of residence time in patient 2.

urea, creatinine, uric acid, glucose, inulin, dextran, and total protein in five CAPD patients. These coefficients were shown to depend on the solute size and should not be considered constant over any appreciable range of molecular sizes. The effects of these parameters on solute transport can be quite complex and simplifying assumptions should be made with care.

Author's note. Figures 2–6, 8–11, 13 and 14 are published with permission of W. Keith Pyle from his Ph.D. dissertation "Mass Transfer in Peritoneal Dialysis."

ACKNOWLEDGMENT

Supported in part by the Artificial Kidney–Chronic Uremia Program of the National Institutes of Health, contract N01-AM-3-2205.

References

1. Popovich, R. P., Moncrief, J. W., Decherd, J. F., Bomar, J. B., and Pyle, W. K.: The definition of a novel portable/wearable equilibrium peritoneal dialysis technique. *Abstr Am Soc Artif Intern Organs* 5: 64, 1976.
2. Popovich, R. P., Pyle, W. K., Moncrief, J. W., Decherd, J. F., and Brooks, S.: Preliminary verification of the low dialysis clearance hypothesis via a novel equilibrium peritoneal dialysis technique. *Trans Aust Conf Heat Mass Transfer* 2: 217, 1977.
3. Popovich, R. P., Moncrief, J. W., Nolph, K. D., Ghods, A. J., Twardowski, Z. J., and Pyle, W. K.: Continuous ambulatory peritoneal dialysis. *Ann Intern Med* 88: 449, 1978.
4. Moncrief, J. W., Rubin, J., Nolph, K. D., and Popovich, R. P.: Additional experience with continuous ambulatory peritoneal dialysis. *Trans Am Soc Artif Intern Organs* 24: 476, 1978.
5. Moncrief, J. W., and Popovich, R. P.: Continuous ambulatory peritoneal dialysis. *Contrib Nephrol* 17: 139, 1979.
6. Oreopoulos, D. G., and Katirzolous, A.: Continuous ambulatory peritoneal dialysis (CAPD): A life sustaining treatment without artifical organs. *Int J Artif Organs* 2(6): 268, 1979.
7. Moncrief, J. W., Popovich, R. P., Nolph, K. D., Rubin, J., Robson, M., Dombros, N., deVeber, G., and Oreopoulos, D. G.: Clinical experience with continuous ambulatory peritoneal dialysis. *J Am Soc Artif Intern Organs* 2(3): 114, 1979.
8. Rubin, J., Nolph, K. D., Popovich, R. P., Moncrief, J. W., and Prowant, B.: Drainage volumes for continuous ambulatory peritoneal dialysis. *J Am Soc Artif Intern Organs* 2(2): 54, 1979.
9. Villarroel, F., Klein, E., and Holland, F.: Solute flux in hemodialysis and hemofiltration membranes. *Trans Am Soc Artif Intern Organs* 23: 225, 1977.
10. Anderson, J. L., and Quinn, J. A.: Restricted transport in small pores: A model for steric exclusion and hindered particle motion, *Biophys J* 14: 130, 1974.
11. Brenner, H., and Gaylos, L. J.: The constrained Brownian movement of spherical particles in cylindrical pores of comparable radius: models of the diffusive and convective transport in membranes and porous media. *J Colloid Interface Sci* 58: 312, 1977.
12. Bird, R. B., Steward, W. E., and Lightfoot, E. N.: *Transport Phenomena,* John Wiley & Sons, New York, 1960.
13. Conte, S. D., and de Boor, C.: *Elementary Numerical Analysis,* 2nd ed. McGraw-Hill, New York, 1965.
14. Brown, K. M.: Computer oriented methods for fitting tabular data in the least squares sense. Fall Joint Computer Conference, National Center for Atmospheric Research, Boulder, Colorado, 1972.
15. Babb, A. L., Johansen, P. J., Strand, M. J., Tenckhoff, H., and Scribner, B. H.: Bidirectional permeability of the human peritoneum to middle molecules. *Proc Eur Dial Transplant Assoc* 10: 247, 1973.

16. Nolph, K. D., Ghods, A. J., Brown, P. A., Miller, F., Harris, P., Pyle, W. K., and Popovich, R. P.: Effects of nitroprusside on peritoneal mass transfer coefficients and microvascular physiology. *Trans Am Soc Artif Intern Organs* **23**: 210, 1977.
17. Villarroel, F., Popovich, R. P., and Nolph, K. D.: Evaluation of permeance in peritoneal dialysis. *J Dial* **2**: 361, 1978.
18. Popovich, R. P., Pyle, W. K., Bomar, J. B., and Moncrief, J. W.: Chronic replacement of kidney function. *AIChE Symp Series, Peritoneal Dialysis* **75**(187): 31, 1979.
19. Villarroel, F.: Kinetics of intermittent and continuous peritoneal dialysis. *J Dial* **1**(4): 333, 1977.
20. Henderson, L. W., and Nolph, K. D.: Altered permeability of the peritoneal membrane after using hypertonic peritoneal dialysis fluid. *J Clin Invest* **48**(6):992, 1969.

CHAPTER EIGHT

Blood Flow to the Peritoneum: Physiological and Pharmacological Influences*

JOHN F. MAHER, M.D.

AN EFFECTIVE RATE OF mass transport by peritoneal dialysis requires adequate blood flow to the dialyzing surface and sufficient area and permeability of the membrane to allow rapid permeation of solutes and rapid diffusion throughout dialysate, which is periodically replaced, thereby maintaining electrochemical gradients.

The recent upsurge of interest in peritoneal dialysis has been accompanied by attempts to augment transport rates by manipulation of each of the resistances. Our studies[1] and those from other laboratories[2-4] have demonstrated the enhancement of peritoneal mass transport that results from splanchnic vasodilation and the restricted transport that vasoconstrictors induce.[5,6] These alterations in blood flow are reflected by changes in the clearance of larger solutes more than of smaller solutes, i.e., by changes in area and permeability, because mass transport is not ordinarily limited by the rate of solute delivery to the membrane. Drugs that affect permeability directly are limited. Examples include furosemide[7] and protamine sulfate.[8] Mass transport can also be augmented by enhanced mixing or more rapid exchange of dialysate[9,10] or by increasing convective transport by increased use of hyperosmotic dialysate.[11,12]

Because of the limited gain in solute transport that can be achieved by modifying the dialysis solution composition or flow rate and the restricted capability to affect peritoneal area or permeability directly, the effect of

---

Professor of Medicine, Director, Division of Nephrology, Uniformed Services, University of the Health Sciences, Bethesda, Maryland

*The opinions or assertions contained herein are the private views of the author and should not be construed as official or as necessarily reflecting the views of the Uniformed Services University of the Health Sciences or Department of Defense. There is no objection to its presentation and publication.

physiological or pharmacological manipulations on peritoneal blood flow rates assumes increased importance in modifying transport rates.

THE PERITONEAL CIRCULATION

The parietal layer of the peritoneum, a small fraction of the total peritoneal surface area, receives its blood supply from the vasculature of the abdominal wall. The visceral peritoneum, the larger portion of the mesothelium, is supplied primarily by branches of the superior mesenteric artery, a major division of the splanchnic circulation.

The mesenteric circulation is remarkable for its size and complexity and, until recently, for the paucity of knowledge about its physiology. Mesenteric arterioles with contractile elements subdivide into precapillaries, the openings of which are controlled by sphincters. In turn, these divide into true capillaries that proceed to venous capillaries, which join to become venules, then muscular venules, and, subsequently, veins. The metarteriole is a central or preferential channel, which is the main controlling unit of capillary flow.[13] Rhythmic, independent, and apparently random movement of the precapillary sphincters is associated with a periodic flush of blood into the capillaries during the relaxation phase. Hyperemia is associated with prolongation of sphincter relaxation, whereas ischemia occurs when closure of the sphincter is persistent. The mesentery is an important vascular space that can function as a storehouse for blood and a site of blood flow regulation.

The systemic circulation can be viewed as a two-compartment model in parallel, that is, the splanchnic and peripheral (mostly muscle) circulations. Distribution among these compartments is influenced by a variety of factors, including exercise, epinephrine, and endotoxemia.[14] The splanchnic vasculature has a resting volume estimated to be about one-third of the blood volume and a blood flow rate that exceeds 1,200 ml/minute in man.[15] Mesenteric blood flow as assessed by flow meter or solute clearance averages about 10% of the cardiac output, or 40 ml/minute/100 g.[13,16] Based on gas clearance measurements, the effective blood flow rate to the peritoneum has been estimated at 60 to 100 ml/minute.[17] At this blood flow rate, solute extraction by diffusion is incomplete, indicating that the capillary wall restricts mass transport[18] and solute delivery is not the major factor limiting removal by peritoneal dialysis.

The pore radii of mesenteric capillaries range from 50 to 110 Å, comparable to those of glomerular capillaries.[19] The capillary filtration coefficient averages 0.17 ml/minute/100 g/ mm Hg, which is close to that of glomerular capillaries and much higher than the capillaries of muscle.[13] Of course, the greater capillary pressure in the glomerular tuft and the larger glomerular surface area result in a higher filtration rate. Based on available data, the ultrafiltration rate through the capillaries supplying the peritoneum should be approximately 3.0 ml/minute. With the instillation of isotonic dialysis solution, increased interstitial pressure causes net absorption of fluid. This is offset by adding dextrose to the dialysis solution, resulting in net ultrafiltration that averages 3.0 ml/minute at a 1.5% dextrose concentratoin. Of course, the diffusion rate of small solutes is much higher than the ultrafiltration rate.

PHYSIOLOGICAL INFLUENCES ON PERITONEAL CIRCULATION

With age, cardiac output and renal blood flow decrease. The effect of age on the peritoneal circulation is incompletely defined, however. Since systemic vascular disease decreases blood flow and peritoneal clearances,[20] it is anticipated that the aging process would also decrease mesenteric blood flow rate. Whether this change is sufficient to alter peritoneal clearances significantly has not been established.

Cardiac output is also a function of body size. Accordingly, unless blood flow distribution is changed, mesenteric blood flow should relate to body size. Since the peritoneal surface area also correlates with body surface area, peritoneal clearances are in fact determined by body size.[21]

Because angiotensin increases mesenteric vascular resistance,[22] stimulation of renin by the erect posture should decrease mesenteric blood flow rate, but probably insufficiently to depress peritoneal clearances. On the other hand, angiotensin may contribute to the low peritoneal clearances observed with malignant hypertension and other ischemic renal diseases.[20] Carotid sinus stimulation has only minor effects on splanchnic resistance, decreasing splanchnic blood flow by 15% of control values,[23] which should be insufficient to depress clearances significantly.

With exercise, splanchnic vascular resistance increases and splanchnic blood flow decreases in patients with heart disease from control values of 1.2 liters/minute to 0.8 liters/minute.[24] These changes correlate with the alteration in systemic arteriovenous oxygen difference. The advent of the technique for ambulatory peritoneal dialysis[25] has stimulated studies now in progress of the quantitative effects of exercise on peritoneal mass transport.

The splanchnic vascular bed also has the capacity to sequester blood, excluding or releasing blood into the circulation as systemic volume changes. With acute loss of 15-20% of blood volume, blood pressure, cardiac output, and heart rate are maintained and splanchnic blood flow rate and splanchnic vascular resistance do not change, but there is a significant fall in splanchnic blood volume from 1.4 to 0.85 liters and a significant decrease in hepatic venous pressure.[26] With overt hemorrhage, peritoneal clearances decrease despite restoration of blood pressure by 1-norepinephrine.[27] Maintenance of normal peritoneal clearance appears to depend both on adequate mesenteric blood flow and blood volume. When superior mesenteric arterial blood flow is reduced to 50-75% of normal, it can be restored to normal by the intra-arterial administration of such vasodilators as glucagon, prostaglandin E_1, or isoproterenol,[28] indicating the role of myogenic vasoconstriction in modulating mesenteric blood volume and flow. With graded hemorrhage, superior mesenteric arterial blood flow is not maintained as well as is renal blood flow until severe hemorrhage has resulted.[13,29] These findings suggest that mesenteric blood flow is as inconstant as is circulation to the skin. Such alterations may induce variations in peritoneal clearances.

As with other vascular beds, local cooling decreases splanchnic blood flow while warming induces hyperemia.[13] Heat transfer across peritoneal capillaries is very rapid, however, so that with intermittent flow of dialysate the effect of temperature is transient.

As portal venous pressure is elevated, the mesenteric vascular resistance increases because of a myogenic response of the arterioles.[30] This effect is blocked by papaverine, but not by procaine. Increased venous pressure distends the mesenteric capillaries, which should increase their permeability. The transmission of the pressure to the arterioles distends them, causing the myogenic response, thereby autoregulating blood flow. Moreover, after exposure of the mesenteric circulation to a vasoconstrictor, the closure of precapillary sphinctors decreases capillary flow and filtration and increases venous pressure.[31] Blood flow is thus redistributed through conduit channels. Arteriovenous oxygen extraction decreases and ^{86}Rb clearance is lower, consistent with a reduction of the capillary surface area.[32] The decrease in mesenteric blood flow rate is then followed by an escape from the vasoconstrictor effects. Blood flow autoregulates as the same vessels then relax.[33] These homeostatic effects may explain, in part, the varying degrees of response observed in different laboratories to pharmacological manipulations of peritoneal transport parameters.

NEURAL AND HORMONAL CONTROL OF MESENTERIC BLOOD FLOW

The mesenteric vasculature is accompanied by autonomic neuroelements from the celiac plexus. The primary means of neurocontrol of the splanchnic vessels is the sympathetic innervation. Sympathetic stimulation constricts the arteriolar smooth muscle, decreasing splanchnic blood flow, and sympathectomy is followed by increased splanchnic perfusion. Parasympathetic innervation of the superior mesenteric artery derives from the vagus nerve. Whether vagal section reduces peritoneal clearances is uncertain.

Epinephrine and norepinephrine may decrease superior mesenteric arterial blood flow rate, but their effects favor muscular and cutaneous vasoconstriction. The resultant increase in blood pressure may actually increase mesenteric perfusion.[13] Acetylcholine, on the other hand, dilates the mesenteric vasculature, but the increased tone and motility that also result from this agent can obscure the hyperemia.[13] Serotonin constricts large splanchnic arteries but relaxes arterioles and precapillary sphincters.[16] Serotonin does not reduce oxygen uptake by the intestine, unlike vasopressin, which also vasoconstricts the mesenteric vessels.

The gastrointestinal hormones are a group of polypeptides that specifically dilate the splanchnic vasculature and induce certain physiological effects.[34] At pharmacological doses, vasodilation is easily recognized as mesenteric blood flow rate may exceed 200% of control values after glucagon administration.[35] Secretin, which is structurally similar, increases superior mesenteric arterial flow and peritoneal clearances to a lesser extent than glucagon.[35,36] Gastrin and cholecystokinin are structurally similar and each increases superior mesenteric arterial blood flow.[35] The increase in mesenteric blood flow rate can be induced after intraduodenal instillation of corn oil, 1-phenylalanine or acid, following a short latency consistent with the physiological release of secretin or cholecystokinin.[37] Similar changes can also be induced by intravenous low doses of these hormones. The endogenous release of cholecystokinin or secretin or their intra-arterial infusion relaxes precapillary sphincters and increases the capillary filtration coefficient from 0.05 to 0.1 ml/minute/mm Hg/100 g.[38] An increase in net osmotic ultrafiltration rate occurs when secretin is given intravenously during peritoneal dialysis, but not when cholecystokinin or glucagon are administered.[36] The capillary filtration coefficient is also increased by 5-hydroxytryptamine.[38] The effects of cholecystokinin and secretin on mesenteric blood flow are additive and are potentiated by theophylline.[39] The vasodilation induced by these hormones is unaffected by α- or β-adrenergic activity and is interpreted to represent direct relaxation of vascular tone, presumably mediated by cyclic AMP. In contrast to these hormones somatostatin and vasoactive intestinal peptide vasoconstrict the splanchnic bed, reducing mesenteric blood flow rates.[35]

The prostaglandins are intimately involved in the fine control of vascular hemodynamics by virtue of their ability to moderate vascular responses.[40] The prostaglandins are a family of 20 carbon unsaturated lipids, which are formed by an enzyme system, present in many tissues, from several precursors, the most common of which is arachidonic acid.[41] Prostaglandins of the E, A, and I series dilate almost all segments of the microcirculation, including arterioles, metarterioles, precapillary sphincters, and venules. This dilatation increases the capillary filtration coefficient, suggesting enhanced permeability or increased capillary surface area or both. The PGF series tends to increase blood pressure primarily by increasing venous constriction.[42] In rabbits undergoing peritoneal dialysis, the intraperitoneal instillation of PGE_1, PGA_1, and especially PGE_2 augment urea and creatinine clearances but do not affect net osmotic ultrafiltration rates, and $PGF_{2\alpha}$ decrease clearances significantly.[43] These changes are in accord with the vasoactive effects of these tissue prostaglandins. Given intravenously, these prostaglandins did not affect peritoneal transport rates, as predicted by their virtually complete degradation during transit through the pulmonary circulation. Prostacyclin (PGI_2) is not degraded in the lung and has a biological half-life of a few minutes. Neither intravenous nor intraperitoneal administration of PGI_2 augmented peritoneal clearances, presumably because widespread vasodilation occurred with no net increase in mesenteric blood flow.[43] Thromboxanes (TXA_2 and TXB_2) are vasoconstrictors that may play a role in the decreased peritoneal clearances, complicating diseases associated with platelet thrombi, a phenomenon that is offset by the antiplatelet aggregating effect of dipyridamole.[44] Both PGE and PGA reduce the vascular responsiveness to various vasoconstrictor stimuli in the mesocecum of the rat. They may mediate bradykinin release, thereby causing compensatory vasodilation, so autoregulating splanchnic blood flow.[40] Inhibition of the prostaglandins prevents this modulation of blood flow, potentiating vasoconstrictor responses. Although deleterious effects on peritoneal blood flow have not been appreciated with the use of prostaglandin synthetase inhibitors, it has recently been recognized that such drugs as the nonsteroidal anti-inflammatory agents, may precipitate ischemic renal failure in susceptable groups of patients.[45]

PHARMACOLOGICAL ALTERATION OF MESENTERIC BLOOD FLOW

A variety of drugs are known to affect the mesenteric circulation and several of these also influence peritoneal mass transport rates.[1] When given intra-arterially or absorbed intraperitoneally, specific vasomotor responses in the splanchnic circulation may be appreciated more readily than when widespread vasoactive effects follow oral or intravenous administration.

Isoproterenol primarily vasodilates the mesenteric circulation, but combined with β-adrenergic blockade by propranolol, it vasoconstricts.[46] In patients with systemic vascular disease and in normal rabbits, intraperitoneal instillation of isoproterenol enhances peritoneal mass transport, increasing clearances by as much as 50% above control values.[47,48]

Phenylephrine vasoconstricts the mesenteric circulation, but after α-adrenergic blockade by phenoxybenzamine, vasodilation results.[46] It is uncertain whether the incidental use of phenylephrine compounds adversely affects peritoneal transport parameters.

Vasoconstriction of the mesenteric circulation by epinephrine depends on α-adrenergic responses, unlike the vasoconstriction of norepinephrine.[46] Because norepinephrine decreases peritoneal clearances significantly, it is a less desirable vasopressor than dopamine for treatment of shock during dialysis.[5] At modest intravenous doses dopamine has little effect on peritoneal mass transport, whereas high doses increase peritoneal solute clearances. A slight increase in ultrafiltration rate is seen at all doses consistent with the more pronounced venular than arteriolar constriction that dopamine induces. Unlike norepinephrine, dopamine increases the distribution of blood flow to the splanchnic and renal circulations.[49,50] When α-adrenergic receptors are blocked by phenoxybenzamine, the increased clearances induced by dopamine are blunted, and when dopaminergic receptors are blocked by haloperidol, the increment is abolished.[5] An initial increase in mesenteric vascular resistance mediated by α-adrenergic receptors is followed by decreased resistance, the vasodilation resulting from a specific direct action on dopamine receptors in the vascular bed.[51]

Nitroprusside increases the fractional distribution of cardiac output to the viscera. Yet, it is ineffective in augmenting peritoneal clearances when given intravenously, presumably because of inducing widespread vasodilation resulting in hypotension. Nitroprusside increases mass transport parameters by as much as 50% when administered intraperitoneally,[1,2,4,52,53] and dilates capillaries, relaxing precapillary sphincters, and opening underperfused capillaries, thereby increasing surface area.[54]

Dipyridamole transiently dilates several vascular beds, including the splanchnic circulation. When added during peritoneal dialysis, modest increments in transport rates occur.[3,44] A more pronounced increment in mass transport occurs in patients with vascular insufficiency associated with platelet thrombi. This effect occurs after vasodilation has abated and is attributed to the antiplatelet aggregating effect.[44]

The mesenteric vasculature also responds to histamine.[16] Following local application of histamine to the mesentery, a pronounced vasodilation is seen accompanied by a marked increase in vascular permeability.[55] What role this effect can or does have in clinical dialysis is uncertain.

The response of the blood flow in the mesenteric circulation as well as in several other vascular beds to perfusion or local serosal application of potassium solutions is of considerable interest. At low concentrations of potassium, as occur with initiation of peritoneal dialysis, vasoconstriction occurs, whereas high potassium concentrations vasodilate, a phenomenon attributed to stimulation of an electrognic Na-K pump.[56] This effect is blocked by ouabain, a potent inhibitor of $NA^+, K^+ - ATPase$.

Local inflammation, as occurs with peritonitis, obviously induces vasodilation, the mechanisms of which need further study. Acute peritonitis is associated with increased solute transport, but a decreased rate of ultrafiltration, which can be explained by predominantly venular dilation reducing the capillary hydrostatic pressure.

Other vasodilators that increase peritoneal mass transport values are tolazoline, an α-adrenergic blocker,[1] and the potent diuretics, furosemide and ethacrynic acid, the effects of which may be unrelated to vasodilation.

SUMMARY

During the past few decades there has been considerable study of the blood flow to the kidney and the effects of drugs, disease, and physiological variables on this circulation. Now that peritoneal dialysis is being used continuously as a substitute for renal function, it behooves nephrologists to learn the effects of these variables on the mesenteric circulation. Potentially decreased transport rates in selected patients can be interpreted correctly and simply returned to normal, and in those with normal values, a simple and safe method to augment transport may be identified and adopted.

It is naive to consider the peritoneum as an inert dialyzing membrane with a blood flow rate as constant as occurs when an extracorporeal pump delivers blood to a hemodialyzer. Rational use of drugs and other physiological manipulations for incidental problems requires an understanding of their effects on blood flow to the peritoneum and on the permeability of the membrane.

References

1. Maher, J. F., Hirszel, P., and Lasrich, M.: An experimental model for study of pharmacologic and hormonal influences on peritoneal dialysis. *Contrib Nephrol* **17:** 131–138, 1979.
2. Nolph, K. D., Ghods, A. J., Brown, P. A., and Twardowski, Z. J.: Effects of intraperitoneal nitroprusside on peritoneal clearances in man with variation of dose, frequency of administration and dwell times. *Nephron* **24:** 114–120, 1979.

3. Ryckelynck, J. P., Pierre, D., DeMartin, A., and Rottembourg, J.: Amélioration des clairances péritonéales par le dipyridamole. *Nouv Presse Med* **7**: 472, 1978.
4. Felt, J., Richard, C. McCaffrey, C., and Levy, M.: Peritoneal clearance of creatinine and inulin during dialysis in dogs: effect of splanchnic vasodilators. *Kidney Int* **17**: 459–469, 1979.
5. Hirszel, P., Lasrich, M., and Maher, J. F.: Augmentation of peritoneal mass transport by dopamine. Comparison with norepinephrine and evaluation of pharmacologic mechanisms. *J Lab Clin Med* **94**: 747–754, 1979.
6. Gutman, R. A., Nixon, W. P., McRae, R. L., And Spencer, H. W.: Effect of intraperitoneal and intravenous vasoactive amines on peritoneal dialysis: study in anephric dogs. *Trans Am Soc Artif Intern Organs* **22**: 570–573, 1976.
7. Maher, J. F., Hohnadel, D. C., Shea, C., DiSanzo, F., and Cassetta, M.: Effects of intraperitoneal diuretics on solute transport during hypertonic dialysis. *Clin Nephrol* **7**: 96–100, 1977.
8. Alavi, H., Lianos, E., and Bentzel, C.: Enhanced peritoneal permeability of the rat by intraperitoneal use of protamine sulfate. *Abstr Am Soc Nephrol* **12**: 110A, 1979.
9. Warden, G. D., Maxwell, J. G., and Stephen, R. L.: Use of reciprocating peritoneal dialysis with a subcutaneous peritoneal catheter in endstage renal failure in diabetes mellitus. *J Surg Res* **24**: 495–500, 1978.
10. Finkelstein, F. O., and Kilger, A. S.: Enhanced efficiency of peritoneal dialysis using rapid small volume exchanges. *ASAIO J* **2**: 103–106, 1979.
11. Henderson, L. W., and Nolph, K. D.: Altered permeability of the peritoneal membrane after using hypertonic peritoneal dialysis. *J Clin Invest* **48**: 992–1001, 1969.
12. Zelman, A., Gisser, D., Whittam, P. J., Parsons, R. H., and Schuyler, R.: Augmentation of peritoneal dialysis efficiency with programmed hyper/hypoosmotic dialysates. *Trans Am Soc Artif Intern Organs* **23**: 203–208, 1977.
13. Grayson, J., and Mendel, D.: *Physiology of the Splanchnic Circulation.* Williams & Wilkins, Baltimore 1965, p. 200.
14. Green, J. F.: Determinants of systemic blood flow. *Int Rev Physiol* **18**: 33, 1979.
15. Hirsch, L. J., and Glick, G.: The splanchnic circulation. *Mod Concepts Cardiovasc Dis* **46**: 17–20, 1977.
16. Lanciault, G., and Jacobson, E. D.: The gastrointestinal circulation. *Gastroenterology* **71**: 851–873, 1976.
17. Aune, S.: Transperitoneal exchange II. Peritoneal blood flow estimated by hydrogen gas clearance. *Scand J Gastroenterol* **5**: 99–104, 1970.
18. Renkin, E. M.: Exchange of substances through capillary walls. In, *Circulatory and Respiratory Mass Transport,* G. E. W. Wolstenholme, Ed. Little, Brown, Boston, 1969, pp. 50–64.
19. Crone, C., and Christensen, O.: Transcapillary transport of small solutes and water. *Int Rev Physiol* **18**: 149–213, 1979.
20. Nolph, K. D., Stoltz, M. L., and Maher, J. F.: Altered peritoneal permeability in patients with systemic vasculitis. *Ann Intern Med* **75**: 753–755, 1971.
21. Elzouki, A. Y. Gruskin, A. G., Polinsky, M. S., Baluarte, H. J. and Prebis, J. W.: Age related changes in urea–C^{14} peritoneal dialysance. *Clin Dial Transplant Forum* **9**: 102–103, 1979.
22. Gross, F., Khairallah, P. A., and McGiff, J. C.: Pharmacology of angiotensin. In *Renal Hypertension,* I. H. Page, and J. W. McCubbin (Eds). Year Book Medical Publishers, Inc., Chicago, 1968.
23. Tyden, F., Samnegard, H., and Thulin, L.: The effects of changes in the carotid sinus baroreceptor activity on splanchnic blood flow in anesthetized man. *Acta Physiol Scand* **106**: 187–189, 1979.
24. Heese, G., Lund-Jacobsen, H., and Hansen, J. F.: Forearm and splanchnic blood flow at rest and during exercise in relation to the systemic arterio-venous oxygen difference in cardiac patients. *Scand J Clin Lab Invest* **37**: 455–459, 1977.
25. Popovich, R. P., Moncrief, J. W., Nolph, K. D., Ghods, A. J., Twardowski, Z. J., and Pyle, W. K.: Continuous ambulatory peritoneal dialysis. *Ann Intern Med* **88**: 449–456, 1978.
26. Price, H. L., Deutsch, S., Marshall, B. E., Stephen, G. W., Behar, M. G., and Neufeld,

G. R.: Hemodynamic and metabolic effects of hemorrhage in man with particular reference to the splanchnic circulation. *Circ Res* **18:** 469–474, 1966.
27. Greene, J. A., Jr., Lapco, L., and Weller, J. M.: Effect of drug therapy of hemorrhagic hypotension on kinetics of peritoneal dialysis in the dog. *Nephron* **7:** 178, 1970.
28. Treat, E., Ulano, H. B., Shanbour, L.S., and Jacobson, E. D.: Selective dilation with prostaglandin E_1, glucagon and isoproterenol of the constricted superior mesenteric artery. *Surg Forum* **22:** 371–373, 1971.
29. Abel, F. L., and Murphy, Q. R.: Mesenteric renal and iliac vascular resistance in dogs after hemorrhage. *Am J Physiol* **202:** 978–980, 1962.
30. Johnson, P. C.: Myogenic nature of increase in intestinal vascular resistance with venous pressure elevation. *Circ Res* **7:** 992–999, 1959.
31. Folkow, B., Lewis, D. H., Lundgren, O., Mellander, S., and Wallentin, I.: The effect of sympathetic vasoconstrictor fibres on the distribution of capillary blood flow in the intestine. *Acta Physiol Scand* **61:** 458–466, 1964.
32. Shepherd, A. P., Mailman, D., Burks, T. F., and Granger, H. J.: Effects of norepinephrine and sympathetic stimulation on extraction of oxygen and ^{86}Rb in perfused canine small bowel. *Circ Res* **33:** 166–174, 1973.
33. Ross, G.: Effects of norepinephrine infusions on mesenteric arterial blood flow and its tissue distribution. *Proc Soc Exp Biol Med* **137:** 921–924, 1971.
34. Rayford, P. L., Miller, T. A., and Thompson, J. C.: Secretin, cholecystokinin and newer gastrointestinal hormones. *N Engl J Med* **294:** 1093, 1157, 1976.
35. Thulin, L., and Samnegård, H.: Circulatory effects of gastrointestinal hormones and related peptides. *Acta Chir Scand (Suppl)* **482:** 73-74, 1978.
36. Maher, J. F., Hirszel, P., and Lasrich, M.: Effects of gastrointestinal hormones on transport by peritoneal dialysis. *Kidney Int* **16:** 130–136, 1979.
37. Fara, J. W., Rubenstein, E. H., and Sonneschein, R. R.: Intestinal hormones in mesenteric vasodilation after intraduodenal agents. *Am J Physiol* **223:** 1058–1067, 1972.
38. Biber, B., Fara, J., and Lundgren, O.: Vascular reactions in the small intestine during vasodilation. *Acta Physiol Scand* **89:** 449–456, 1973.
39. Farah, J. W.: Effects of gastrointestinal hormones on vascular smooth muscle. *Am J Dig Dis* **20:** 346–353, 1975.
40. Messina, E. J., Weiner, R., and Kaley, G.: Prostaglandins and local circulatory control. *Fed Proc* **35:** 2367–2375, 1976.
41. Heinemann, H. O., and Lee, J. B.: Prostaglandin and blood pressure control. *Am J Med* **61:** 681–695, 1976.
42. Friedman, W. F., Molony, D. A., and Kirkpatrick, S. E.: Prostaglandins: physiological and clinical correlations. *Adv Pediatr* **25:** 151–204, 1978.
43. Maher, J. F., Hirszel, P., and Lasrich, M.: Modulation of peritoneal transport rates by prostaglandins. *Adv Prostaglandin Thromboxane Res* **6:** 695–699, 1980.
44. Maher, J. F., Hirszel, P., Abraham, J. E., Galen, M. A., Chamberlin, M., and Hohnadel, D. C.: Effect of dipyridamole on peritoneal mass transport. *Trans Am Soc Artif Intern Organs* **22:** 219–223, 1977.
45. Kimberly, R. P., Bowden, R. E., Keiser, H. R., and Plotz, P. H.: Reduction of renal function by newer nonsteroidal anti-inflammatory drugs. *Am J Med* **64:** 804–807, 1978.
46. Swan, K. G., and Reynolds, D. G.: Adrenergic mechanisms in the canine mesenteric circulation. *Am J Physiol* **220:** 1179–1785, 1971.
47. Brown, S. T., Ahearn, D. J., and Nolph, K. D.: Reduced peritoneal clearances in scleroderma increased by intraperitoneal isoproterenol. *Ann Intern Med* **78:** 891–894, 1973.
48. Maher, J. F., Shea, C., Cassetta, M., and Hohnadel, D. C.: Isoproterenol enhancement of peritoneal permeability. *J Dial* **1:** 319–331, 1977.
49. Robie, N. W., and McNay, J. L.: Comparative splanchnic blood flow effects of various vasodilator compounds. *Circ Shock* **4:** 69–78, 1977.
50. Angehrn, W., Schmidt, E., Althaus, F., Niedermann, K., and Rothlin, M.: Effect of dopamine on hepatosplanchnic blood flow. *J. Cardiov Pharmacol* **2:** 257–265, 1980.
51. Higgins, C. B., Millard, R. W., Braunwald, E., and Vatner, S. F.: Effects and mechanisms of action of dopamine on regional hemodynamics in the conscious dog. *Am J. Physiol* **225:** 432–437, 1973.

52. Villarroel, F., Popovich, R. P., and Nolph, K. D.: Evaluation of permeance in peritoneal dialysis. *J Dial* **2**: 361–368, 1978.
53. Raja, R. M., Kramer, M. S., and Rosenbaum, J. L.: Enhanced clearance with intraperitoneal nitroprusside in high flow recirculation peritoneal dialysis. *Trans Am Soc Artif Intern Organs* **24**: 133–135, 1978.
54. Nolph, K. D., Ghods, A., Brown, P., Miller F., Harris, P., Pyle, K., and Popovich, R.: Effects of nitroprusside on peritoneal mass transfer coefficients and microvascular physiology. *Trans Am Soc Artif Intern Organs* **23**: 210–217, 1977.
55. Wayland, H.: Transmural and interstitial molecular transport. In *Proceedings of CAPD: an International Symposium,* M. Legrain, Ed. Excerpta Medica, Amsterdam, 1980, pp. 18–27.
56. Haddy, F.: The mechanism of potassium vasodilation. In *Mechanisms of Vasodilation,* P. M. Vanhoutte, and I. Leusen, Eds. S. Karger, Basel, 1978, pp. 200–205.

CHAPTER NINE

Pharmacokinetics of Co-Trimoxazole Using the Peritoneal Route: Consequence for the Treatment of Peritonitis in Patients Maintained on Peritoneal Dialysis

E. SINGLAS, Ph.D.

J. N. COLLIN, Ph.D.

J. ROTTEMBOURG, M.D.

M. LEGRAIN, M.D.

A. de MARTIN, M.D.

PERITONITIS REMAINS THE MAJOR limiting factor in the successful use of continuous ambulatory peritoneal dialysis (CAPD). Prompt, powerful, and safe antimicrobial treatment is required. Adequate prescription of any drug proposed to treat peritonitis in patients on CAPD requires a good knowledge of pharmacokinetic characteristics of the drug considered, including peritoneal transfer.

Pharmacokinetics of Co-Trimoxazole (CT) using either the oral or the peritoneal route were studied in 24 patients of both sexes, 16–76 years of age, with terminal renal failure. Mean residual creatinine clearance was 1.5 ml/minute (range 0 ± 4 ml/minute). Eighteen patients were on intermittent peritoneal dialysis, six on CAPD.

Trimethoprim (TMP) and sulfamethoxazole (SMZ) were determined using the same methods as Rieder et al.[1]

Protocol I: A single oral dose of 4 mg/kg of TMP and 20 mg/kg of SMZ was given to 10 noninfected patients at the beginning of a 12-hour peritoneal dialysis session using a semiautomatic cycling machine. Plasma concentration was highest at 4 hours for TMP (1.81 mcg/ml ± 0.29) and 6 hours for SMZ (26.5 mcg/ml ± 5.8). Pharmacokinetic characteristics are given in Table 1. The elimination of the drug through the peritoneum during the 12 hours was

Laboratoire de Pharmacocinétique Clinique et Service de Néphrologie, Groupe Hospitalier Pitié-Salpêtrière, Paris, France

TABLE 1.
Co-Trimoxazole: Pharmacokinetic Characteristics in Terminal Renal Failure in 10 Patients on Peritoneal Dialysis. Mean Values

K_e^a (hour^{-1})	$T_{1/2}^a$ (hour)	AUC^a (μg/ml/hour)	Plasma Clearance (ml/minute)	V_d^a (liter/kg)	Protein Binding (%)
Sulfamethoxazole (20 mg/kg)^b					
0.0534	18.1	902	26.2	0.55	48.0
±0.0142	±3.5	±118	±5.7	±0.07	±1.4
Trimethoprim (4 mg/kg)^b					
0.0342	23.7	77.3	66.2	2.2	34.7
±0.0056	−4.0	±22.8	±11.5	±0.5	±1.1

^{a} K_e: Elimination constant; $T_{1/2}$: half-life of elimination; AUC: area under curve; V_d: volume of distribution.
^{b} Drugs given orally in single dose.

very low. The mean peritoneal dialysance was 5.1 ml/minute for TMP and 1.2 ml/minute for SMZ.

Protocol II: A peritoneal lavage was performed in 13 patients during 12 hours, using a semiautomatic cycling machine. Five patients had clinical symptoms of peritonitis confirmed by bacteriological controls. The dialysate flow was 3 liters per hour; 1.5 liters was introduced into the cavity at each cycle and 16 mg of TMP and 80 mg of SMZ were added to each liter of the dialysate.*

Absorption rate of TMP and SMZ through the peritoneum is high: 90% of TMP and 40% of SMZ perfused into the peritoneum cavity were absorbed. It increased in patients with peritonitis, reaching 93% for TMP and 55% for SMZ. During the peritoneal irrigation, a continuous increase of plasma concentration of TMP and SMZ was observed until the 12th hour. The highest plasma concentrations were observed in the infected group. They were similar, with a delay of about 6 hours, to those observed after a single oral dose of CT according to protocol I. The high rate of peritoneal absorption of TMP and SMZ is the consequence of a high concentration gradient between the dialysate and the body fluids.

Protocol III: Six patients with bacterial peritonitis in relation with CAPD were treated according to the following schedule: continuous peritoneal lavage was performed during the first 2 days, 40 liters per day were perfused using a semiautomatic cycling machine, with 16 mg of TMP and 80 mg of SMZ being added to each liter of irrigating fluid. Neither oral nor parenteral CT was administered during this period. After 48 hours, CAPD was resumed using four to five 2-liter plastic bags per day. CT treatment was maintained for 2 weeks, using exclusively the oral route at a dose of 4 mg of TMP and 20

---

*Co-Trimoxazole solutions delivered in ampoules of 10 ml were kindly supplied by Roche Laboratories.

TABLE 2.
CAPD Peritonitis

Causes of Infection	
Staphylococcus epidermidis	14
Staphylococcus aureus	6
Enterococcus	5
Streptococcus	7
Moraxella	3
Aseptic peritonitis	21
	56[a]

[a] In 375 patient-months.

mg of SMZ per kg of body weight. Plasma concentrations after 48 hours of peritoneal irrigation, performed with the cycling machine, were 3.8 ± 0.3 mcg/ml for TMP and 29 ± 3.2 mcg/ml for SMZ. The subsequent exclusive oral administration of CT maintained a mean plasma concentration of 4.2 mcg/ml of TMP and 35 mcg/ml of SMZ. Such concentrations are superior to the bactericidal concentration and well below the toxic concentration of SMZ estimated at 150 mcg/ml.

DISCUSSION

Results concerning the peritoneal transfer of TMP and SMZ during protocol I, II, and III support the intraperitoneal administration of CT to treat efficiently peritoneal infections occurring in patients treated with CAPD. This route, used exclusively, offers both immediate high concentration of the antibacterial agent in the peritoneal cavity and early adequate plasma concentration. The adjunction of CT given by mouth is unnecessary in the absence of septicemia and can induce excessive plasma concentrations. In most cases after 2 days of peritoneal lavage with CT added to the dialysate, the oral route can be used exclusively with an appropriate schedule, taking into account the absence of renal elimination and the very low peritoneal clearance of the drug. If on clinical and bacteriological grounds, continuous peritoneal administration of CT is required for more than 48 hours, the administration of CT using the peritoneal route must be decreased by half.

Forty-seven patients with terminal renal failure have been treated since August 1978 with CAPD. Fifty-six episodes of peritoneal infection have been recorded over 375 patient-months, including 21 aseptic peritonitis. Causes of infection are given in Table 2. The therapeutic regimen described in protocol III has been considered as a first choice in all cases, treatment being started before the results of the routine bacteriological investigations. In two patients in whom potential resistance of bacteria to CT was suspected from previous infection episodes, other antibiotics were used from the beginning. In the 21 cases with "aseptic" peritonitis treatment was stopped after 2 days if no bacterial growth was found in two consecutive daily fluid samples. The treatment of 33 cases of bacterial peritonitis was successful in 26 cases, with a mean duration of hospitalization of 4.7 days. CT failed to cure infection due to *Staphylococcus epidermidis* in four cases and *Staphylococcus aureus* in three cases, which required other antibiotic therapy. With this latter group, the mean duration of hospitalization was 9.5 days.

SUMMARY

In conclusion the low peritoneal clearance of TMP and SMZ is not in favor of treatment of peritonitis with Co-Trimoxazole when the oral route is used exclusively. The good peritoneal reabsorption of both TMP and SMZ during peritoneal administration leads to adequate plasma TMP and SMZ concentrations. In our experience the treatment of peritonitis as a complication of CAPD with Co-Trimoxazole as a first choice, using exclusively the peritoneal route for 2 days and subsequently the oral route for 2 weeks, has proved rapidly successful in 78% of cases with bacterial peritonitis.

References

1. Rieder, J., Schwartz, D. E., Fernex M., Bercan, T., Brodwall, E. K., Blumberg, A., Cottier, P., and Scheittlin, W.: Pharmacokinetics of the antibacterial combination sulfamethoxazole plus trimethoprin in patients with normal or impaired kidney function. *Antibiot Chemother* **18:**148–198, 1974.
2. Rottembourg, J., Jacq, D., Singlas, E., and N'Guyen, M.: Medical management of peritonitis in continuous ambulatory peritoneal dialysis. In: *CAPD:* M. Legrain, Ed., *Proceedings of an International Symposium,* Excerpta Medica, Amsterdam, 1980, pp. 330–339.

CHAPTER TEN

Peritoneal Dialysis Limitations and Continuous Ambulatory Peritoneal Dialysis

KARL D. NOLPH, M.D.

MICHAEL I. SORKIN, M.D.

PERITONEAL UREA CLEARANCES ARE LOW

MAXIMUM UREA CLEARANCES during peritoneal dialysis usually do not exceed 30 ml/minute, even with very high dialysis solution flow rates.[1,2] At clinical flow rates of 2–4 liters/hour, urea clearances are usually below 25 ml/minute. Since its early beginnings, these low urea clearances and accordingly the long treatment periods required to control blood urea nitrogen (BUN) have limited the growth and development of peritoneal dialysis probably more than any other factor. Although the debate continues as to the molecular size of the most important uremic toxins, most dialysis programs strive for maintenance of the BUN below 100 on good protein intakes. It would appear that intermittent peritoneal dialysis cannot provide such control with less than 40 hours of treatment per week when residual renal urea clearances fall below 1 ml/minute.[3]

Continuous ambulatory peritoneal dialysis (CAPD) increases treatment time to the maximum.[4-12] That is, treatment becomes essentially continuous. With CAPD dialysis solution, drainage volumes are usually 8–10 liters per day and thus imply maximum urea clearances of only 5.5–6.9 ml/minute (well below values possible during peritoneal dialysis with more rapid dialysis solution flow rates). The total time commitment of the patient to technical maneuvers with four 2-liter exchanges per day becomes essentially four 30-minute periods or 2 hours per day. This represents 14 hours per week and

---

Division of Nephrology, Department of Medicine, University of Missouri Medical Center and VA Hospital, Columbia, Missouri

is similar to treatment time requirements for hemodialysis. Thus, although the treatment is continuous, the time demand away from "freedom" is nearly one-third of that required for intermittent peritoneal dialysis.

It is the intent of this chapter to describe the peritoneal dialysis system and to explain its limitations. We will also review the evidence that CAPD is the best method available to overcome these peritoneal dialysis limitations.

THE PERITONEAL DIALYZER IS PROBABLY A CAPILLARY KIDNEY

Most solutes removed during peritoneal dialysis probably move from peritoneal capillaries into the peritoneal cavity.[1,2] Some net solute movement may take place from peritoneal lymphatics, but the extent of participation of these "fibers" is unknown. As in extracorporeal hollow fibers dialyzers, the blood path consists of multiple separate and distinct cylindrical channels.

A man-made hollow fiber dialyzer has relatively high urea clearances, which can easily exceed 100–150 ml/minute. What are the major factors that account for these differences in the efficiency of small solute removal in peritoneal and man-made capillary kidneys?

MAJOR DIFFERENCES BETWEEN PERITONEAL AND HOLLOW FIBER DIALYZERS

Table 1 summarizes major differences between peritoneal and hollow fiber dialyzers.

Studies to date would suggest that urea clearances in peritoneal dialysis are limited mainly by the peritoneal interstitial resistance and stagnant fluid films in the peritoneal cavity.[13]

Gas diffusion studies suggest that effective peritoneal capillary flow may be 2–3 times maximum urea clearances, offering no major limitation to peritoneal urea clearances.[2]

Wayland[14,15] has found that following the intravenous administration of sodium fluorescein to rats, a major portion of this small molecular weight solute (monitored visually) moves quickly (1–5 seconds) across mesenteric capillary walls into the interstitium. In contrast, fluorescent labeled albumin is held up almost entirely by the vascular walls for indefinite periods.

In our own laboratories we have subjected efficient hollow fiber dialyzers to the stagnant fluid film conditions of peritoneal dialysis. Even in the absence of a mesothelium and interstitium, hollow fiber small solute clearances decrease dramatically in seconds when operated in a 2-liter pool of dialysate.[2] This is true even with aggressive mixing and/or rapid cycling of the dialysis solution greater than possible under clinical circumstances. In contrast, in the hollow fiber dialyzer used properly, urea clearance would appear to be limited primarily by blood flow and actually approaches values near blood flow into the dialyzer under usual clinical conditions.

Both anatomical and kinetic studies would suggest that the peritoneum has relatively large pores with a mean pore diameter greater than 40 Å.[16–23]

TABLE 1.
Major Differences between Peritoneal and Hollow Fiber Dialyzers

Peritoneal Dialysis	Hollow Fiber Dialysis
Urea clearance limited mainly by interstitium and fluid films in peritoneal cavity. Maximum $C_{urea} \simeq 30$, capillary flow 70 ml/minute.	Urea clearance limited mainly by flood flow. Maximum $C_{urea} > 150$, capillary flow >200 ml/minute.
Relatively large mean pore diameter (>40 Å) and thin capillary walls (1-2 μm) with measurable albumin removal	Relatively small mean pore diameter (20 Å) and thick capillary walls (16-30 μm). Albumin transport miniscule.
Internal capillary diameter 5-10 μm.	Internal capillary diameter 200-215 μm.
Unknown numbers of capillaries involved with low pore density (<0.2% of endothelial surface) and small total pore area.	7,000-20,000 capillaries with high pore density and large total pore area.
Numbers of capillaries perfused and permeability susceptible to physiological and drug manipulation.	Number of capillaries perfused and permeability relatively fixed.
Low dialysate flow (8 liters/day-4 liters/hour).	High dialysate flow (>12 liters/hour).
Blood membrane interaction with vascular injury.	Deposition of platelets, fibrin, and white blood cells, complement activation.
Interstitium and mesothelium separate capillaries from dialysis solution (30-100 μm from capillary lumen to dialysate)	Direct capillary and dialysis solution contact (16-30 μm from capillary lumen to dialysate).
Transmembrane hydrostatic pressure (TMP) 40 mm Hg at arteriolar end of capillaries.	TMP, 100-600 mm Hg.
Dialysate osmolality (340-490) high in glucose.	Dialysate osmolality (280-300) low or no glucose
Maximum ultrafiltration rate is 12 ml/minute at start of hypertonic exchange.	Maximum ultrafiltration rate 20-30 ml/minute at high TMP

Endothelial intercellular channels may represent effective pores across the thin capillary walls (1-2 μm).[16-23] Albumin is removed during clinical peritoneal dialysis, suggesting that capillaries do permit some large proteins to migrate across the capillary wall under usual peritoneal dialysis conditions. Wayland has shown that the topical application of vasodilators, such as nitroprusside and histamine to rat mesentery, can result in seconds in a visible, almost explosive, leaking of fluorescent labeled albumin across the capillary walls of the peritoneal microcirculation.[14,15] In hollow fiber dialyzers, mean pore diameter appears to be much smaller and capillary walls much thicker.[24] Large proteins are not removed to any significant extent.

Internal capillary diameters are much smaller in the peritoneal microcirculation than in hollow fiber dialyzers. The implications of this are not clear, except that stagnant fluid film resistances within the capillary lumen should be quite small.

The number of capillaries participating in peritoneal exchange is unknown. Pappenheimer[20] suggested that endothelial intercellular channels represent only 0.2% of the endothelial surface. Thus, the effective pore area of the peritoneal membrane may be a very tiny fraction of total peritoneal surface. In contrast, hollow fiber dialyzers have a very high pore density and a large pore area. It is possible that the small total pore area of the peritoneum to some extent limits all clearances. If there were more of these relatively large pores in the peritoneal system, protein losses could be disastrous.

The peritoneal system has the unique characteristics of variability in 1) the number of capillaries perfused at any one time, 2) the permeability from capillary to capillary, 3) permeability differences from the arteriolar to the venous end of the capillary, and 4) changes in permeability in any one capillary from moment to moment.[14,15,21,25-27] For example, it would appear that vasodilatation, whether physiological or drug induced, results in increased numbers of capillaries perfused, opens capillaries that are more permeable, and may selectively alter permeability in certain sections of capillaries. For example, nitroprusside and histamine seem to widen intercellular gaps in small venules.[14,15] In hollow fiber dialyzers the number of capillaries perfused changes only slightly with fiber clotting, and fiber permeability is more homogeneous and fixed.

In peritoneal dialysis, dialysis solution flow rate is low, ranging from 8 to 10 liters per day in CAPD to usually no more than 4 liters/hour with automatic cycling. In contrast, during hollow fiber dialysis, dialysis solution flow rates in excess of 12 liters/hour are not uncommon. Limitations on peritoneal urea clearances are often ascribed to low dialysis solution flow rates. This is certainly the case in CAPD; however, we now know that even with the most rapid cycling, peritoneal dialysis clearances in excess of 30 ml/minute are unusual and not explained by dialysate flow rate.

Peritoneal dialysis uses a biological membrane. Blood membrane interaction should occur only with vascular injury. In contrast, during hollow fiber dialysis, platelets and white blood cells are deposited on the membrane and complement is activated.[28-30]

The total distance from the capillary lumen to dialysis solution is relatively far in peritoneal dialysis, since solutes must cross the interstitium and mesothelium. Even though capillary walls are thicker in hollow fiber dialyzers, the total distance from capillary lumen to dialysis solution is much shorter.

Transmembrane hydrostatic pressure in peritoneal capillaries at the afferent end is probably near 40 mm of mercury.[19] At the venular end of capillaries, oncotic pressure presumably exceeds transmembrane hydrostatic pressure. Thus, ultrafiltration during peritoneal dialysis is achieved primarily by adding glucose to dialysis solution and generating osmotic pressure. It is not known whether the osmotic pressure increases actual ultrafiltration across the proximal capillary wall or mainly decreases reabsorption in the distal capillary and venule.[31] Dialysis solutions with hollow fiber dialyzers may have little or no glucose added.

The maximum ultrafiltration rate seen during peritoneal dialysis has been reported to be 12 ml/minute during the first few minutes of a hypertonic (4.25% dextrose) exchange.[31] In hollow fiber dialysis, in contrast, sustained ultrafiltration rates in excess of 20–30 ml/minute can be maintained at high transmembrane pressure.

IMPLICATIONS OF PERITONEAL DIALYSIS CHARACTERISTICS FOR CAPD

First, it is unlikely that inherent limitations in the peritoneal system will ever permit urea clearances much in excess of 30 ml/minute. If it is true that weekly clearances of small solutes are important in controlling uremic toxicity, intermittent peritoneal dialysis will be doomed to long treatment times in the indefinite future. CAPD capitalizes on the unique location and anatomical characteristics of peritoneal dialysis and overcomes inefficiency with time.

Second, weekly peritoneal clearances of large solutes during CAPD are very high. Actual minute-to-minute clearances of solutes in the molecular weight range of 5,000 daltons may actually approach those during hollow fiber dialysis so that with the continuous nature of CAPD, weekly clearances are 5–6 times those with hollow fiber dialysis.[4,5] For even larger solutes, such as albumin, the ratio of weekly clearances with CAPD to weekly clearances with hollow fiber dialyzers approaches infinity. Thus, the limitations on the number of exchanges per day required for CAPD may depend primarily on small solute clearances. Preliminary reports of patients who do well on five exchanges per day, but not four exchanges per day, or similarly, patients who do well on four exchanges per day, but not three exchanges per day, would support the idea that small solute clearances are important in controlling uremic toxicity.[32–34] The symptoms that appear as the number of exchanges is reduced are often nausea, vomiting, and decreased appetite. These findings would support the recent arguments of Gotch[34] that small molecular weight solutes may have an important influence on appetite and nutritional health.

Third, massive destruction of the peritoneum might still be compatible with weekly clearances of larger solutes on CAPD well above those achieved on a weekly basis with hemodialysis. This is true since they may be many times higher in CAPD as compared to hemodialysis with an intact peritoneum. As long as small solute clearances approach the flow rates of dialysis solution, weekly clearances of small solutes may remain relatively unaltered. it would appear that it would take massive destruction of the peritoneal membrane before CAPD would become clinically inadequate.

SUMMARY

The inherent problems of stagnant fluid films and interstitial resistance perhaps coupled with low total pore area make low urea clearances a fixed characteristic of peritoneal dialysis. CAPD overcomes inefficiency with time. Preliminary reports suggesting that three or even four exchanges are not enough per day in some patients support the arguments that small molecular weight toxins may be important.

ACKNOWLEDGMENTS

Supported in part by U.S. Public Health Service grant numbers 1AM5 2216, NIH 1 AM62211, NIH 1AM7 2217, and CRC RR 0028711.

References

1. Nolph, K. D.: Peritoneal dialysis. In *Replacement of Renal Function by Dialysys*, W. Drukker, E. M. Parson and J. F. Maher, Eds. Martinus Nijhoff Medical Division, The Hague, 1978, pp. 277–321.
2. Nolph, K. D., Popovich, R. P., Ghods, A., J. and Twardowski, Z.: Determinants of low clearances of small solutes during peritoneal dialysis. *Kidney Int* 13: 117, 1978.
3. Ahmad, S., Shen, F., Gallagher, N.M., et al.: Intermittent peritoneal dialysis: status reassessed. *Am Soc Artif Intern Organs* 3: 36, 1979.
4. Popovich, R. P., Moncrief, J. W., Nolph, D. D., Ghods, A. J., Twardowski, Z. J., and Pyle, W. K.: Continuous ambulatory peritoneal dialysis. *Ann Int Med* 88: 449–456, 1978.
5. Nolph, K. D., Popovich, R. P., and Moncrief, J. W.: Theoretical and practical implications of continuous ambulatory peritoneal dialysis. *Nephron* 21: 117–122, 1978.
6. Moncrief, J. W., Nolph, K. D., Rubin, J., et al.: Additional experience with continuous ambulatory peritoneal dialysis (CAPD). *Trans Am Soc Artif Intern Organs* 24: 476–483, 1978.
7. Oreopoulos, D. G., Robson, M., Faller, B., et al.: Continuous ambulatory peritoneal dialysis: a new era in the treatment of chronic renal failure. *Clin Nephrol* 11(3): 125–128, 1979.
8. Moncrief, J. W.: Continuous ambulatory peritoneal dialysis. *Dial Transplant* 8(11): 1077–1080, 1979.
9. Lindsay, R.: A comparison of CAPD and hemodialysis. In *CAPD: Proceedings of an International Symposium*. M. Legrain, Ed. Excerpta Medica, Amsterdam, 1980.
10. Fuchs, C.: Technique of continuous ambulatory peritoneal dialysis (CAPD). *Nieren- und Hockdruck-krankheiten* 5: 183–187, 1979.
11. Dorn, D.: Clinical observations with continuous ambulatory peritoneal dialysis (CAPD). *Nieren- und Hockdruck-krankheiten* 5: 188–192, 1979.
12. Schuenemann, B., Falda, Z., Mergerian, H., et al.: Clinical experience with continuous ambulatory peritoneal dialysis. *Nieren- und Hockdruck-krankheiten* 5: 193–197, 1979.
13. Nolph, K. D.: CAPD—a logical approach to peritoneal dialysis limitations (a comparison of the peritoneal dialysis system and hollow fiber kidneys). *J Nephrol-Urol-Andrology* (in press).
14. Wayland, H., and Silberber, A.: Blood to lymph transport. *Microvasc Res* 15: 367–374, 1978.
15. Wayland, H.: Action of histamine on the microvasculature. In *CAPD: Proceedings of an International Symposium*, M. Legrain, Ed. Excerpta Medica, Amsterdam, 1980.
16. Karnovsky, M. J.: The ultrastructural basis of capillary permeability studies with peroxides as a tracer. *J Cell Biol* 35: 213, 1967.
17. Cotran, R. S.: The fine structure of the microvasculature in relation to normal and altered permeability. In *Physical Bases of Circulatory Transport: Regulation and Exchange*, E. B. Reeve, and A. C. Guyton, Eds. W. B. Sauders, Philadelphia, 1967, pp. 249–275.
18. Karnovsky, M. J.: The ultrastructural basis of transcapillary exchanges. In *Biological Interfaces: flows and exchanges*. Little, Brown & Co., Boston, 1968, pp. 64–95.

19. Renkin, E. M.: Exchange of substances through capillary walls: circulatory and respiratory mass transport. In *Ciba Foundation Symposium,* G. E. W. Wolstenholme, Ed. Little, Brown & Co., Boston, 1969, pp. 50–66.
20. Pappenheimer, J. R.: Passage of molecules through capillary walls. *Physiol Rev* **33:** 387, 1953.
21. Nolph, K. D., Ghods, A., Brown, P., Miller, F., Harris, P., Pyle, K., and Popovich, R.: Effects of nitroprusside on peritoneal mass transfer coefficients and microvascular physiology. *Trans Am Soc Artif Intern Organs* **23:** 210, 1977.
22. Gosselin, R. E., and Berndt, W. O.: Diffusional transport of solutes through mesentery and peritoneum. *J Theor Biol* **3:** 487, 1962.
23. Nagel, W., and Kuschinsky, W.: Study of the permeability of isolated dog mesentery. *Eur J Clin Invest* **1:** 149, 1970.
24. Green, D. M., Antwiler, G. D., Moncrief, J. W., Decherd, J. F., and Popovich, R. P.: Measurement of the transmittance coefficient spectrum of cuprophan. *Trans Am Soc Artif Intern Organs* **22:** 627–636, 1976.
25. Miller, F. N., Nolph, K. D., Harris, P. D., *et al.*: Microvascular and clinical effects of altered peritoneal dialysis solutions. *Kidney Int* **15:** 630–639, 1979.
26. Miller, F. N., Joshua, I. G., Harris, P. D., *et al.*: Peritoneal dialysis solutions and the microcirculation. In *Today's Art of Peritoneal Dialysis,* Vol. 17 of *Contributions to Nephrology,* A. Trevino-Becerra and F. Boen, Eds. S. Karger, Basel, 1979, pp. 51–58.
27. Miller, F. N., Wiegman, D. L., Joshua, I. G. *et al.*: Effects of vasodilators and peritoneal dialysis solution on the microcirculation of the rate cecum. *Proc Soc Exp Biol Med* **161:** 605–608, 1979.
28. Jensen, D. P., Brubaker, L. H., Nolph, K. D., Johnson, C. A., and Nothum, R. J.: Hemodialysis coil-induced transient neutropenia and overshoot neutrophilia in normal man. *Blood* **41:** 399–498, 1973.
29. Ahearn, D. J., Marshall, J. W., Nothum, R. J. Esterly, J. A., Nolph, K. D., and Maher, J. F.: Morphologic studies of dialysis membranes—adherence of blood components of air rinsed coils. *Trans Am Soc Artif Intern Organs* **19:** 435, 1973.
30. Marshall, J. W., Ahearn, D. J., Nothum, R. J., Esterly, J., Nolph, K. D., and Maher, J. F.: Adherence of blood components to dialyzer membranes: morphological studies. *Nephron* **12:** 157–170, 1974.
31. Rubin, J., Nolph, K. D., Popovich, R. P., Moncrief, J., and Prowant, B.: Drainage volumes during CAPD. *Trans Am Soc Intern Organs* **2:** 2, 1979.
32. Maher, J. F., and Nolph, K. D.: Resistance to diffusion in dialyzers. *Clin Nephrol* **1:** 333–335, 1974.
33. Nolph, K. D., and Maher, J. F.: Clinical and laboratory evaluation of coil dialyzers. In *Renal Dialysis,* D. Whelpton, Ed. Sector Publishing, London, 1974, pp. 105–122.
34. Gotch, F. A.: A quantitative evaluation of small and middle molecule toxicity in therapy of uremia. *Dial Transplant* **9:** 183–194, 1980.

CHAPTER ELEVEN

Metabolite Generation and Clearance Variation in Long-Term CAPD

DAVID H. RANDERSON, M.Sc., Ph.D.

PETER C. FARRELL, Ph.D., D.Sc.

INTRODUCTION

HIGH ATTRITION RATES AMONG peritoneal dialysis (PD) patients on maintenance dialysis therapy have often been ascribed to negative nitrogen balance resulting from high protein and amino acid losses to the dialysis fluid. The occurrence of a depletion syndrome has been reported by both Palmer et al.[1] and Tenckhoff.[2] In contrast, Linder and Tenckhoff[3] reported positive nitrogen balance in six chronic PD patients during four study periods of 7 days each in a metabolic ward. These authors suggested that patients should be able to compensate for obligatory protein losses by maintaining a dietary protein intake (DPI) of at least 1 g/kg/24 hours.

Continuous ambulatory peritoneal dialysis (CAPD) patients, because they undergo continuous dialysis, may have higher protein and amino acid losses than intermittent peritoneal dialysis (IPD) patients, putting them at increased risk of negative nitrogen balance. Furthermore, urea clearance on CAPD is about 60% of that of routine hemodialysis (HD) clearance and yet CAPD patients have suprisingly low steady-state urea serum levels, approximately 20 mm/liter,[4] suggestive of a number of possibilities. The patients could be anabolic, lacking in sufficient DPI, or the DPI could be acceptable with increased nitrogen losses in the stools.

A further complication of long-term PD has more recently been suggested by Finkelstein et al.[5] They noted a loss of small molecule clearance with long-term IPD, although Rubin et al.[6] have recently reported a contrary result for long-term CAPD patients. The latter patients are exposed to fluid in the abdomen for up to 168 hours per week, compared to 30 to 40 hours for

---

Centre for Biomedical Engineering, The University of New South Wales, Kensington, N.S.W., Australia

IPD patients and, in addition, the incidence of peritonitis in CAPD patients is between 2–4 times that observed in IPD patients.[4] Both these factors could conceivably result in greater deterioration of peritoneal permeability in CAPD patients.

As part of a prospective evaluation of the place of CAPD in the management of chronic renal failure, urea and creatinine generation rates have been measured to provide feedback on DPI and possible changes in skeletal muscle mass, respectively. Peritoneal clearances, as characterized by the over-all mass transfer coefficient (MTC) for a spectrum of solutes, have been determined at 3–4 monthly intervals during more than 12 months of CAPD.

MATERIALS AND METHODS

Three detailed evaluations for urea and creatinine generation rates and peritoneal permeability clearances[7] have been performed on 10 long-term CAPD patients during 10 months of CAPD. The third evaluations were performed at an average of 42 ± 2 weeks (range 34–51 weeks). Table 1 gives the average times from commencement of CAPD for the three evaluations, along with mean residual renal function. Two of the patients were anephric. Five patients were female, and the average age was 46 ± 5 (range 13–64) years. Peritonitis during the study period averaged one episode every 18 patient-weeks (54% aseptic, 33% gram-positive). Two patients had no peritonitis during the study period.

Since the third evaluation, three patients died (two due to causes unrelated to PD and one with peritonitis) and one transferred to HD due to recurrent aseptic peritonitis. The remaining six patients underwent a fourth evaluation at 56 ± 4 (42–68) weeks (Table 1). Four of these patients were female, and the average age was 41 ± 8 (13–64) years. Peritonitis for this remaining group averaged one episode every 39 patient-weeks (44% aseptic, 44% gram-positive). Two still have had no peritonitis.

Solute generation rates (urea and creatinine) were obtained by measuring total urinary and dialysis output over a 24–30-hour period with compensation for changes in serum levels. Protein catabolic rate (PCR, g/kg/24 hours) was obtained from net urea generation rate (G_u, mM/minute) by assuming nitrogen balance and applying the correlation developed by Gotch[8]:

$$\text{PCR} = 9.35\,(28 \times G_u + 1.5)/W$$

where W(kg) is the patient's weight.

Protein levels in dialysate were also measured and added to PCR to give an estimate of DPI with the inherent assumption that the patients are in nitrogen balance.

Solute clearance was obtained by measurement of the total amount of solute removed per exchange dividend by the mean time of the exchange and the mean serum solute level.[9,10] Clearance provides a comparison between the efficiency of CAPD, other modes of dialysis therapy, and the natural kidneys. However, because it decreases with dwell time and is influenced by ultrafiltration, it provides little indication of membrane viability. The initial clear-

TABLE 1.
Study Periods and Residual Renal Function[a]

	Evaluations			
	1	2	3	4
Group A: Ten Patients with Three Evaluations Completed				
Period on CAPD (weeks)	7 ± 1	23 ± 3	42 ± 2	
Residual creatinine clearance				
(ml/minute)	1.7 ± 0.4	1.1 ± 0.4	0.9 ± 0.2	
Group B: Six Patients with Four Evaluations Completed				
Period on CAPD (weeks)	6 ± 2	21 ± 3	39 ± 3	56 ± 4
Residual creatinine clearance				
(ml/minute)	1.5 ± 0.6	0.8 ± 0.4	1.0 ± 0.6	0.7 ± 0.4

[a] The patients in Group B are also included in Group A.

ance, or MTC, is a more sensitive measure of membrane properties, since it is a function of peritoneal permeability, surface area, and blood flow rate, and it is independent of dialysis regimen. Theoretical models can be applied to serially obtained data to optimize model and experimental data correlation and provide the MTC.[9,10]

Clearance and MTC data for the endogenous solutes urea and creatinine and the exogenously administered radiolabeled vitamin B_{12} were obtained on the second day of solute generation studies. On the day of the study, patients took no antihypertensive drugs and fasted before and during the evaluation. The second daily exchange was the test exchange. However, a 1.5% dextrose-containing fluid was also used in the first exchange to reduce carry-over effects induced by hypertonic solutions. The 1.5% test solution was prewarmed to 37 °C and during infusion a blood sample was taken for assay.

Immediately after infusion of dialysate 7 ml were withdrawn after *in situ* mixing. Samples were then taken half-hourly. After exactly 4.5 hours fluid was drained back into the sack, subsampled, and the volume noted. A final blood sample was taken during drainage.

Patients participating in the study were all volunteers and methodology was approved by the University of New South Wales Committee for Experimental Procedures Involving Human Subjects, in compliance with the principles of the World Medical Association as enunciated in the Declaration of Helsinki.

Significance of data was assessed by analysis of variance.

RESULTS AND DISCUSSION

An assessment of patient nutritional status is given in Table 2. None of the parameters presented for either Group A (10 patients evaluated three times) or Group B (six patients evaluated four times) showed statistical significance ($p > 0.10$). Serum urea levels remained stable during the study periods.

TABLE 2.
Urea and Protein Turnover

	Evaluations			
	1	2	3	4
Group A[a]				
Serum urea (mM/liter)	19.9 ± 1.8	20.1 ± 1.4	17.8 ± 1.9	
Urea generation (μM/minute)	129 ± 12	140 ± 11	105 ± 14	
PCR (g/kg/24 hours)	0.84 ± 0.07	0.90 ± 0.13	0.76 ± 0.10	
Dialysate protein (g/kg/24 hours)	0.23 ± 0.04 (n = 9)	0.20 ± 0.02	0.16 ± 0.01 (n = 9)	
DPI (g/kg/24 hours)	1.09 ± 0.08	1.10 ± 0.15	1.00 ± 0.11	
Serum albumin (g/liter)	30 ± 1	32 ± 1	28 ± 2	
Group B[b]				
Serum urea (mM/liter)	20.0 ± 2.2	18.9 ± 2.2	17.7 ± 2.4	17.9 ± 0.4
Urea generation (μM/minute)	113 ± 17	126 ± 9	102 ± 15	82 ± 10
PCR (g/kg/24 hours)	0.96 ± 0.08	1.04 ± 0.20	0.86 ± 0.15	0.72 ± 0.09
Dialysate protein (g/kg/24 hours)	0.25 ± 0.03	0.19 ± 0.04	0.19 ± 0.02	0.21 ± 0.01
DPI (g/kg/24 hours)	1.20 ± 0.10	1.23 ± 0.22	1.05 ± 0.16	0.94 ± 0.11
Serum albumin (g/liter)	29 ± 1	29 ± 1	25 ± 2	29 ± 3

[a] Mean ± S.E.M. (n = 10).
[b] Mean ± S.E.M. (n = 6).

There was a drop off in average DPI with a concomitant decrease in albumin levels for patients of both groups at the third evaluation. Four of the patients were in poor dietary status for a variety of reasons. One was depressed following spouse's death, one had a protracted upper respiratory tract infection, one had recurrent sterile peritonitis (and transferred to HD), and the other was disinterested in improving his situation, electing to cease dialysis altogether. The first two of these patients continued to the fourth evaluation but showed little change in DPI. Another patient showed evidence of protein-calorie malnutrition at the fourth evaluation (serum albumin 19 g/liter) and another had a recurrent yeast peritonitis unresponsive to treatment. The latter patient refused either abdominal surgery or transfer to HD on religious grounds and subsequently died. Thus, at the 13-month mark, four of our six patients were in danger of protein depletion and required careful

TABLE 3.
Creatinine Excretion and Weight

	Evaluations			
	1	2	3	4
Group A[a]				
Serum creatinine (m*M*/liter)	0.75 ± 0.03	0.80 ± 0.03	0.75 ± 0.04	
Creatinine excretion (mg/kg/24 hours)	13.3 ± 1.9	15.0 ± 1.6	12.5 ± 1.6	
Weight (kg)	58.2 ± 6.0	61.4 ± 6.2	63.0 ± 6.1	
Group B[b]				
Serum creatinine (m*M*/liter)	0.76 ± 0.05	0.76 ± 0.04	0.72 ± 0.03	0.79 ± 0.02
Creatinine excretion (mg/kg/24 hours)	14.4 ± 3.0	15.8 ± 2.3	14.4 ± 2.6	13.5 ± 1.1
Weight (kg)	46.5 ± 4.0	49.0 ± 4.5	50.8 ± 4.6	51.8 ± 5.2

[a] Mean ± S.E.M. ($n = 10$).
[b] Mean ± S.E.M. ($n = 6$).

dietary management to avoid wasting. Five of the six patients are still ongoing and will be further assessed at 18 months of CAPD therapy.

Creatinine excretion data and patient weights are presented in Table 3. Weight gain in Group A was highly significant ($p < 0.001$) but of lesser significance in Group B ($p < 0.025$). Changes in creatinine excretion were not significant in either group.

The stability of creatinine excretion data is suggestive of no change in muscle mass with increased fat deposition. Furthermore, any possible nutritional problems have not resulted in muscle wasting. Patient weight changes

TABLE 4.
Solute Clearance

	Evaluations			
	1	2	3	4
Group A[a]				
Urea (ml/minute)	6.4 ± 0.5	6.5 ± 0.5	6.7 ± 0.3	
Creatinine (ml/minute)	5.4 ± 0.4	5.5 ± 0.3	5.7 ± 0.3	
Vitamin B_{12} (ml/minute)	3.9 ± 0.5	3.5 ± 0.5	3.3 ± 0.2	
Group B[b]				
Urea (ml/minute)	6.0 ± 0.7	6.2 ± 0.8	6.5 ± 0.4	5.8 ± 0.6
Creatinine (ml/minute)	5.0 ± 0.5	5.5 ± 0.6	5.9 ± 0.3	5.2 ± 0.4
Vitamin B_{12} (ml/minute)	4.0 ± 0.8 ($n = 5$)	2.7 ± 0.6	3.6 ± 0.5	2.9 ± 0.3

[a] Mean ± S.E.M. ($n = 10$).
[b] Mean ± S.E.M. ($n = 6$). Dwell time 4.5 hours.

TABLE 5.
Mass Transfer Coefficient

	Evaluations			
	1	2	3	4
Group A[a]				
Urea (ml/minute)	26.8 ± 2.8	24.4 ± 1.8	24.3 ± 1.8	
Creatinine (ml/minute)	15.2 ± 2.1	13.6 ± 1.3	14.1 ± 1.6	
Vitamin B_{12} (ml/minute)	6.2 ± 0.9 ($n = 9$)	5.9 ± 0.9	4.6 ± 0.5	
Group B[b]				
Urea (ml/minute)	23.0 ± 0.7	27.1 ± 2.4	24.6 ± 2.4	22.6 ± 1.8
Creatinine (ml/minute)	12.5 ± 1.9	15.2 ± 1.9	14.6 ± 0.8	14.1 ± 1.3
Vitamin B_{12} (ml/minute)	7.1 ± 1.0 ($n = 5$)	5.5 ± 1.6	5.1 ± 0.9	4.9 ± 0.7

[a] Mean ± S.E.M. ($n = 10$).
[b] Mean ± S.E.M. ($n = 6$).

also appear to have stabilized at the 10-month point, with negligible gain beyond that. There is no clear explanation for this observation and further patient monitoring is needed.

Serial clearance data are presented in Table 4. Contrary to other data on IPD patients,[5] we have seen no evidence of falling clearances for the smaller solutes. This is in agreement with the data of Rubin *et al.*[6] Vitamin B_{12} clearances appear to display some tendency to fall, but the data did not reach a level of statistical significance. More follow-up data will be collected on this parameter.

The MTC, as mentioned, is the only reliable marker for peritoneal viability.[10] Table 5 shows that MTCs for urea and creatinine have not changed over 13 months of CAPD. Once again, vitamin B_{12} has shown a tendency to fall but the data are still not significantly different from period to period.

CONCLUSIONS

These data indicate that nutritional considerations are of prime importance with CAPD patients, as they are with IPD patients. Although patients can maintain positive nitrogen balance and avoid muscle wasting by sustaining a dietary protein intake of 1.2 g/kg/24 hours, any condition that causes a drop in DPI can rapidly lead to nitrogen depletion due to dialysate protein and amino acid losses.

Patients do put on weight, at least in the initial months of CAPD, and this seems to be due to fat deposition rather than muscle gain. However, this has yet to be confirmed.

No loss of peritoneal viability has been observed in 13 months of CAPD. Although follow-up studies are proposed, the data presented here suggest that

CAPD should be efficacious, from the viewpoint of solute removal, for long-term treatment of end-stage renal failure.

References

1. Palmer, R. A., Newell, J. E., Gray, E. J., and Quinton, W. E.: Treatment of chronic renal failure by prolonged peritoneal dialysis. *N Engl J Med* **274:** 248, 1966.
2. Tenckhoff, H.: Home peritoneal dialysis. In *Clinical Aspects of Uremia and Dialysis.* S.G. Massry and A.L. Sellers, Eds. Charles C Thomas, Springfield, Ill. 1976, pp. 583–615.
3. Lindner, A., and Tenckhoff, H.: Nitrogen balance in patients on maintenance peritoneal dialysis. *Trans Am Soc Artif Intern Organs* **16:** 255, 1970.
4. Randerson, D. H., and Farrell, P. C.: Clinical assessment of CAPD. *Dial Transplant* (in press).
5. Finkelstein, F. O., Kliger, A. S., Bastl, C., and Yap, P.: Sequential clearance and dialysance measurements in chronic peritoneal dialysis patients. *Nephron* **18:** 342, 1977.
6. Rubin, J., Nolph, K., Arfania, D., Brown, P., and Prowant, B.: Follow-up of peritoneal clearances in patients undergoing continuous ambulatory peritoneal dialysis. *Kidney Int* **16:** 619, 1979.
7. Farrell, P. C., and Randerson, D. H.: Membrane permeability changes in long-term CAPD. *Trans Am Soc Artif Intern Organs* **26:** 197, 1980.
8. Gotch, F. A.: A general review of the progress made in the technical aspects of hemodialysis in the last four years. In *Recent Advances in Biomedical Engineering.* Technical Aspects of Renal Dialysis, Newcastle, Del., 1976.
9. Randerson, D. H., and Farrell, P. C.: Kinetic modelling applied to continuous ambulatory peritoneal dialysis. *Proc Aust Conf Chem Eng* **7:** 36, 1979.
10. Randerson, D. H., and Farrell, P. C.: Mass transfer studies of the human peritoneum. *Am Soc Artif Intern Organs J* (in press).

CHAPTER TWELVE

CAPD: Nutritional Concerns—Have We Learned from the Experiences in the 1960s and 1970s?

MICHAEL J. BLUMENKRANTZ, M.D.

THE 1960s WAS THE DECADE in which maintenance peritoneal dialysis was first attempted on a large scale. Since each treatment usually required an abdominal puncture, dialysis was often performed infrequently, that is, every 6–10 days. Unless the patient had significant residual renal function, this frequency of dialysis was often inadequate and patients remained uremic. Due to anorexia, nutrient intake was often insufficient during the interdialytic period. In order to minimize azotemic symptoms, protein intake was restricted. During the long (36–40 hours), often uncomfortable, dialysis procedure, most patients had little desire to eat. The combination of insufficient dialysis and inadequate nutrient intake were major factors contributing to the frequently observed rapid development of malnutrition and wasting. Peritonitis occurred frequently as a result of abdominal punctures and breaks in the sterile system by the repeated manual exchange of bottles of dialysate. This led to catabolism, increased dialysate protein loss, and further decrease in food intake. These factors compounded the patient's nutritional demise.

In the 1970s, the development of the permanent Tenckhoff peritoneal catheter and automated equipment enabled intermittent peritoneal dialysis to be performed at more frequent intervals. However, as in the 1960s, the same combination of factors, that is, inadequate dialysis and insufficient nutrient intake, often resulted in failure of patients to thrive. All patients at a particular center were usually placed upon a standardized peritoneal dialysis regimen, as has been customary in most hemodialysis units. For intermittent peritoneal dialysis the regimen usually consisted of three or four 10-hour treatments each week. For most patients undergoing hemodialysis, the failure

---

Medical and Research Services, Veterans Administration, Wadsworth Medical Center, Los Angeles, California

to individualize the quantity of dialysis therapy does not have adverse consequences; 4 or 5 hours of hemodialysis thrice weekly, in general, appears to be adequate. Compared with hemodialysis, peritoneal dialysis is very inefficient for removal of small molecules. Even with the exchange of 4 liters of dialysate each hour, peritoneal urea clearances average only 25 ml/minute. In contrast, with currently available hemodialysis equipment, urea clearances can approach 170–190 ml/minute.

The fact that residual renal function contributes to clearance of middle molecular weight compounds has long been recognized. With peritoneal dialysis, residual renal function contributes significantly to small molecular clearance as well. For example, an endogenous urea clearance of 1 ml/minute (1.44 liters/day or 10 liters/week) is equal to urea clearance of approximately 6–7 hours of intermittent peritoneal dialysis (Table 1).

In many centers, no account was made for residual renal function when the amount of intermittent peritoneal dialysis was prescribed. In addition, the number of hours that peritoneal dialyses was performed was most often not increased as residual renal function decreased; patients were generally maintained on a fixed schedule.

The failure to individualize peritoneal dialysis therapy often has serious consequences. Even if physicians and dietitians prescribe abundant dietary protein and calories, if the amount of dialysis is insufficient the patient may become anorectic and actual protein and calorie intake will fall. The relationship between the amount of weekly clearance and the patient's appetite, protein intake and serum urea nitrogen (SUN) is often not appreciated. It has been claimed that anuric diabetic patients with a SUN averaging 80 mg/dl receiving only 25 hours of peritoneal dialysis per week were ingesting 1.5 g protein/kg of body weight/day; in actuality inspection of the patient SUN values and weekly renal and dialysate clearances suggest that the patients were probably only eating 0.7–0.8 g/kg/day.

The end result of inadequate dialysis and insufficient nutrient intake is often the gradual development of malnutrition, tissue wasting, and a general failure to thrive. A decrease in peritoneal clearance is frequently invoked as the cause. This may well occur; however, the decrease in total clearance is

TABLE 1.

Effect of Change in Renal Urea Clearance of 1 ml/minute on CAPD or Intermittent PD Requirements

Renal urea clearance of 1 ml/minute ≃ 1.44 liters/day ≃ 10 liters/week
1. With CAPD, 10 liters of additional effluent dialysate/week necessary to maintain same urea clearance
2. With IPD peritoneal urea clearance = 25 ml/minute[a] = 1.5 liters/hour
10 liters/week / 1.5 liters/hour = 6.6 hours/week of additional intermittent PD for same urea weekly clearance[b]

[a] Average clearance of patient undergoing PD, 1.5% dextrose, 4 liters/hour exchange rate.
[b] This estimate is an approximation; other factors influence number of additional hours required.

most often *not* due to a decrease in membrane permeability (ml/minute) but rather to an inadequate duration (minutes) of dialysis.

An apparently puzzling observation is often the failure of the SUN to rise. The SUN is the result of the relationship between protein intake and weekly urea clearance. In a stable patient, a given level of SUN (for example, 80 mg/dl) can result from two very different processes: 1) sufficient dialysis (total urea clearance, both peritoneal and renal) and an adequate protein intake, or 2) insufficient dialysis in patients eating a low protein intake. It is probable that if a patient has an SUN of 80 mg/dl as a result of the latter process, he may do poorly.

We are now in the 1980s and a new technique for peritoneal dialysis, CAPD, shows great promise. However, we are already beginning to see the same circumstances that contributed to the problems with peritoneal dialysis in the 1960s and 1970s. In many centers, all patients receive four exchanges per day; other centers advocate three exchanges per day for everyone. Again, we are seeing a failure to individualize therapy. It should be apparent that whereas a 50-kg woman with a glomerular filtration rate (GFR) of 2–3 ml/minute may do very well with three exchanges a day, an anuric 85-kg man will be underdialyzed with this regimen; he may require five or even six exchanges per day to enable him to ingest enough protein for his daily needs, for example, 1.2 g/kg or 100 g/day.

Clearance is dependent on the amount of dialysate drainage per week or per day and not the number of bags instilled. Four exchanges per day may result in 8.5 liters/day of effluent dialysate in one patient and 11 liters/day in another patient who uses predominately "4.25%" dialysate.

In patients undergoing CAPD, the total daily urea clearance should be ascertained and the dialysis regimen individualized so that sufficient dialysis is provided for the patient to have the appetite to ingest a sufficient amount of protein intake. Total daily urea clearance in liters/day is defined as the sum of renal urea clearance plus peritoneal urea clearance [effluent dialysate volume × (dialysate urea/serum urea)].

The assessment of adequacy of dialysis is multifaceted and complex. However, most nephrologists would agree that a patient who actually has the appetite to ingest 1.2–1.3 g protein/kg normalized body weight/day (which is the probable recommended dietary allowance for a peritoneal dialysis patient) is not uremic and is probably being adequately dialyzed. A nomogram is currently being prepared that will depict the relationship between SUN, dietary protein intake and total daily urea clearance. A stable patient having a daily urea clearance of 11 liters/day and a SUN of 80 mg/dl is ingesting approximately 90 g of protein/day. This intake is probably adequate for a 75-kg man. If the daily urea clearance is decreased to 6.5 liters/day, the patient may still maintain an SUN of 80 mg/dl; however, his protein intake will have to decrease to 60 g/day and he may have problems in the long run.

In summary, the amount of peritoneal dialysis must be individualized, depending on protein intake, residual urea clearance, and total dialysate outflow. If we do not individualize therapy, I suspect that the long-term results with many of our CAPD patients (especially large anuric men) will again be poor. If we do not learn from the past, then in the 1980s many nephrologists may again conclude that peritoneal dialysis "does not work."

ACKNOWLEDGMENTS

Supported in part by USPHS Contract AM-5-2218, USPHS CRC Grant RR 865, and VA Research Funds.

CHAPTER THIRTEEN

Caloric Intake and Nitrogen Balance in Patients Undergoing CAPD*

G. M. GAHL	R. SCHURIG
H. v. BAEYER	H. BECKER
R. RIEDINGER	M. KESSEL
B. BOROWZAK	

INTRODUCTION

CONTINUOUS AMBULATORY PERITONEAL DIALYSIS (CAPD) is characterized by considerable glucose absorption from the dialysate and by obligatory dialysate protein loss of approximately 70 g per week.[1-3] Very early it was recognized that both facts might have great impact on the metabolic and nutritional status of the CAPD patient.[1-4] Glucose uptake from the dialysate serves as a considerable source of extra energy intake. It was assumed that weight gain, frequently encountered in CAPD patients, was attributed to this extra energy intake.[1,3] On the other hand, the glucose absorption via the peritoneal route, by negatively affecting appetite, might interfere with oral caloric intake and in particular with protein intake. However, high protein intake is mandatory in CAPD to compensate for the obligatory dialysate protein loss. Very early it was speculated that CAPD patients may be anabolic if protein intake of 1.0 g/kg body weight or more per day is provided.[2] This hypothesis, derived from clinical observations, was recently confirmed by Giordano et al.,[5] who demonstrated positive nitrogen balance in seven of eight CAPD patients. However, this study was undertaken under clinical conditions, the patients being admitted to a metabolic ward.

Department of Nephrology, Freie Universität Berlin, Klinikum Charlottenburg, West Germany
*The article entitled "Outpatient Evaluation of Dietary Intake and Nitrogen Removal in Continuous Ambulatory Peritoneal Dialysis," which appears in the May 1981 issue Vol. 94, No. 5, of the *Annals of Internal Medicine,* is based partially on this presentation.

Dietary surveys in our patients often revealed a striking discrepancy between actual and recommended dietary—caloric as well as protein—intake, although the patients were repeatedly instructed about their dietary requirements. Therefore a study was initiated in stable CAPD patients:

1) to provide information on actual dietary intake as compared to recommended intake with emphasis on protein intake;
2) to determine the rate of glucose absorption from the dialysate and its relation to total caloric intake;
3) to evaluate nitrogen balance.

In contrast to the study of Giordano et al.[5] our study was performed on an outpatient basis, since it was felt that this might be more relevant for long-term conclusions than a study under artificial clinical conditions.

PATIENTS AND METHODS

Five clinically stable patients are included in this study. They have been on CAPD for periods of 5–11 months. Three patients were transferred from intermittent peritoneal dialysis (IPD) after 15–28 months; two patients were primarily admitted for CAPD. Clinical data are listed in Table 1. Patients appeared adequately dialyzed and had steady-state laboratory data prior to the study (Table 2). At the time of the study, there were no signs of gastrointestinal disorders, including diarrhea.

CAPD was performed as previously described.[3] In general, 6 liters of 1.5% glucose dialysate and 2 liters of 4.25% glucose dialysate (Baxter-Travenol, Deerfield, Ill.) were exchanged per day. One patient exchanged only 4.6 liters per day. The patients were informed about the purpose of the study. This was performed for a period of 2 weeks, without hospitalization of the patients. In order to evaluate dietary intake and nitrogen balance, two identical meals were prepared by the patients or their spouses each time throughout the 2-week period and the duplicate was collected for analysis every day. Each meal was carefully recorded for calculation of protein and caloric content. It was homogenized and kept frozen until analyzed. Feces were not collected,

TABLE 1.
Clinical Data

Patient	Age (years)	Sex	Diagnosis	GFR[a] (ml/minute)	Urine Volume (ml/day)	Months on CAPD
1	62	F	Glomerulonephritis	0.1	33	11
2	59	F	Pyelonephritis	0	0	10
3	59	M	Nephrosclerosis	1.2	320	5
4	57	M	Diabetic nephropathy	3.1	1,170	6
5	77	M	Pyelonephritis	0.6	265	7

[a] Endogenous creatinine clearance (ml/minute × 1.73 m^2).

TABLE 2.
Serum Chemistries

Patient	Creatinine (mg/dl)	BUN (mg/dl)	Total Protein (g/dl)	Albumin (g/dl)	Transferrin (mg/dl)	C_3 Complement[a] (mg/dl)	C_4 Complement[b] (mg/dl)
1	9.6	57	6.2	3.6	215	74	29
2	9.3	49	6.7	4.3	240	107	36
3	9.0	56	8.4	4.2	290	95	67
4	10.7	45	7.8	3.9	250	106	34
5	10.5	49	6.7	2.7	150	132	76

[a] Normal C_3 complement is 69-130 mg/dl.
[b] Normal C_4 complement is 18-32 mg/dl.

since patients otherwise would have refused to participate in the study. Stool nitrogen losses were estimated according to data from the literature,[6] as were nitrogen losses through the skin, which were related to body surface area.[7,8] Nitrogen loss through the lungs was not considered.

Urine and dialysate outflow were collected and analyzed at 24-hour periods for urea, creatinine, uric acid, proteins, total nitrogen, and glucose. Dialysate inflow volume and glucose content were carefully recorded. Daily nitrogen balance was calculated as the difference between nitrogen intake and the sum of nitrogen content of urine and dialysate and estimated fecal and skin nitrogen loss in each individual.

Laboratory methods

Urea, creatinine, uric acid, and serum protein were measured using standard laboratory methods. Glucose was determined using the hexokinase method. Transferrin, C_3 and C_4 complements, were measured using the radial immunodiffusion technique, and dialysate protein concentration was measured by a modified Biuret method.[9] Total nitrogen was determined using the micro-Kjeldahl method.

Diets

Patients were instructed to ingest a high-caloric diet providing a protein intake of 1.2–1.5 g/kg body weight per day. The importance of this diet was regularly emphasized when the patients were examined in the outpatient clinics by the CAPD staff prior to the study. In addition a dietitian instructed the patients about their dietary requirements. The patients themselves estimated their caloric and protein intake as being adequate and according to our recommendations. During the 2-week study period patients were instructed to adhere to the same eating habits as prior to the study.

RESULTS

Table 3 demonstrates daily dialysate volume, ultrafiltration, glucose content of dialysate inflow, and the total amount of glucose absorbed per day. Minor

TABLE 3.
Dialysate Volume, Ultrafiltration, and Glucose Absorption from Dialysate (Mean ± Sx)

Patient	Dialysate Volume (liter/day)	Average Ultra-filtration (ml/day)	Glucose Content of Instilled Dialysate (g/day)	Glucose Absorption (g/day)	Absorption Rate (% of Administered Dialysate Glucose)
1	4.6	1,026 ± 350	72.85 ± 15.55	49.92 ± 11.66	68.5
2	8.0	1,172 ± 461	228.17 ± 26.41	173.04 ± 21.88	75.8
3	8.0	1,436 ± 313	174.91 ± 16.92	127.74 ± 12.11	73.0
4	8.0	1,306 ± 288	184.17 ± 21.41	136.13 ± 20.79	73.9
5	8.0	378 ± 358	133.75 ± 24.87	116.91 ± 21.75	87.4

variations in glucose content of dialysate inflow are due to the fact that patients occasionally varied the ratio of 1.5 to 4.25% glucose dialysate according to individual ultrafiltration requirements. Patient 5 only very occasionally used the high osmolar dialysate. This patient exhibited the highest rate of glucose absorption; accordingly ultrafiltration was considerably lower than in the other patients. On an average, the absorbed dialysate glucose provided a peritoneal caloric intake of approximately 700 kcal/day.

Table 4 shows body weight, daily nitrogen and protein intake, and, in addition, oral plus peritoneal caloric intake. It can be seen that the mean daily protein intake was less than 1.0 g/kg body weight in all patients. The average daily caloric intake exceeded 40 kcal/kg body weight only in patient 2.

Daily nitrogen balance of patient 2 during the 2-week study period is shown in Figure 1. It is evident that nitrogen intake varied considerably from day to day. This could be demonstrated in all patients. Mean daily nitrogen balance of patients 1–5 are shown in Figure 2. It is obvious that nitrogen balance was slightly positive in four of five patients. Cumulative nitrogen balance of the 2-week period in the anabolic patients was 16–27 g.

TABLE 4.
Body Weight, Mean Daily Nitrogen, Protein and Total Caloric Intake

Patient	Body Weight (kg)	Patient Ideal Body Weight[a] (%)	Nitrogen (g/day) (mean ± Sx)	Nitrogen (g/body weight) (mean ± Sx)	Protein (g/kg)	Total Caloric Intake (Oral + Peritoneal) (kcal)	(kcal/kg)
1	38.7	82	5.46 ± 1.18	0.14 ± 0.03	0.88	1,265	32.7
2	42.6	108	6.51 ± 1.54	0.15 ± 0.03	0.96	1,875	44.0
3	65.4	90	7.72 ± 1.42	0.12 ± 0.02	0.74	1,754	26.8
4	82.4	135	9.37 ± 1.87	0.12 ± 0.02	0.71	2,360	28.6
5	62.6	94	7.73 ± 1.95	0.12 ± 0.03	0.77	1,872	29.9

[a] According to Metropolitan Life Insurance tables.

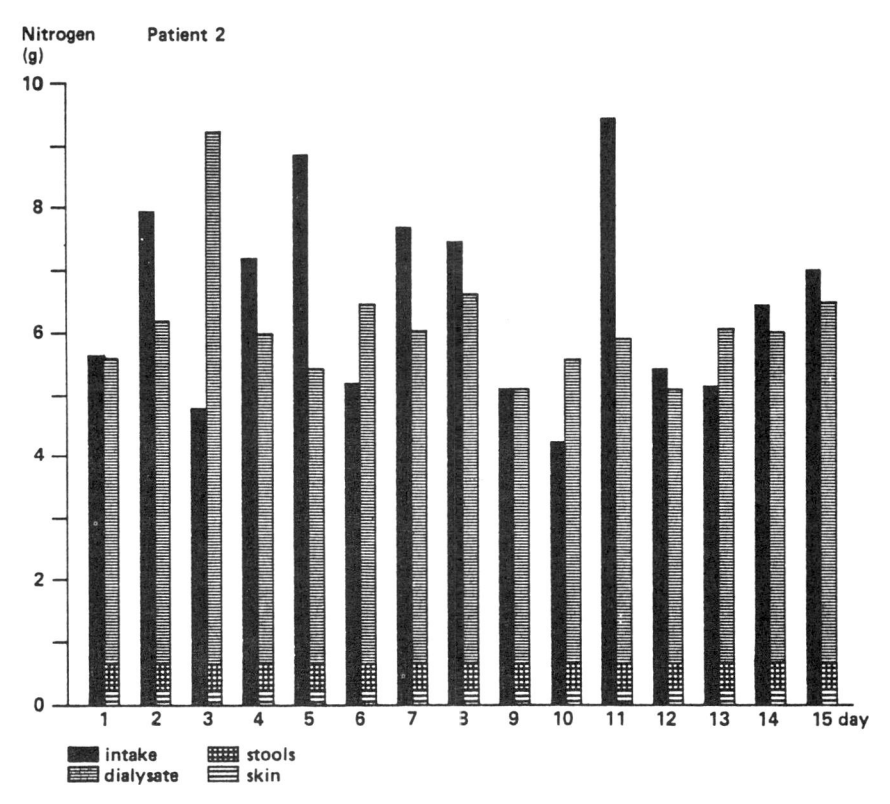

Figure 1. Daily nitrogen balance (g/day) of an individual patient during the 2-week study period. Note the variations of nitrogen intake from day to day.

COMMENT

The data of our study indicate that total energy intake, including the calories originating from the absorbed dialysate glucose, was 30–40 kcal/kg body weight. Thus total energy intake per day appeared adequate. The glucose absorbed from the peritoneum provided approximately 30% of the total caloric intake per day. Consequently, dietary intake was only 20–30 kcal/kg body weight. In spite of this remarkably low dietary intake, patients had the impression that their appetite was good. This observation supports our earlier experience in CAPD that patients often tended to overestimate their daily dietary intake, although they had been repeatedly informed about the significance of their dietary requirements.

The low protein intake of 0.7–0.9 g/kg body weight per day in the present study correlated with the low total dietary intake. Apparently the glucose absorbed from the dialysate results in a reduction of appetite, thus giving rise to low protein intake. This observation indicates that low protein intake may represent another potential risk of glucose absorption from the dialysate. Our

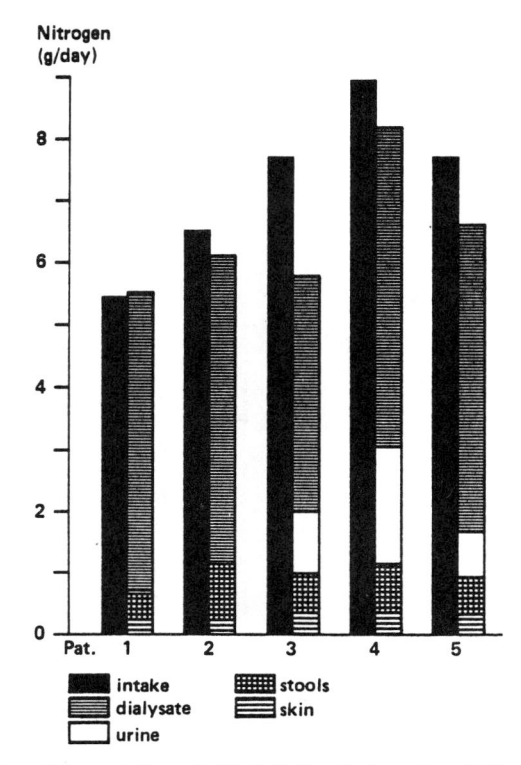

Figure 2. Mean nitrogen balance (g/day) during the 2-week period in patients 1 to 5.

data show that in spite of the low protein intake and in spite of dialysate protein loss of approximately 10 g/day, nitrogen balance was slightly positive in four patients; patient 5 was in nitrogen equilibrium. These data support the clinically derived hypothesis of Popovich et al.[2] that CAPD patients may be anabolic.

Recently Giordano et al.[5] described positive nitrogen balance in CAPD patients who ingested a high caloric diet providing a protein intake of 1.2 g/kg body weight per day. These authors concluded that this protein intake is safe in the majority of patients, at least when they are in a clinically steady state and free of complications. Our data show that CAPD patients may be anabolic even with a protein intake of less than 1.0 g/kg body weight per day. However, it should be emphasized that the patients in our study were clinically in a steady state. It is obvious that the protein intake observed in our study is inadequate to maintain CAPD patients anabolic or at least at a nitrogen equilibrium in the long run, since intercurrent illnesses, such as peritonitis, are associated with significant catabolism. On an empirical basis, in particular with regard to CAPD-associated protein loss, our patients were recommended to adhere to a daily protein intake of 1.2–1.5 g/kg body weight. Based on the findings of the present study it is concluded that this in fact must be guaranteed in order to maintain patients in good clinical and nutritional conditions for many years. Apparently more effort in dietary care is required to achieve this goal.

SUMMARY

A 2-week study was undertaken in five CAPD patients to evaluate dietary intake, glucose absorption from the dialysate, and nitrogen balance. The study was carried out on an outpatient basis, while the patients ingested their usual diet. Balance studies were performed at 24-hour periods. The results indicate that patients greatly overestimate their caloric and protein intake, which was 0.75–0.95 g/kg body weight per day. In spite of this low protein intake nitrogen balance was slightly positive in four of five patients. Dialysate glucose contributed considerably to total caloric intake, since approximately 75% of the dialysate glucose were absorbed independently from total glucose administered. It is concluded that CAPD patients need to be periodically monitored for eating habits, i.e., caloric and protein intake.

ACKNOWLEDGMENTS

The authors thank Professor R. Averdunk for laboratory advice and Mrs. M. Schmid for skillful technical assistance. Parts of this study were supported by the "Deutsche Forschungsgemeinschaft," Bonn-Bad Godesberg (Ke 170/4).

References

1. De Santo, N. G., Capodicasa, G., Senatore, R., Cicchetti, T., Damiano, M., Torella, R., Giugliano, D., Improta, L., and Giordano, C.: Glucose utilization from dialysate in patients on continuous ambulatory peritoneal dialysis (CAPD). *Int J Artif Organs* **2:** 119, 1979.
2. Popovich, R. P., Moncrief, J. W., Nolph, K. D., Ghods, A. J., Twardowski, Z. J., and Pyle, W. K.: Continuous ambulatory peritoneal dialysis. *Ann Intern Med* **88:** 449, 1978.
3. Gahl, G. M., Becker, H., Schurig, R., Pustelnik, A., v. Baeyer, H., and Kessel, M.: Kontinuierliche ambulante Peritonealdialyse (CAPD). *Schweiz Med Wschenschr* **109:** 1990, 1979.
4. Oreopoulos, D. G.: The coming of age of continuous ambulatory peritoneal dialysis (CAPD). *Dial Transplant* **8:** 460, 1979.
5. Giordano, C., De Santo, N. G., Pluvio, M., Di Leo, V. A., Capodicasa, G., Cirillo, D., Esposito, R., and Damiano, M.: Protein requirement of patients on CAPD: a study on nitrogen balance. *Int J Artif Organs* **3:** 11, 1980.
6. Lindner, A., and Tenckhoff, H.: Nitrogen balance in patients on maintenance peritoneal dialysis. *Trans Am Soc Artif Intern Organs* **16:** 255, 1970.
7. Sirbu, E. R., Margen, S., and Calloway, D. H.: Effect of reduced protein intake on nitrogen loss from the human integument. *Am J Clin Nutr* **20:** 1158, 1967.
8. Calloway, D. H., Odell, A. C. F., and Margen, S.: Sweat and miscellaneous nitrogen losses in human balance studies. *J Nutr* **101:** 775, 1971.
9. Weichselbaum, T. E.: An accurate and rapid method for the determination of protein in small amounts of blood and plasma. *Am J Clin Pathol* **10:** 40, 1946.

CHAPTER FOURTEEN

Acid-Base Studies in Continuous Ambulatory Peritoneal Dialysis

B. P. TEEHAN, M.D., F.A.C.P.

G. A. REICHARD, Ph.D.

M. H. SIGLER, M.D., F.A.C.P.

C. R. SCHLEIFER, M.D.

M. C. CUPIT, R.N.

A. C. HAFF, M.S.

ANY FORM OF DIALYSIS THERAPY for end-stage renal failure must achieve certain goals in order to receive general clinical acceptance. Typically, these include control of waste product metabolites at nontoxic levels, volume homeostasis, and control of divalent cation levels. Neutral hydrogen ion balance is also recognized as an important goal. Continuous ambulatory peritoneal dialysis (CAPD) results in acceptable levels of blood urea nitrogen (BUN) and creatinine, an edema-free normotensive state, and significant calcium uptake from dialysate, along with reduced need for phosphate binders. It has generally been assumed that acid-base control is also satisfactory, but this aspect of the uremic state is not considered in several recent large series.[1-4] Since it has been shown that hemodialysis can achieve both neutral hydrogen ion balance and repair of base deficits,[5] it is important to determine whether or not CAPD can achieve similar results.

We have noticed a tendency toward mild chronic metabolic acidosis in our CAPD patients (Table 1). We therefore undertook a study of the parameters that determine acid-base balance in CAPD. To accomplish this, we modified the model used by Gotch et al.[5] in hemodialysis. The major determinants of acid-base balance in this model are lactate uptake, or base gain, dialysate bicarbonate and base equivalent (organic anion) loss, metabolic hydrogen ion generation and net renal acid excretion. Each of these parameters, except net renal acid excretion, was studied in a group of stable CAPD patients and base balance was calculated in those with no residual renal function.

The results indicate that lactate uptake from dialysate is efficient (70%) but is often exceeded by the sum of dialysate bicarbonate loss and hydrogen

Haverford Dialysis Unit, Lankenau Hospital, Philadelphia, Pennsylvania

TABLE 1.
CAPD Acid-Base Profile

Patient	pH	pCO$_2$ (mm Hg)	CO$_2$ Content (mmole/liter)	Anion Gap (mmole/liter)	Primary Acid-Base Disorder
C.T.	7.43	32[a]	20[a]	15[a]	Metabolic acidosis, respiratory alkalosis
L.M.	7.34[a]	37	20[a]	20[a]	Metabolic acidosis
C.W.	7.31[a]	33[a]	15[a]	17[a]	Metabolic acidosis
T.D.	7.41	33[a]	21[a]	17[a]	Metabolic acidosis, respiratory alkalosis
T.D.	7.38	35[a]	20[a]	19[a]	Metabolic acidosis
R.H.	7.42	36	23	16[a]	Metabolic acidosis, respiratory alkalosis
T.M.	7.33[a]	45	23	11	Metabolic & respiratory acidosis
R.H.	7.42	39	28	8[a]	Normal
H.R.	7.34[a]	43	21[a]	19	Metabolic acidosis, respiratory acidosis
W.H.	7.45	39	26	14	Normal
Mean ± S.D.	7.38 ± 0.05	37 ± 4	22 ± 4	16 ± 4	
Normal	7.37–7.45	34–46	22–27	10–14	

[a] Abnormal values.

ion generation, thus resulting in a modest base deficit in the average CAPD patient. Since metabolic hydrogen ion generation was normal (≤ 1 mEq/kg/day) and organic anion loss was small (≈ 4 mmole/day), lactate flux and dialysate bicarbonate loss were the major factors determining acid-base balance. Base balance is relatively easy to measure in these patients and therefore it may serve as a rational basis for increasing dialysate lactate concentration or supplementing base administration with oral bicarbonate or citrate.

METHODS

The method used to determine acid-base balance is an adaptation of the model proposed by Gotch et al.[5] for hemodialysis. It is based on the hypothesis that in the absence of renal function, metabolic hydrogen ion generation and the dialysate fluxes of base and base equivalents are the major determinants of acid-base balance in dialysis patients. The over-all base balance in a CAPD patient is summarized in Equation (1).

$$\text{Base Balance} = \Sigma J_{\text{lac}} - (\Sigma J_{\text{HCO}_3^-} + \Sigma J_{\text{OA}} + G_{\text{H}^+}), \qquad (1)$$

where base balance is expressed in mmole/day; ΣJ_{lac} equals lactate uptake in mmole/day; $\Sigma J_{\text{HCO}_3^-}$ equals dialysate bicarbonate loss in mmole/day; ΣJ_{OA} equals dialysate organic acid anion losses in mmole/day; G_{H^+} equals metabolic hydrogen ion generation, in mEq/day. Simply stated, base balance equals base gain (ΣJ_{lac}) minus base loss ($\Sigma J_{HCO_3^-} + \Sigma J_{OA}$) plus H^+ gain (G_{H^+}).

The present study was undertaken over single 24-hour periods in stable CAPD outpatients consuming *ad libitum* diets and not on alkali supplements. On the day of the study, arterial blood was drawn one hour after the first morning exchange was instilled into the peritoneal cavity. All dialysate was collected during the next 24 hours and arterial blood samples were repeated at the same time on the second day. Dialysate was pooled anaerobically and the total volume was measured. Lactate, beta-hydroxybutyrate, acetoacetate, pO_2, pCO_2, pH, HCO_3^-, and urea nitrogen levels were measured in all blood and dialysate samples. In addition, electrolytes were measured in all blood samples.

Both the D and L isomers of the racemic mixture used in commercial dialysate were measured in all samples. Specific enzymatic methods were used for those[6] and for each of the organic acid anions.[7] The Instrumentation Laboratory blood gas analyzer was used for the determination of pH, pCO_2, and pO_2 in both blood and dialysate. Bicarbonate levels were calculated from pH and pCO_2, both in blood and dialysate. D- and L-lactate were measured in each of five bags of fresh dialysate; D-lactate level was 17.58 ± 0.3 mmole/liter and L-lactate level was 18.01 ± 0.42 mmole/liter. The mean value of 8 volume measurements in the 2-liter Dianeal bags was 2.063 ± 0.004 liters. Thus, the mean value for total lactate load per exchange is 73.4 mmole.

Total lactate uptake (ΣJ_{lac}) is calculated from Equation (2):

$$\Sigma J_{lac} = V_{Di} (C_{Di} \text{ D-lac} + C_{Di} \text{ L-lac}) - V_{Do} (C_{Do} \text{ D-lac} + C_{Do} \text{ L-lac}), \quad (2)$$

where V_{Di} and V_{Do} are 24-hour dialysate inflow and outflow volumes, respectively, and C_{Di} and C_{Do} are dialysate inflow and outflow concentrations, respectively.

Bicarbonate flux consists of dialysate bicarbonate losses only and this is easily calculated from Equation (3).

$$J_{HCO_3^-} = V_{Do} \cdot C_{Do} \text{ HCO}_3^- \quad (3)$$

Metabolic hydrogen ion generation (G_{H^+}) was estimated from the protein catabolic rate (PCR), which in turn was calculated from the rate of urea nitrogen appearance or the urea nitrogen generation rate (G_u). G_u, expressed in g/24 hour, was calculated from 24-hour dialysate and urinary urea nitrogen losses plus any change in BUN times urea volume of distribution, where the latter equals body weight in kilograms times 0.58, plus 2 liters. The close correlation between G_u and PCR, where

$$PCR = (G_u + 1.7)/0.154 \quad (4)$$

has been established and emphasized by Borah *et al.*[8] and appears to be valid over a broad range of protein catabolic rates. The estimation of G_{H^+} from PCR is based on the fact that the net production of nonvolatile acid will be determined primarily by the level or protein intake in this group of patients.[5] Gotch *et al.*[5] reviewed the available acid-base literature in an attempt to identify studies in which both net acid excretion and nitrogen balance were measured. From a limited number of papers, 53 individual studies were found from which a relationship between G_{H^+} and PCR could be determined. This yielded the following equation:

$$G_{H^+} = 0.77 \text{ PCR} \tag{5}$$

with a standard deviation of $\pm 35\%$.

Finally, the major organic acid anion removed during CAPD is beta-hydroxybutyrate, with smaller amounts of acetoacetate also lost. Total 24-hour dialysate losses (ΣJ_{OA}) were calculated from Equation (6):

$$J_{OA} = V_{Do}(C_{Do}\,\beta\text{-OHB} + C_{Do}\,\text{Acac}), \tag{6}$$

where β-OHB and Acac represent beta-hydroxybutyrate and acetoacetate, respectively.

Combining Equations (2)–(6) above, we have the basic expression, Equation (7), used to determine base balance in CAPD patients from the various determinants that are measured directly.

$$\begin{aligned}\text{Base Balance} = &\,[V_{Di}(C_{Di}\,\text{D-lac} + C_{Di}\,\text{L-lac}) - V_{Do}(C_{Do}\,\text{D-lac} \\ &+ C_{Do}\,\text{L-lac})] - \left[0.77\,\frac{G_u + 1.7}{0.154} + V_{Do}C_{Do}\text{HCO}_3^- \right.\\ &\left. + V_{Do}(C_{Do}\,\beta\text{-OHB} + C_{Do}\,\text{Acac})\right]. \end{aligned} \tag{7}$$

RESULTS

Lactate uptake from dialysate and plasma lactate levels are shown in Table 2. There is no significant difference in total lactate uptake whether calculated

TABLE 2.
Comparison of D(−) and L(+) Lactate Isomers During CAPD

Patient	L(+)+D(−) (mmole/day)	L(+)×2 (mmole/day)	% Lactate Uptake D(−)	% Lactate Uptake L(+)	Plasma Lactate D(−) (m/mole/liter)	Plasma Lactate L(+) (mmole/liter)
T.D.	203	207	68	71	0.1	1.6
T.D.	207	210	70	72	0.1	1.3
T.D.	226	220	80	76	0.2	2.1
C.T.	171	166	81	76	—	—
L.M.	275	277	74	76	—	—
C.W.	182	183	83	84	0.10	2.0
W.M.	188	183	89	84	0.2	0.9
R.H.	234	236	80	81	0.1	0.8
H.R.	190	192	65	66	0.1	1.7
Mean ± S.D.	208 ± 32	208 ± 33	77 ± 8	76 ± 6	0.1 ± 0.05	1.5 ± 0.5

from the sum of the two isomers or twice the usually measured L isomer. Lactate uptake expressed as a percentage of the amount infused is virtually identical for the two isomers also, suggesting that the peritoneal membrane does not distinguish between the naturally occurring L isomer and the D isomer in the racemic dialysate. Plasma levels of L($-$) lactate (1.5 ± 0.05 mmole/liter) are elevated above control values (1.0 ± 0.1 mmole/liter), while for D lactate the plasma levels are much lower (0.1 ± 0.05 mMol/liter). The modest evaluation of the L isomer may be due to the daily dialysate lactate load superimposed on endogenous lactate, L($+$), production, whereas the much lower level of the D isomer suggests efficient metabolism via a non-LDH enzyme system (probably D-2-hydroxy acid dehydrogenase) to pyruvate and, ultimately, to CO_2 and H_2O.[9]

Total lactate uptake correlated with the number of exchanges but tended to be more efficient (uptake/dose) with fewer exchanges and prolonged dwell times. The dialysate:plasma lactate ratio was 8.8 in those with five exchanges/day, but only 2.4 in those with three daily exchanges. Lactate uptake did not correlate with body surface area.

Dialysate bicarbonate loss closely approximated lactate uptake, 192 ± 29 vs 212 ± 29 mmole/day, respectively. Bicarbonate loss correlated with dialysate outflow rate ($r = 0.72$, $p < 0.01$) and dialysate bicarbonate levels achieved 94% of plasma levels. The mean plasma:dialysate bicarbonate ratio (1.7) was significantly less than the mean dialysate:plasma lactate ratio (4.6), indicating more complete equilibration for bicarbonate than lactate. Thus, bicarbonate loss in dialysate proved to be a major determinant of base balance in these patients.

Dialysate losses of beta-hydroxybutyrate and acetoacetate were small, 4.1 ± 1.9 and 1.0 ± 0.3 mmole/day, respectively. Plasma levels of both organic anions were normal; beta-hydroxybutyrate = 0.5 mmole/liter and acetoacetate = 0.1 mmole/liter. There was no difference between diabetic and nondiabetic patients. In addition to organic acid anion loss in dialysate, total anion loss was estimated from the difference between total measured cations and anions in expended dialysate in six patients. (Cations: Na, K, Ca, and Mg; anions: lactate, bicarbonate, chloride, β-OHB, and Acac.) This yielded an "anion gap" of 36 ± 17 mmole/day. The presumed composition of this gap includes protein, sulfates, phosphates, and, perhaps, small amounts of unmeasured organic anions, such as pyruvate and urate. The impact of these unmeasured anions on acid-base balance in CAPD patients is uncertain, but at a mean dialysate pH of 7.32 ± 0.05 ($n = 9$), there would be no significant H^+ removal with these anions.

Metabolic hydrogen ion generation (G_{H^+}) was 50 ± 17 mEq/day ($N = 12$), or 0.75 mEq/kg/day. This was derived from PCR as reflected by the rate of urea appearance. Mean PCR in this group of patients was 65 g/day or 1 g/kg/day. Although there is a substantial inherent error (±17.5 mEq/day) in estimating G_{H^+} from PCR, the over-all contribution of G_{H^+} to base balance is sufficiently small so that the results are not significantly altered.

Since net renal acid excretion was not measured in these patients, base balance was calculated only in those with no residual renal function. These results are shown in Table 3. Seven balance studies conducted over 24-hour

TABLE 3.
Base Balance in CAPD

Patient	Lactate Uptake (mmole/day)	HCO$_3^-$ Loss (mmole/day)	β-OHB Loss (mmole/day)	Acac Loss (mmole/day)	G_{H^+} (mEq/day)	Base Balance (mMol/day)
T.D.	211	196	1.5	1.0	55	−42.5
T.D.	206	230	1.5	1.0	40	−66.5
L.M.	275	211	5.9	2.0	79	−22.9
C.W.	185	139	0.8	0.8	35	+9.5
R.H.	193	184	5.1	1.0	30	−27.0
J.E.	234	198	5.4	1.0	46	−16.4
L.M.	238	198	4.7	0.9	53	−18.6
Mean	220	194	3.6	1.1	48	−26.4
± S.D.	± 31	± 28	± 2.2	± 0.4	± 16	± 23.5

periods in five patients show a mean daily net base loss of 26.4 ± 23.5 mmole. Only one patient (C.W.) was in a modest positive base balance, 9.5 mmole/day. During the balance study, mean (±S.D.) values for arterial blood gases in these patients were pH = 7.36 ± 0.03, pCO$_2$ = 34 ± 1.6, and calculated HCO$_3^-$ = 20 ± 2.5 mmole/liter. Each value is at or just below the lower limits of normal, indicating a mild chronic metabolic acidosis. The disproportionately low pCO$_2$ in this group indicates that a primary and independent respiratory alkalosis is also present. This is accounted for by one patient with scleroderma and another with moderate fluid overload who was studied twice. However, in the absence of this respiratory "overcorrection" mean pH for the group would be lower, thereby emphasizing the presence of metabolic acidosis.

DISCUSSION

The major determinants of acid-base balance in chronic hemodialysis have been identified and quantified by Gotch et al.[5,10] in a series of detailed and elegant studies. This group was able to demonstrate neutral hydrogen ion balance on acetate dialysis and a modest positive base balance on bicarbonate dialysis. Since there was a tendency toward chronic metabolic acidosis in our CAPD patients, we adapted their model to study acid-base balance in these patients. Lactate uptake and dialysate bicarbonate loss were found to be the major determinants, with hydrogen ion generation and dialysate organic anion loss playing lesser roles.

The significance of these studies lies in the relationship between chronic metabolic acidosis and bone disease. Chronic metabolic acidosis is an invariable consequence of end-stage renal failure. Although often mild and asymptomatic in chronic dialysis patients, it may cause lethargy and anorexia, which were not apparent until the pH is corrected with base supplements. The role of chronic metabolic acidosis in causing a negative calcium balance and contributing to uremic osteodystrophy, however, is of greater concern. In a group of nondialysis patients with chronic stable renal acidosis (serum $HCO_3^- = 18.7 \pm 3.2$ mmole/liter), Litzow et al.[11] demonstrated significant daily negative calcium balance that was completely corrected by alkali therapy and restoration of serum bicarbonate to normal (27.4 ± 2.1 mmole/liter). It is important to note that serum bicarbonate levels remained stable but low in these and other studies[12] in spite of a continued positive hydrogen ion balance. The negative base balance (26.4 ± 23.5 mmole/day) found in the present study is equivalent to positive hydrogen ion balance. The fact that serum HCO_3^- remains stable (20 ± 2.5 mmole/liter) in spite of a daily negative base balance simply suggests that, at some point, buffering of added hydrogen ion is accomplished by a moiety other than bicarbonate, presumably alkaline bone salts.

Although net calcium uptake from dialysate has been demonstrated in CAPD patients,[3] it is not known whether these patients are in negative or positive calcium balance. Furthermore, experience with CAPD has not been long enough yet to know whether these patients will be prone to osteopenia or not. The tendency toward chronic metabolic acidosis and the negative base balance (positive H^+ balance) demonstrated by the present study suggests that they may be in negative calcium balance. This question could be resolved with calcium balance studies on a metabolic ward.

Since the negative base balance in these patients is modest, it could be corrected by an increase in dialysate lactate concentration or by oral supplements of bicarbonate or citrate. Therapeutic manipulation of the other determinants of acid-base balance would not be appropriate since G_{H^+} can be reduced only by decreasing protein intake and reduction of dialysate bicarbonate loss would require a decrease in 24-hour dialysate volume and a resultant decrease in over-all clearance.

ACKNOWLEDGMENT

We wish to acknowledge the constructive comments of Frank A. Gotch, M.D., during the preparation of this manuscript.

References

1. Popovich, R. P., Moncrief, J. W., Nolph, K. D., et al.: Continuous ambulatory peritoneal dialysis. *Ann Intern Med* **88**: 449, 1978.
2. Oreopoulos, D. G., Khana, R., McCready, W., et al.: Continuous ambulatory peritoneal dialysis in Canada. *Dial Transplant* **9**: 224, 1980.
3. Moncrief, J. W., Nolph, K. D., Rubin, J., et al.: Additional experience with continuous ambulatory peritoneal dialysis (CAPD). *Trans Am Soc Artif Intern Organs* **24**: 476, 1978.
4. Oreopoulos, D. G., Robson, M., Izatt, S., et al.: A simple and safe technique for continuous ambulatory peritoneal dialysis (CAPD). *Trans Am Soc Artif Intern Organs* **24**: 484, 1978.
5. Gotch, F. A., Sargent, J. A., Keen, M. L., et al.: The solute kinetics of intermittent dialysis therapy. Annual Report, NIAMDD, 1979, NOI-AM-4-2202.
6. Holroyde, C. P., Axelrod, R. S., and Skutches, C. L.: Lactate metabolism in patients with colorectal cancer. *Cancer Res* **39**: 4900, 1979.

7. Reichard, G. A., Owen, O. E., Haff, A. C., *et al.:* Ketone body production and oxidation in fasting obese humans. *J Clin Invest* **53:** 408, 1974.
8. Borah, M. F., Schoenfeld, P. Y., Gotch, F. A., *et al.:* Nitrogen balance during intermittent dialysis therapy of uremia. *Kidney Int* **14:** 491, 1978.
9. Brin, M.: The synthesis and metabolism of lactic acid isomers. *Ann N Y Acad Sci* **119:** 942, 1965.
10. Gotch, F. A., and Sargent, J. A.: Measurement of H^+ balance (H^+b) during acetate and bicarbonate dialysis (AD, BD) therapy. *Kidney Int* **16:** 887, 1979.
11. Litzow, J. R., Lemann, J., and Lennon, E. J.: The effect of treatment of acidosis on calcium balance in patients with chronic azotemic renal disease. *J Clin Invest* **46:** 280, 1967.
12. Goodman, A. D., Lemann, J., Lennon, E. J., *et al.:* Production, excretion, and net balance of fixed acid in patients with renal acidosis. *J Clin Invest* **44:** 495, 1965.

CHAPTER FIFTEEN

Finding the Uremic Molecule(s)

JONAS BERGSTRÖM, Professor, M.D.

A CONSIDERABLE NUMBER OF organic compounds are present in raised concentrations in uremic plasma, but only for a few of them has a toxic role been established. Presumably several compounds may act synergistically as toxins, each being present in concentrations not being toxic per se. Experiments with various hemodialysis regimens have given controversial results with regard to toxicity of small and middle molecules. However, new modalities of treatment, such as CAPD and hemofiltration and a number of *in vitro* studies, lend support to the middle molecule (MM) hypothesis. Systematic attempts to purify, identify, characterize, and synthetize MM compounds are now under way in several laboratories. Some of the most recent works published in this field are now reviewed.

The chemical theory of causation of the uremic syndrome begins with Prévost and Dumas,[1] who discovered that removal of the kidneys led to a rise in blood urea concentration. It would appear to be a relatively simple task to find out what is toxic in uremia, presupposing that toxic substances that accumulate in the body fluids of the uremic patient are those that are normally excreted in the urine. However, the problem has proved not to be a simple one, and despite more than 150 years of research, it has not been possible to explain all uremic toxic manifestations by accumulation of known compounds. Accordingly, the search for uremic toxins continues.

In Table 1 criteria are listed that should be fulfilled by a uremic toxin of clinical importance. However, only a few substances fulfill these criteria (Table 2). In total, hundreds of compounds have now been found to accumulate in the plasma of uremic patients or found to be present in uremic dialysate.[2] Hence, it appears that uremic plasma contains a grossly abnormal mixture of several compounds and we know very little about how these compounds may interact on vital biological processes.

It is against this background that we should look on individual uremic toxins. There is evidence that certain compounds, known to accumulate in uremia, may induce toxic effects *in vitro,* when present together in the

Huddinge University Hospital, Huddinge, Sweden

TABLE 1.
Criteria to be Fulfilled by a Uremic Toxin

1. The compound should be chemically identified and specifically and quantitatively measurable in biological fluids.
2. The plasma level and tissue concentrations of the compound should be higher in uremic than in nonuremic patients.
3. High concentrations should be related to specific uremic symptoms.
4. Toxic effects should be obtained in human subjects, experimental animals, or in an appropriate *in vitro* system at concentrations comparable to those found in the body fluids of uremic patients.

medium, which are not found when these compounds are present alone. A classic study by Lascelles and Taylor[3] showed that combinations of metabolites (urea, magnesium, acetoin, 2-3-butylene glycol, sulfate, creatinine, creatine, p-cresol, and guanidine) inhibit respiration in cerebral slices, each metabolite being present in a concentration not being inhibitory per se. Combinations of metabolites (urea, creatinine, guanidinosuccinic acid, and methylguanidine) cause depression in cardiac output and myocardial oxygen extraction in the isolated and perfused heart, which may not be obtained with each of the compounds alone.[4] This raises the question of whether testing of uremic compounds has to be made in a "uremic" environment.

TABLE 2.
Uremic Toxins

A. Established	B. Suspected
Water	Creatinine
Sodium	Methylguanidine
Potassium	Guanidinosuccinic acid
Hydrogen ions	Other guanidines
Inorganic phosphate	Amino acids
Urea	Amines
Parathyroid hormone	Phenols
Renin	Indoles
	Aromatic oxyacids
	Pseudouridine
	cAMP
	Uric acid
	Oxalic acid
	Magnesium
	Arsenic
	Myoinositol
	Middle molecules
	Glucagon
	Growth hormone
	Natriuretic hormone
	Acid mucopolysaccharides
	RNase

A controversial question concerns the molecular size of the most important uremic toxins. The controversy started many years ago with the observation that patients on intermittent dialysis did not develop neuropathy as readily as hemodialysis patients, in spite of having much lower weekly clearance of small molecules, such as urea and creatinine.[5,6] Based on clinical observations in hemodialysis patients, the MM hypothesis was introduced[7] according to which uremic peripheral neuropathy is caused by accumulation of compounds of molecular weight 500–5,000 daltons. Such molecules are less readily dialyzed through conventional dialysis membranes in the artificial kidney but permeable through the peritoneal membrane, which has a larger pore size. Numerous investigations followed, applying various dialysis strategies, designed to increase or decrease small and middle molecules independently, relating these changes to the symptomatology of the patient.[8] Some studies appeared to support the hypothesis, whereas other studies seemed to refute it. The reason for this may again be that uremia is multifactorial, both small and middle molecules being toxic. Depending on the design of the experiment, one may appear to be more important than the other type of molecule.

In conclusion, I believe that the indirect approach to studying uremic toxicology by applying different hemodialysis strategies has come to a dead end, if not combined with direct measurements of toxic small and middle molecules.

Nevertheless, new indirect evidence for MM playing a role as uremic toxins has been presented recently. It was shown that platelet function, which was abnormal in hemodialysis patients, was normal in peritoneal dialysis patients.[9,10] The remarkable good clinical results with continuous ambulatory peritoneal dialysis (CAPD) regarding control of uremic symptoms, weight gain, improvement in hemoglobin concentration, and general well-being[11,12] are in favor of the MM hypothesis; this form of treatment is relatively inefficient for removing small molecules, but more efficient than any other form of dialysis treatment for removing MM. Hemofiltration is a technique for blood purification which, in contrast to hemodialysis, is nondiscriminatory for small and middle molecules, and thus more efficient for eliminating MM than hemodialysis. Better control of hypertension (not related to extracellular fluid control) was reported with hemofiltration than with hemodialysis, which was assumed to be due to more efficient removal of a MM, which interferes with sympathetically mediated vascular tone.[13] Other beneficial effects of hemofiltration have been reported (improvement in blood lipids, decrease in peripheral neuropathy), but these results have not been substantiated in controlled studies.[14]

As emphasized earlier in this review, there still are good reasons to believe that various MM may be important uremic toxins. Using quantitative chromatographic methods, we have found in a prospective study that uremic patients with infection, edema, vomiting, and malnutrition have significantly higher mean concentrations of MM in plasma than patients without major symptoms. No such difference was found for urea and creatinine.[15,16] We also found that CAPD patients had lower levels of MM in plasma than hemodialysis and intermittent peritoneal dialysis patients.[17]

The search for uremic toxins, using biochemical methodology, still goes on in many laboratories. It appears that studies in this field are less common today than a few years ago, despite new and powerful analytical techniques now available, which could help to resolve some of the problems encountered in separation and identification of uremic toxins, such as high performance liquid chromatography, coupled gas chromatography, mass spectrometry, and isotachophoresis. The most recent candidates of small molecular size are choline,[18] β-aminoisobutyric acid,[19] polyamines,[20] and myoinositol.[21,22] Although toxicity of these compounds is suspected, there is still no convincing proof that they are clinically important. The polyamines (putrescine, spermine, and spermidine) are strongly basic derivates of basic amino acids, which are readily bound to protein. There is evidence that spermidine may be attached to a strongly basic peptide, found in uremic plasma.[23] Polyamines have a number of biological effects (impaired glucose transport, participation in RNA and DNA synthesis, binding of vitamin B_6) and might well account for some of the abnormalities in uremia, although this has not yet been proved. Myoinositol is a candidate for a uremic neurotoxin with some *in vitro* effects on ganglion cells in tissue culture. Cyclic AMP has also been found elevated in uremic plasma, and there is a possible association with the platelet defect in uremia.[24,25] Larger molecules, such as ribonuclease[26] and acid mucopolysaccharides,[27] are also new but not established candidates for uremic toxins.

Some groups are now in the process of identifying individual MM compounds. It was recently reported by the Necker group in Paris that ultrafiltrate from dialysis patients with polyneuropathy contains an acid polyol with carbohydrate structure ($C_{22}H_{45}O_{30-40}$).[17]

Lutz[23] isolated four basic peptides by partition chromatography and paper electrophoresis with a molecular weight range of 1,300–1,800 daltons, and determined the molar ratios of the individual amino acids but not the amino acid sequences. One contained spermidine, and one a guanidine group and an amino sugar derivative. They were strongly protein bound, showed evidence of insulin-binding capacity and one of them inhibits insulin stimulation of lipoprotein lipase.

Remarkable new achievements have been reported by Abiko and co-workers in Japan.[28–30] Using ultrafiltration, gel filtration, and ion exchange chromatography, they were able to isolate two peptides from plasma of severely uremic patients. Both peptides were subjected to amino acid sequence determination and were later on synthesized. One is a heptapeptide, which corresponds to position 13 through 19 of β-microglobulin, the other is a tryptophan-containing pentapeptide, corresponding to position 123 through 127 of the β-chain of fibrinogen. Both peptides have an inhibiting effect on rosette formation between human lymphocytes and sheep erythrocytes *in vitro,* suggesting that they might cause or contribute to the impaired immune response in uremia. These are the first reports in which the complete structure of new biologically active MM peptides are given and in which it was possible to show that they consist of fragments of known proteins.

Our own work on separation and characterization of MM fractions prepared by ultrafiltration, gel chromatography, and gradient elution ion exchange chromatography continues. A group of acid, ultraviolet (UV) absorbing MM fractions are now subjected to further separation by high voltage electrophoresis and isotachophoresis. We have shown that three of these fractions contain amino acids after hydrolysis, indicating that they consist of peptide material.[15] By using isotachophoresis it was revealed that each of these three fractions (7a, 7b, and 7c) consisted of at least two different compounds with different UV absorption and mobility.[31] We have now concentrated our effort on fraction 7c, which is found to be very high in some patients with toxic uremic symptoms. Fraction 7c was isolated from ultrafiltrate obtained in dialysis patients, where peak 7c was very high in plasma. Isotachophoresis showed that this fraction consisted almost entirely of one single compound, which was confirmed by high-voltage electrophoresis. After hydrolysis, glycine was the only amino acid recovered. The C-terminus was glycine, but the N-terminus was blocked by two groups in sequence, which could be separated by partial hydrolysis.[32] Although we have not yet been able to identify the blocking groups on the N-terminus, our results reveal that we have identified a new compound, which contains glycine.

ACKNOWLEDGMENT

This work has been supported by USPHS contract MO1-AM-2-2215 from the National Institute of Arthritis, Metabolism and Digestive Diseases, Bethesda, Maryland.

References

1. Prévost, A. L., and Dumas, J. A.: Examen du sang et de son action dans les divers phénomènes de la vie. *Ann Chim Phys* **23**: 90, 1821.
2. Bergström, J., and Fürst, P.: Uraemic toxins. In *Replacement of Renal Function by Dialysis,* W. Drukker, F. M. Parsons, and J. F. Maher, Eds. Martinus Nijhoff Medical Division, The Hague, 1978, p. 334.
3. Lascelles, P. T., and Taylor, W. H.: The effect upon tissue respiration in vitro of metabolites which accumulate in uraemic coma. *Clin Sci* **31**: 403, 1966.
4. Scheuer, J., and Stezoski, S. W.: The effect of uremic compounds on cardiac function and metabolism. *J Mol Cell Cardiol* **5**: 287, 1973.
5. Scribner, B. H.: Discussion. *Trans Am Soc Artif Intern Organs* **11**: 29, 1965.
6. Tenckhoff, H., and Curtis, F. K.: Experience with maintenance hemodialysis in the home. *Trans Am Soc Artif Intern Organs* **16**: 90, 1970.
7. Babb, A. L., Farrell, P. D., Uvelli, D. A., and Scribner, B. H.: Hemodialyzer evaluation by examination of solute molecular spectra. *Trans Am Soc Artif Intern Organs* **18**: 98, 1972.
8. Bergström, J., Fürst, P., and Zimmerman, L.: Uremic middle molecules exist and are biologically active. *Clin Nephrol* **11**: 229, 1979.
9. Lindsay, R. M., Moorthy, A. V., Koens, F., and Linton, A. L.: Platelet function in dialyzed and non-dialyzed patients with chronic renal failure. *Clin Nephrol* **4**: 52, 1975.
10. Lindsay, R. M., Friésen, M., Koens, F., Linton, A. L., Oreopoulos, D., and de Veber, G.: Platelet function in patients on long-term peritoneal dialysis. *Clin Nephrol* **6**: 335, 1976.
11. Popovich, R. P., Moncrief, J. W., Nolph, K. D., Chods, A. J., Twardowski, Z. J., and Pyle, W. K.: Continuous ambulatory peritoneal dialysis. *Ann Intern Med* **88**: 449, 1978.
12. Robson, M. D., Oreopoulos, D. G., Clayton, S., Izatt, S., Rapoport, A., and de Veber, G. A.: Comparison of intermittent with continuous peritoneal dialysis. *Proc Eur Dial Transplant Assoc* **15**: 197, 1978.

13. Levy, S. P., Stone, R. A., Ford, C. A., Beans, E., and Henderson, L. W.: The influence of hemodiafiltration on blood pressure regulation. *Trans Am Soc Artif Intern Organs* **13**: 691, 1977.
14. Bergström, J.: Ultrafiltration without dialysis for removal of fluid and solutes in uremia. *Clin Nephrol* **9**: 155, 1978.
15. Bergström, J., Fürst, P., and Zimmerman, L.: A study of uremic toxicology. Annual Report, NIH Contract NO1-AM-2-2215, 1979.
16. Bergström, J., Alvestrand, A., Asaba, H., Fürst, P., Yahiel, V., and Zimmerman, L.: Uremic middle molecules. In *Controversies in Nephrology, Vol. 1,* G. E. Schreiner, J. F. Winchester, W. Mattern, and B. F. Mendelson, Eds. Georgetown University, Washington, D.C., 1979, p. 425.
17. Man, N. K., Cueille, G., Zingraff, J., Drueke, T., Jungers, P., Sausse, A., Boudet, J. L., and Funck-Brentano, J. L.: Evaluation of plasma neurotoxin concentration in uraemic polyneuropathic patients. *Proc Eur Dial Transplant Assoc* **15**: 164, 1978.
18. Rennick, B., Acara, M., Hysert, P., and Mookerjee, B.: Choline loss during hemodialysis: homeostatic control of plasma choline concentration. *Kidney Int* **10**: 329, 1976.
19. Blumberg, A., Esslen, E., and Bürgi, W.: Myoinositol—a uremic neurotoxin? *Nephron* **21**: 186, 1978.
20. Campbell, R., Bartos, F., Bartos, D., and Grettie, D.: The uremic hyperpolyaminemic perturbations: An hypothesis. In *Controversies in Nephrology, Vol. 1,* G. E. Schreiner, J. F. Winchester, W. Mattern, and B. F. Mendelson, Eds. Georgetown University, Washington, D.C., 1979, p. 435.
21. Clements, R. S., De Jesus, P. V., and Winegrad, A. T.: Raised plasma myoinositol levels in uraemia and experimental neuropathy. *Lancet* **I**: 1137, 1973.
22. Liveson, J. A., Gardner, J., and Bornstein, M. B.: Tissue culture studies of possible uremic neurotoxins: myoinositol. *Kidney Int* **12**: 131, 1977.
23. Lutz, W.: Chemical compositions and rate of passage across semipermeable membranes of basic peptides isolated from peritoneal dialysis fluid from patients with chronic renal failure. *Acta Med Pol* **17**: 137, 1976.
24. Bartelson, N. M., Basil, T., and Lavender, A. L.: 3′,5′-cyclic AMP levels in hemodialysis patients. Seventh Annual Meeting of the American Society of Nephrology, 1974, p. 7.
25. Schneider, W., and Jutzler, G. A.: Implications of cyclic adenosine 3′,5′-monophosphate in chronic renal failure. *N Engl J Med* **291**: 155, 1974.
26. Rabin, E. Z., Tattrie, B., Algom, D., Freedman, M., Saunders, F., and Roncari, D. A. K.: Ribonuclease activity in renal failure: evidence for toxicity. Ninth Annual Meeting of the American Society of Nephrology, 1976, p. 22.
27. Friman, C., Storgårds, E., Juvani, M., and Kock, B.: The glycosaminoglycans (mucopolysaccharides) in plasma in patients with renal insufficiency. *Clin Nephrol* **8**: 435, 1977.
28. Abiko, T., Kumikawa, M., Higuchi, H., and Sekino, H.: Identification and synthesis of a heptapeptide in uremic fluid. *Biochem Biophys Res Commun* **84**: 184, 1978.
29. Abiko, T., Onodera, I., and Sekino, H.: Isolation, structure and biological activity of the Trp-containing pentapeptide from uremic fluid. *Biochem Biophys Res Commun* **89**: 813, 1979.
30. Abiko, T., Kumikawa, M., and Sekino, H.: Inhibition effect of rosette formation between human lymphocytes and sheep erythrocytes by specific heptapeptide isolated from uremic fluid and its analogs. *Biochem Biophys Res Commun* **86**: 945, 1979.
31. Zimmerman, L., Baldesten, A., Bergström, J., and Fürst, P.: Isotachophoretic separation of middle molecule peptides in uremic body fluids. *Clin Nephrol* **13**: 183, 1980.
32. Zimmerman, L., Fürst, P., Bergström, J., and Jörnvall, H.: A new glycine containing compound with a blocked amino group from uremic body fluids. *Clin Nephrol* **14**: 107, 1980.

CHAPTER SIXTEEN

Further Experience with the Use of Amino Acid Containing Dialysate (Amino-Dianeal) in Peritoneal Dialysis

D. G. OREOPOULOS, M.D., Ph.D., F.R.C.P.(C.), F.A.C.P.

J. W. BALFE, M.D., F.R.C.P. (C)

R. KHANNA, M.D.

P. CRASSWELLER, M.D.

L. GOTLOIB, M.D.

H. RODELLA, B.Sc.

G. ZELLERMAN, M.S.B.I.D., ENG.

L. BRANDES, B.Sc.

W. McCREADY, M.B., M.R.C.P.

R. OGILVIE, Ph.D.

H. HUSDAN, Ph.D.

INTRODUCTION

AS THE LONG-TERM EXPERIENCE with patients maintained on continuous ambulatory peritoneal dialysis (CAPD) increases, two areas of major concern emerge: recurrent peritonitis and nutritional aspects. Recurrent peritonitis is already decreasing in frequency and new technological improvements are undoubtedly going to reduce it still further to acceptable levels. The nutritional aspects that are the cause for concern are hypertriglyceridemia, obesity, and persistent hypoalbuminemia, with a simultaneous decrease in serum transferrin and C_3 levels. Although the exact pathogenesis of these complications has not yet been defined, it is possible that the continuous

---

Departments of Medicine, Urology and Clinical Biochemistry and the Metabolic-Renal Laboratory, Toronto Western Hospital, Ontario, Canada, and the Division of Nephrology, Hospital for Sick Children, Toronto, Ontario, Canada

dextrose absorption (150–200 g/day) from the dialysate may be responsible for the first two and continuous daily removal of protein with CAPD responsible for the third. In addition, enhanced hepatic synthesis of proteins, resulting from the hypoproteinemia, may be contributing to the increased triglyceride levels.

If, indeed, dextrose in the dialysate is contributing to these complications, one should consider the use of another osmotic agent. In the past we have proposed the use of a mixture of amino acids instead of dextrose.[1] Since the average amino acid molecular weight is around 100 daltons, one would expect that osmotically they will be approximately twice as effective when compared with an equal concentration of dextrose, which has molecular weight of 180 daltons. Indeed, actual measurements of the osmolality of dialysate solutions containing amino acids instead of dextrose confirmed this reasoning.[1]

The potential advantages of using an amino acid containing dialysate are 1) elimination of all the side effects of dextrose, and 2) enhancement of protein synthesis and thus replacement of protein losses and improvement of hypoproteinemia with all its consequences.

In this paper we describe further experiences with the use of an amino acid containing dialysate in animals and human beings maintained on CAPD.

MATERIALS, METHODS, AND RESULTS

Experiments in rabbits

Three normal New Zealand rabbits (females 3–4 kg) were maintained on CAPD through a special Silastic peritoneal catheter. To avoid the strong tendency to clot in the dialysate, an omentectomy was performed on the animals prior to catheter implantation and in addition 20,000 units of heparin per liter was added to the dialysate. The animals were permanently connected to a modified automatic cycler* and 300 ml of dialysate was delivered every 6 hours. To avoid twisting of the tubing connecting the animals to the cycler, they were restrained in special cages, which prevented excessive movement but allowed free access to food and water.

One animal was dialysed with Dianeal 2.5 g% (control) and the other two with Amino-Dianeal solution containing 1 g% amino acid and 0.5 g% dextrose.

Figure 1 shows the changes in total serum proteins and Figure 2, the changes in 12-hour fasting levels of serum triglycerides. Although the duration of the experiment was short (2 weeks) all animals showed a marked decrease in serum protein, probably as a result of increased protein losses, not compensated for by an increased protein intake (since rabbits are vegetarian animals). However, the percent decrease in serum proteins from the baseline was smaller in the animals dialysed with the Amino-Dianeal solution than

---

*American Medical Products Corporation.

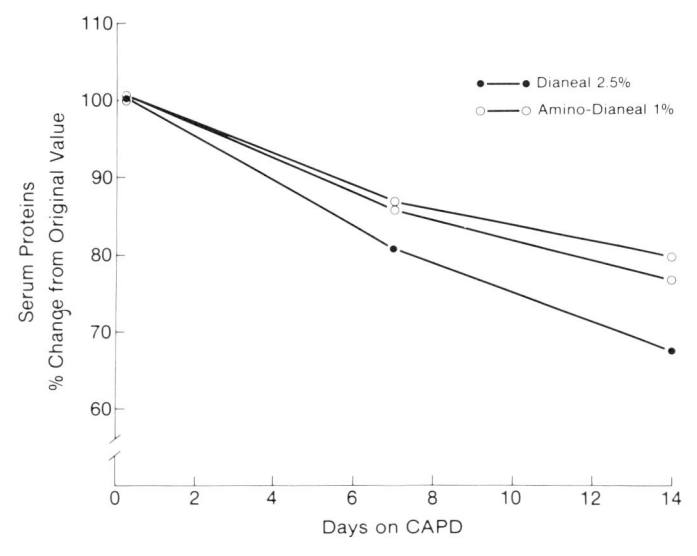

Experience with Amino Acid in Peritoneal Dialysis 111

Figure 1. Changes in total serum protein among three rabbits maintained on CAPD. The control animal was dialysed with dextrose (2.5%) Dianeal solution and the study animals with Amino-Dianeal (1%) solution.

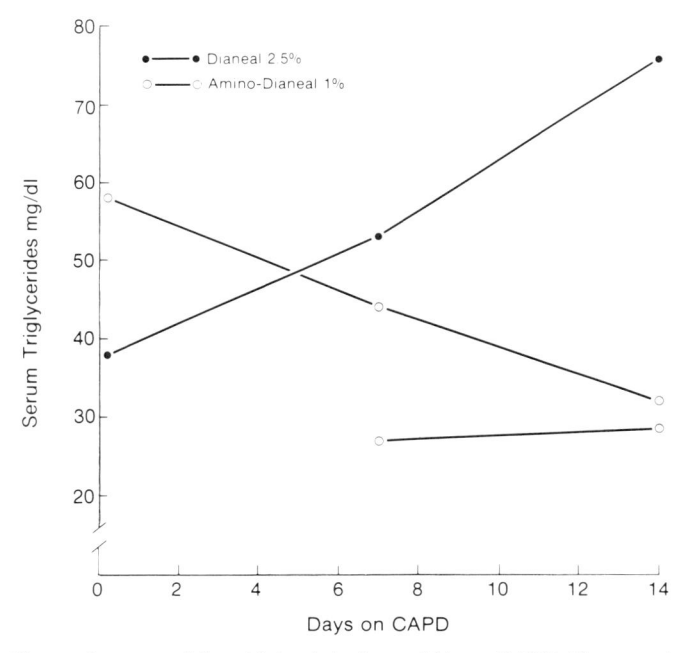

Figure 2. Changes in serum triglyceride levels in three rabbits on CAPD. The control animal was dialysed with dextrose (2.5%) Dianeal solution and the study animals with Amino-Dianeal (1%).

with the control dialysate (Dianeal). The changes in serum triglyceride levels between the control and the study animals were even more marked: increased in the control animal, decreased in one of the study animals, and remained low in the other, in which baseline values were not available. Similar experiments are presently being performed with a larger number of animals.

Experience with human beings

Since we have had no previous experience with human trials of this type, we used these solutions in only two patients who were not eating, were severely malnourished, and had severe hypoproteinemia. Other treatment modalities were neither available nor indicated.

Patient I. E.L., a 10-month old baby, had been on CAPD since the age of 4 months suffering from end-stage renal disease secondary to congenital oxalosis. She was dialysed using 300-ml exchange volumes. During the months prior to starting on amino acids, she refused to eat and developed marked hypoproteinemia and edema and was failing to thrive. Because of her refusal to eat, a nasogastric tube was used to give her 600 ml of formula (Prosobee R) containing 6.8 g/dl of carbohydrate and 2.5 g/dl of protein. In addition, it was decided to start her on daily exchanges of dialysate containing 1.5 g% dextrose and 1 g% amino acids. Initially, all four exchanges contained amino acids, but because on this regimen her blood urea nitrogen (BUN) increased to 120–130 mg%, it was decided to use only one of the four daily exchanges with amino acids, while the other three contained dextrose (Dianeal, 2.5 g% or 4.25 g%). Figures 3, 4, and 5 show the changes in BUN, serum

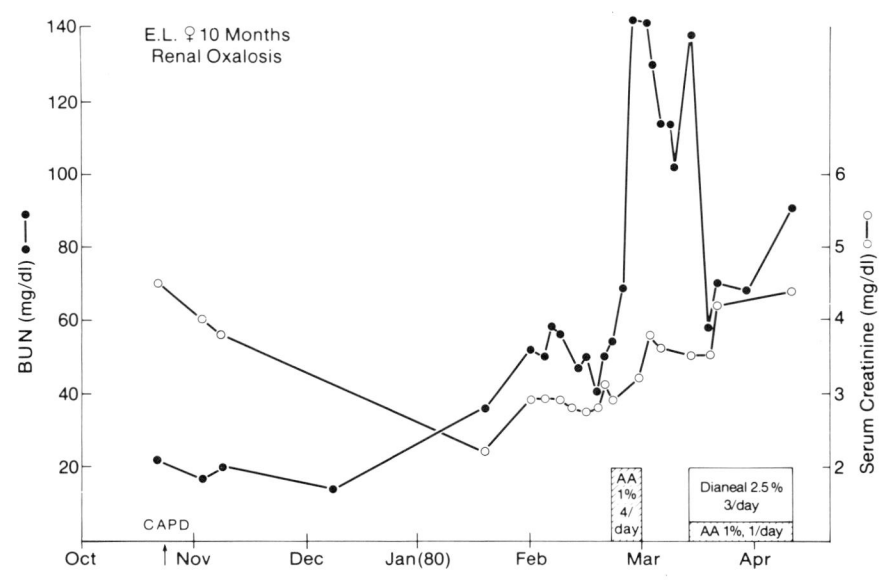

Figure 3. Patient E.L. Changes in BUN and serum creatinine before and after the use of Amino-Dianeal exchanges.

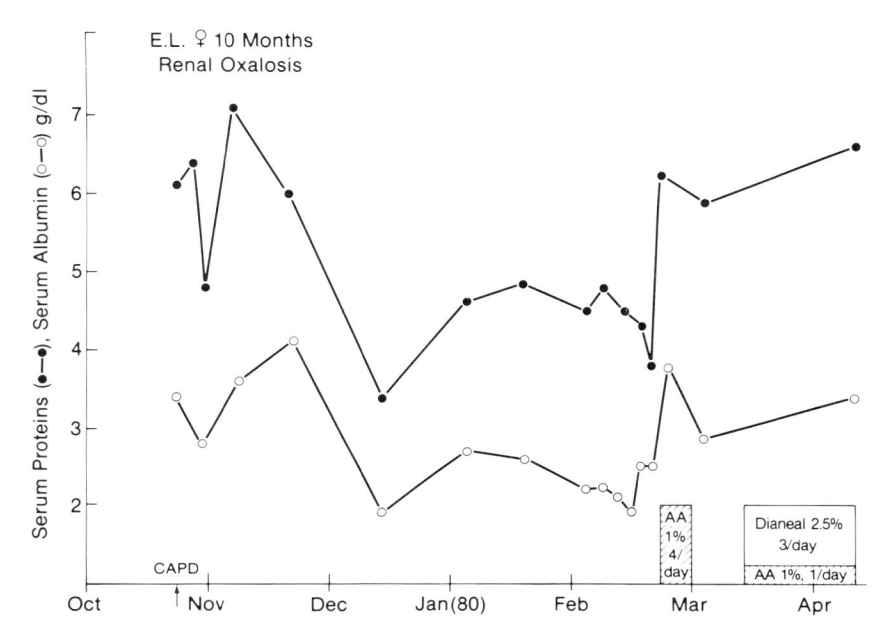

Experience with Amino Acid in Peritoneal Dialysis 113

Figure 4. Changes in serum proteins and albumin before and during the use of Amino-Dianeal solutions in patient E.L.

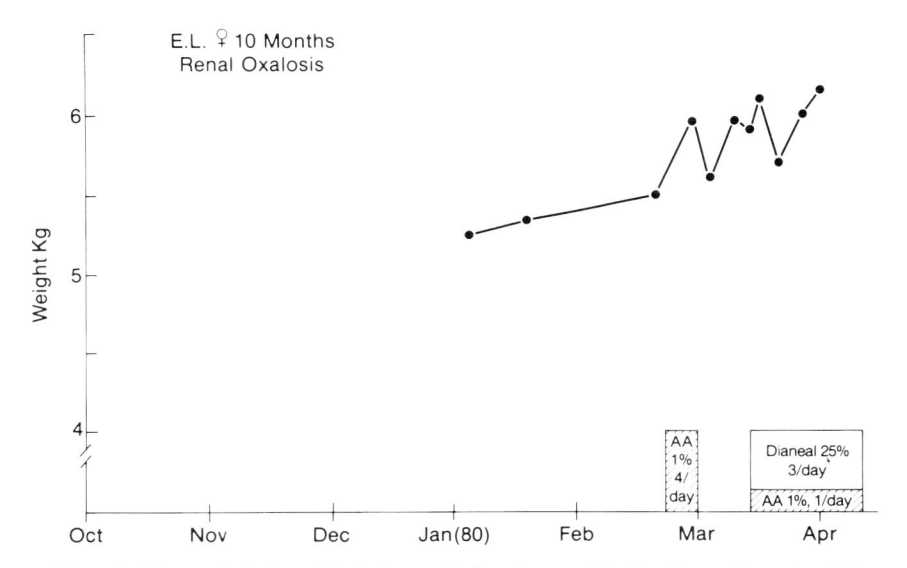

Figure 5. Changes in body weight before and after the use of Amino-Dianeal in patient E.L.

creatinine, total protein, albumin, and weight before and during the use of Amino-Dianeal. The combination of the improved dietary intake with the nasogastric tube feeding and the use of amino acids probably caused the increase in BUN, which leveled around 80 mg%. The child's weight has increased without edema and her general appearance improved. Because she still refuses to eat, the nasogastric tube feeding has been continued.

The amount of ultrafiltration with the Amino-Dianeal was, on average, 14 ml per exchange, similar to that of the Dianeal exchanges. The removal of urea and creatinine was similar in both solutions.

Patient II. R.N., a 60-year-old man, suffering from chronic glomerulonephritis and hypertension had been on chronic intermittent peritoneal dialysis since 1974 and on CAPD since 1978. During the last year he had been plagued with recurrent attacks of pneumonia, chronic obstructive lung disease, and hypothyroidism. During the last few months, he has been losing weight and developed hypoproteinemia and hypoalbuminemia. He was started on one out of four exchanges per day with Amino-Dianeal (0.8%) for 4 days, and, since his BUN increased only slightly, he was changed to two to four exchanges a day. The other two were Dianeal. Figure 6 shows the changes in his BUN and weight during the first 10 days of this regimen. Table 1 shows the amount of ultrafiltration, BUN, and creatinine removed with both Amino-Dianeal and the Dianeal solution. There were no significant differences.

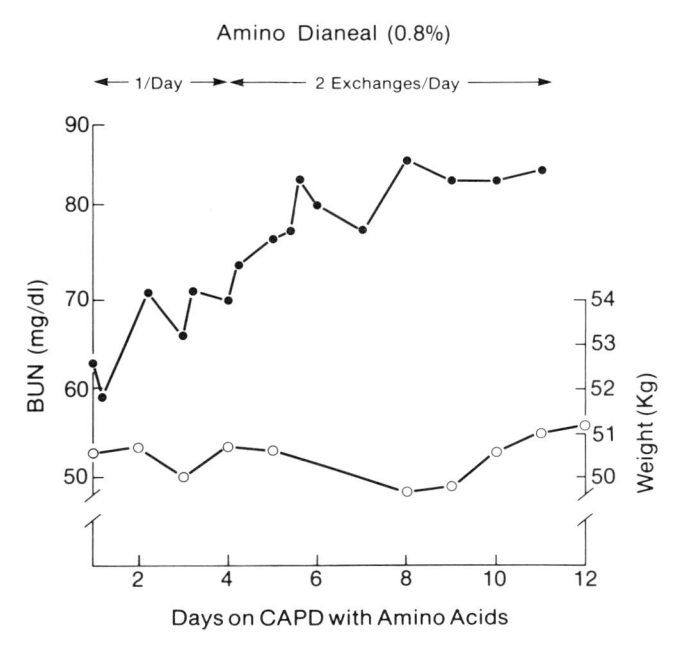

Figure 6. Changes in BUN and weight during the use of Amino-Dianeal dialysate in patient R.N.

TABLE 1.

Comparison of Ultrafiltration Rates and Amounts of Urea, Creatinine and Protein Removed Between Dianeal and Amino-Dianeal Solutions

	2-Liter Exchanges	
	Amino-Dianeal (0.8%-6 hours) [$\bar{x}$ (n)]	Dianeal (1.5%-4 hours) [$\bar{x}$ (n)]
Ultrafiltration (ml)	227 (9)	278 (9)
Protein (g)	1.59 (6)	1.39 (6)
Creatinine (mg)	205 (6)	185 (6)
BUN (g)	1.74 (10)	1.74 (10)

DISCUSSION

Our experience with the animals indicates that the use of amino acids may reduce the rate of hypoproteinemia and at the same time may prevent hypertriglyceridemia in rabbits maintained on CAPD.

With human beings, our experience indicates that the amino acids are as effective osmotic agents as dextrose and do not interfere with the removal of BUN and creatinine. At least two exchanges per day were well tolerated by one patient without producing unacceptable BUN levels.

Further studies will be required to establish the proper concentration of the amino acids and the number of daily exchanges required in these patients.

ACKNOWLEDGMENTS

We would like to thank Ms. Betty Kellman and the personnel of the animal laboratory of the Toronto Western Hospital for their assistance and Mrs. Fyzina Razack for her assistance in the preparation of the manuscript.

Part of this work was supported by the National Institutes of Health (Contract No. N01-8-2213) and the Physician Services Incorporated Foundation of Ontario.

Reference

1. Oreopoulos, D. G., Crassweller, P., Kartirtzoglou, A., Zellerman, G., Rodella, H., and Vas, S.: Amino acids as an osmotic agent (instead of dextrose) in continuous ambulatory peritoneal dialysis. In *CAPD: Proceedngs of an International Symposium.* M. Legrain, Ed. Excerpta Medica, Amsterdam, 1980.

CHAPTER SEVENTEEN

Additives in CAPD*

F. CANTAROVICH, M.D.

J. PÉREZ LOREDO, M.D.

C. CHENA, M.D.

M. REICHART, M.D.

J. TIZADO, B.Ch.

L. CASTRO, M.D.

D. BRANA, M.D.

V. JULIANELLI, M.D.

MATERIALS AND METHODS

THREE DIFFERENT TREATMENT MODALITIES were used (Table 1).

1. Control Period. Mode A was three daily exchanges, 2,000 ml each, with an 8-hour dwell time. The total infused volume was 6,000 ml/day. The morning and afternoon exchanges were 2% dextrose dialysis solution and the overnight exchange with 4.5%. Five patients (residual clearance average 0.9 ml/m) received mode A during a mean of 17.9 days (6–33) of control.
2. Control Period. Mode B was two daily exchanges, 2,000 ml each, with a 12-hour dwell time. The total infused volume was 4000 ml/day, both exchanges with 4.5% dextrose concentration. Two of the five patients received mode B, average 26 days (18–34).
3. "Additives" Period. Mode C was similar to mode B but 150 to 250 ml of mannitol 15% and 150 to 250 ml of dextran 6% (M.W. 70,000) were included in each exchange. The infused volume of exchange was 2,300–2,500 ml and 24-hour volume was 4,600–5,000 ml. Four patients received mode C during an average of 22 days (13–41). The fifth patient was not included in this period because of a residual clearance above 1 ml/m.

Infused and drained volumes, daily ultrafiltration rates, body weight, and daily diuresis were measured. Comparison of infused and consecutive drained

---

Military Central Hospital, Buenos Aires (1426), Argentina
*This preliminary report shows our first short-term experience in using mannitol and dextran added to dialysate solution in CAPD, in order to obtain an increase of water and metabolite removal.[1,2]

TABLE 1.
Three Different Treatment Modalities with CAPD

Mode	Exchanges (per day)	Volume Infused (ml/day)	ml per exchange	Dextrose Concentration 4.5 g%	Dextrose Concentration 2 g%	Total Daily (g)	Additives (ml/day)
A	3	6,000	2,000	2,000	4,000	170	—
B	2	4,000	2,000	4,000	—	180	—
C	2	4,887 (4600-5000)	2,443 (2,300-2,500)	4,000	—	180 Mannitol 300-500 Dextran 300-500	

volumes and dwell times was possible when ultrafiltration by liter infused and ultrafiltration by liter infused related to dwell times were considered.

Table 2 shows the five patients included in this study and the days of follow-up on each mode of treatment. One patient (case 1) received the three modes of treatment. Four patients received A and C modes (cases 1, 2, 3, and 4). One patient was treated with A and B modes.

Dietary intake recorded was 1.1 g/kg/day. Serum urea, serum creatinine, and hematocrit were done.

TABLE 2.
Patients and Days in Each Treatment Modality

Patients[a]		Sex	Age (years)	Diagnosis	Mode A[b]	Mode B[c]	Mode C[d]
1	N.M.	F	20	GNC (Kr = 0.8 ml/m)	6	18	13
2	J.A.	M	65	Nephrosclerosis (Kr = 0.7 ml/m)	19	—	19
3	M.Ch.	M	24	CGN (Kr = 0.2 ml/m)	13	—	41
4	M.Q.	F	59	Nephrosclerosis (Kr = 0.7 ml/m)	33	—	18
5	V.Z.	M	60	Diabetes (Kr = 2.1 ml/m)	18	34	—
				Total Days	89	52	91
				Mean	17.8	26	22.7

[a] (Kr $\bar{X}$ 0.9 ml/m ± 0.7).
[b] Three exchanges/day of 2000 cc of 2%, 2%, and 4.5% dextrose.
[c] Two exchanges/day of 2000 cc of 4.5% dextrose.
[d] Two exchanges/day of 2300-2500 cc of 4.5% dextrose with mannitol (150-250 cc) plus dextran (150-250 cc).

RESULTS

The comparison of results between A and B, B and C, and A versus C are shown in Tables 3, 4, and 5.

Table 3 shows the results in two patients who received A and B modes of treatment with a mean duration of 12 and 26 days, respectively. Case 1 had been 6 days on A and 18 days on B. Case 5 had been 18 days on A and 34 days on B. The differences of the drained volumes between A and B modes would be related with the different infused volumes. The values related with the ultrafiltration ability (ultrafiltration by day, ultrafiltration by liter, and ultrafiltration by liter infused considering dwell time) did not show significant differences.

The analysis of these data show that two daily exchanges with hypertonic solution (4.5%) are as useful on ultrafiltration capacity as three exchanges (two 2% dextrose and one 4.5%). Nevertheless, the daily drained volume with this mode was not adequate enough to obtain appropriate peritoneal clearances. No differences in body weight and urine output were seen.

Table 4 compares the results obtained with mode B (18 days) and mode C (13 days) in case 1. It shows that mode C has major ultrafiltration ability, attending the values of ultrafiltration by liter and ultrafiltration by liter and dwell time.

Table 5 shows the results obtained in four patients (case 1, 2, 3, and 4) with mode A of treatment, average 17 days (6–33), and mode C of treatment, average 22.7 days (13–41). The ultrafiltration daily rate, the ultrafiltration by liter, and the ultrafiltration by liter and dwell time were larger on mode C.

TABLE 3.
Comparison of Results in Patients 1 and 5

	Mode A[a]		Mode B[b]		
Vol. infused (ml/day)	6,000	$n = 24$	4,000	$n = 52$	$p < 0.001$
Vol. drained (ml/day)	6,576 ± 776	$n = 24$	4,425 ± 186	$n = 52$	$p < 0.001$
Ultrafil. by day (ml/day)	576 ± 776	$n = 24$	425 ± 186	$n = 52$	NS
Ultrafil. by liter infused (ml/liter)	95 ± 129	$n = 24$	105 ± 46	$n = 52$	NS
Ultrafil. by liter infused and dwell time (ml/liter/minute)	0.199 ± 0.27	$n = 24$	0.146 ± 0.154	$n = 52$	NS
Diuresis (ml/day)	365 ± 255	$n = 19$	508 ± 485	$n = 39$	NS
Body weight (kg)	57.9 ± 1.3	$n = 13$	58 ± 9.3	$n = 34$	NS
Mean days	12		26		
Dwell time (hours)	8		12		

[a] Three exchanges.
[b] Two exchanges.

TABLE 4.
Comparison of Results in Patient 1

	Mode B[a]		Mode C[b]		p
Vol. infused (ml/day)	4,000	$n = 18$	4,946 ± 87	$n = 13$	>0.001
Vol. drained (ml/day)	4,611 ± 339	$n = 18$	6,492 ± 385	$n = 13$	>0.001
Ultrafil. by day (ml/day)	611 ± 339	$n = 18$	1,546 ± 385	$n = 13$	>0.001
Ultrafil. by liter infused (ml/liter)	152 ± 84	$n = 18$	312 ± 77	$n = 13$	>0.001
Ultrafiltration by liter infused and dwell time (ml/liter/minute)	0.211 ± 0.117	$n = 18$	0.433 ± 0.106	$n = 13$	>0.001
Diuresis (ml/day)	230 ± 66	$n = 17$	415 ± 189	$n = 13$	>0.001
Body weight (kg)	48.7 ± 1.1	$n = 17$	50.3 ± 1.0	$n = 13$	>0.001
Mean days	18		13		
Dwell time (hours)	12		12		

[a] Two exchanges.
[b] Two exchanges with additives.

The larger daily drained volume on mode A was related with the volume infused.

Mode C has a better ultrafiltration capacity than exchanges of dialysate solution without additives. There was also an increase in urine output on mode C.

Humoral and clinical controls during the three periods did not show underdialysis symptoms in this short-term study (Table 6).

TABLE 5.
Comparison of Results in Patients 1, 2, 3, and 4

	Mode A[a]		Mode C		
Vol. infused (ml/day)	6,000	$n = 71$	4,887 ± 74	$n = 91$	$P < 0.001$
Vol. drained (ml/day)	6,538 ± 391	$p = 71$	5,747 ± 569	$p = 91$	$P < 0.001$
Ultrafil. by day (ml/day)	538 ± 391	$p = 71$	860 ± 518	$p = 91$	$P < 0.001$
Ultrafil. by liter infused (ml/liter)	89 ± 65	$p = 71$	174 ± 105	$p = 91$	$P < 0.001$
Ultrafil. by liter infused and dwell time (ml/liter/minute)	0.186 ± 0.135	$p = 71$	0.241 ± 0.146	$p = 91$	0.01
Diuresis (ml/day)	221 ± 87	$p = 47$	352 ± 103	$p = 80$	$P < 0.001$
Body weight (kg)	61.3 ± 9.4	$p = 63$	60.9 ± 8.2	$p = 85$	NS
Mean days	17.7 (6–33)		22.7 (13–41)		
Dwell time (hours)	8		12		

[a] Three exchanges.
[b] Two exchanges with additives.

TABLE 6.
Humoral Control

Patient	Prestudy Serum Urea (mg/dl)	Prestudy Serum Creatinine (mg/dl)	Prestudy Hematocrit (vol %)	Period A Serum Urea	Period A Serum Creatinine	Period A Hematocrit	Period B Serum Urea	Period B Serum Creatinine	Period B Hematocrit	Period C Serum Urea	Period C Serum Creatinine	Period C Hematocrit
1	150	12.4	16	136 3 ± 25.5	9.0 3 ± 1.7	22.6 3 ± 2.8	117.5 2 ± 45.9	4.9 2 ± 0.9	29	85.7 4 ± 13.3	7.3 3 ± 1.3	27
2	190	8.5	28	168.5 2 ± 33.2	10.6 2 ± 2.5	23 2 ± 7.0	—	—	—	145.8 5 ± 18.3	9.0 5 ± 2.6	19
3	117.5 2 ± 45.9	17.7 2 ± 0.2	13	232.1 9 ± 76.8	13.4 9 ± 1.7	19.3 3 ± 1.1	—	—	—	184 33 ± 44.1	12.9 33 ± 2.1	18 3 ± 3.4
4	111	5.6	28	146.2 5 ± 31.0	7.3 5 ± 1.8	27.6 3 ± 0.5	—	—	—	140.8 6 ± 15.4	7.0 6 ± 0.80	30
5	212	6.5	26	84.5 2 ± 21.9	3.9 2 ± 0.1	27	170	4.6 2 ± 0.0	29.6 3 ± 0.5	—	—	—
Mean	156.1 n = 6 ± 44.2	10.1 n = 5 ± 4.9	22.2 n = 5 ± 7.1	153.4 n = 5 ± 53.6	8.8 n = 5 ± 3.5	23.9 n = 5 ± 3.4	143.7 n = 2 ± 37.1	4.8 n = 2 ± 0.2	29.3 n = 2 ± 0.4	139 n = 4 ± 40	9.0 n = 4 ± 2.6	23.5 n = 4 ± 5.9

CONCLUSIONS

The analysis of the results of this short-term study suggest these preliminary conclusions:

1. Dextran and mannitol added to the dialysate, on two daily CAPD exchanges, regardless of dextrose concentration, give significantly larger ultrafiltration rates than three or two daily exchanges without additives.
2. The study showed that two daily CAPD exchanges with additives gives a weekly urea clearence of around 40 liters.
3. Theoretically, three daily CAPD exchanges with additives would give a weekly urea clearence similar to that obtained with four exchanges without additives.
4. The infused volumes of hypertonic solution and the additives were well tolerated by all patients.

In this short period of time no side effects were seen.

A long-term follow-up study is under way in our department with the intention of evaluating the clinical possibilities of these different modalities of treatment, with special regard to the side effects of the additives in relation with serum osmolality, acid-base status, volemia, hepatic impairment, coagulation studies, and nitrogen waste products removal.

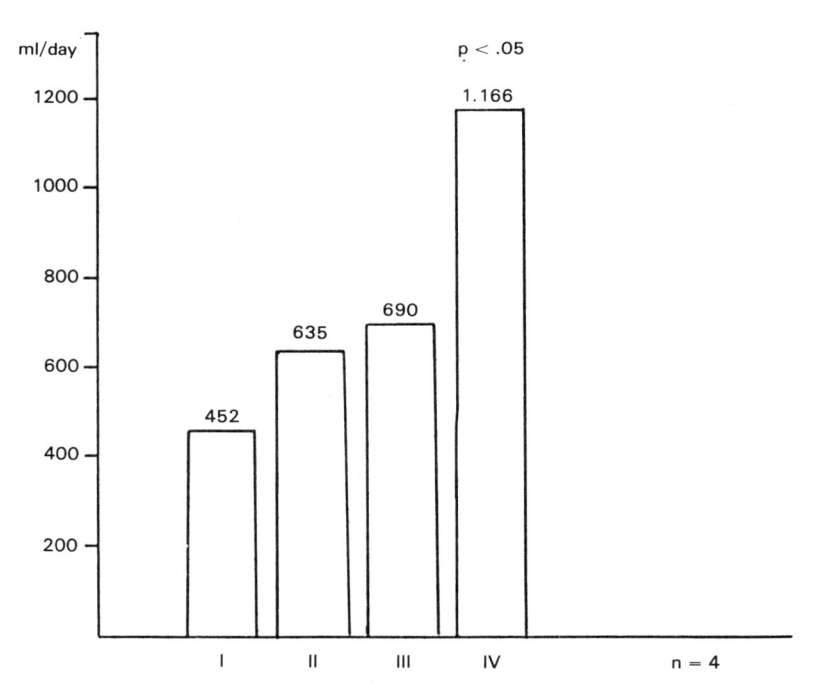

Figure 1. Daily ultrafiltration rate. I: dextrose 4%; II: dextrose 4% + mannitol; III: dextrose 4% + dextran; IV: dextrose 4% + mannitol + dextran.

ADDENDUM

A long-term double-blind protocol to evaluate the results obtained with different additives in CAPD dialysate solutions is in course.

A short-term protocol performed in a 61-year-old patient (Kr 1.02, S.D. = ±0.34, ml/m, *n*: 4), who had a peritonitis 30 days before the study, is presented.

Dialysate solutions. 1) Dialysate plus dextrose 4%; 2) dialysate plus dextrose 4%; with mannitol 15%, 250 ml; 3) dialysate plus dextrose 4%; with dextran 70 6% 250 ml; and 4) dialysate plus dextrose 4%; with dextran 250 ml plus mannitol 250 ml.

Two daily exchanges of 2,500 ml of dialysate were used. Every two days different solutions were utilized. It was an 8 day study. The previous treatment of the patient was CAPD with three daily exchanges.[3]

TABLE 7

Results of a Short-Term Study of a 61-Year-Old Patient

	Dialysate Plus 4% Dextrose	Dialysate Plus 4% Dextrose Plus Mannitol	Dialysate Plus 4% Dextrose Plus Dextran	Dialysate Plus 4% Dextrose Plus Dextran and Mannitol
Serum urea (mg/dl)	101 S.D. ± 4.0	97 S.D. ± 9.4	95.7 S.D. ± 3.4	85.7 S.D. ± 4.6
Serum creatinine (mm/dl)	5.2 S.D. ± 0.3	6.0 S.D. ± 0.1	5.3 S.D. ± 0.7	4.7 S.D. ± 0.1
Serum sodium (mEq/liter)	141 S.D. ± 2	141 S.D. ± 1	141 S.D. ± 2.5	141 S.D. ± 1
Serum potassium (mEq/liter)	4.9 S.D. ± 0.5	4.4 S.D. ± 0.1	4.9 S.D. ± 0.3	4.9 S.D. ± 0.3
Hematocrit (vol %)	22.5 S.D. ± 0.5	19.5 S.D. ± 0.5	22.5 S.D. ± 1	21.7 S.D. ± 0.5
S.osm. (mOsm/liter)	284 S.D. ± 2	309 S.D. ± 7	294 S.D. ± 10	296 S.D. ± 9
Dial. osm. input (mOsm/liter)	507	545	473	508
Dial. osm. output (mOsm/liter)	283 S.D. ± 13	303 S.D. ± 2	294 S.D. ± 8	305 S.D. ± 13
Drained vol. (ml/day)	5.452 S.D. ± 460	5.635 S.D. ± 332	5.690 S.D. ± 224	6.166 S.D. ± 508
Loss protein (g/day)	1.15 S.D. ± 0.05	1.05 S.D. ± 0.05	1.0 S.D. ± 0.1	1.67 S.D. ± 0.13
Dial. urea (mg/dl)	89 S.D. ± 1.4	86.7 S.D. ± 12	89.5 S.D. ± 7	87.5 S.D. ± 17
Dial. creatinine (mg/dl)	4.4 S.D. ± 0.3	4.1 S.D. ± 0.4	4.0 S.D. ± 0.2	4.3 S.D. ± 0.2
Dial. sodium (mEq/liter)	141 S.D. ± 1	140 S.D. ± 1	139 S.D. ± 3	141 S.D. ± 1.1
Dial. potassium (mEq/liter)	3.1 S.D. ± 0.2	3.6 S.D. ± 0.1	3.6 S.D. ± 0.1	3.4 S.D. ± 0.1
D/P Urea	0.88	0.89	0.93	1.02
Ur. perit. clear. (ml/minute)	3.2	3.3	3.6	4.4
Urine output (ml/day)	500	880	775	620
Body weight (kg)	60.3	61.2	61.1	60.2

Results

The daily ultrafiltration rate is higher when the dialysate IV is used ($p < 0.05$) (Fig. 1).

The urea peritoneal clearance improved significantly with the dialysate IV (Table 7).

The D/P urea ratio with this solution was 1.02 and the drained volume was the highest obtained (6.166 S.D. = ±508 ml).

The results in serum and dialysate osmolalities, the values of hematocrit, urea, creatinine, and potassium, and the body weight and diuresis provide several speculations that would be answered after a long-term follow-up with this procedure.

References

1. Gjessing, I.: The use of dextran as dialysin fluid in peritoneal dialysis. *Acta Med Scand* **185**: 237–239, 1969.
2. Jirka, J., and Kotkova, E.: Peritoneal dialysis by iso-oncotic dextran solution in anaesthetized dogs. Intraperitoneal fluid volume and protein concentration in the irrigation fluid. *Proc Eur Dial Transplant Assoc* **4**: 141–145, 1967.
3. Cantarovich, F., Perez Loredo, J., Chena, C., *et al.:* CAPD three daily exchanges, 1980. Unpublished.

CHAPTER EIGHTEEN

CAPD: Three Daily Exchanges

F. CANTAROVICH, M.D.

J. PÉREZ LOREDO, M.D.

C. CHENA, M.D.

R. WILBERG, M.D.

J. VERNETTI, M.D.

C. CORREA, M.D.

J. TIZADO, B.Ch.

AFTER THE FIRST REPORT of Popovich et al.,[1] continuous ambulatory peritoneal dialysis (CAPD) is becoming another alternative for the treatment of end-stage renal disease (ESRD).[2-8]

Actually the efforts of clinical investigators are mainly directed to: 1) improve the efficiency of the method, 2) control the major complication: peritonitis, 3) obtain the best adaptation and comfort for the patients, and 4) reduce the cost of this treatment (in general efforts) to achieve a better control of the national budgets for ESRD programs.

Following these concepts, since February 1979 we have had a CAPD program in our department.[9]

Regardless of residual glomerular filtration rate (GFR), all the patients received, from the beginning of the treatment, three daily exchanges of peritoneal dialysate solution, and in this chapter we show our general results and a follow-up of six patients that exceed 8 months with this treatment modality (8–13 months, average 9.33 months).

MATERIALS AND METHODS

Twenty-six patients with a mean residual GFR of 2.38 S.D. 1.9 ml/minute were included in the program: nine females and 17 males, aged 12–79 years (mean 46.1).

Two of the 26 patients were previously on regular hemodialysis treatment and 24 received CAPD as initial dialytic therapy.

Military Central Hospital, Buenos Aires (1426), Argentina

Technique

A Silastic catheter was inserted in the abdominal cavity following Tenckhoff's technique.[10]

Until March 1980 rigid containers were used; afterward plastic bags were available.

The dialysate solution composition was: sodium, 134 mEq/liter; chlorine, 101 mEq/liter; magnesium, 1.1 mEq/liter; calcium, 4 mEq/liter; lactate, 38 mEq/liter; and glucose 2 and 4.5 g% ml.

Each of the three daily exchanges consisted of 2 liters of dialysate solution and was carried out at 8 AM, 3 PM, and 10 PM. The 8 AM and 3 PM exchanges with 2 g% of glucose and the overnight solution with 4.5 g%.

The training period for patients and relatives was about 4 weeks.

Controls

Serum urea, creatinine, sodium, and potassium determinations were done weekly in the first month; afterward they were performed monthly, together with calcium, phosphorus, uric acid, cholesterol, albumin, and hematocrit. Total lipid and triglyceride determinations were done every 3 months. Electromyography for assessment of peripheral motor nerve conduction were obtained every 3 months. Also audiograms and electroencephalograms were done.

Diet

The clinical record revealed a daily average intake of 40 kcal/kg/day (including 900 kcal from the glucose of the dialysate) and a mean protein daily intake of 1.40 g/kg/day.

RESULTS

The experience with the 26 patients comprises a total of 105.5 patient-months (Table 1). Seventeen patients were transferred to hemodialysis for the following reasons: 5, catheter blockage; 2, no compliance with the treatment; 1, hydrocele; 9, peritonitis.

Two improved their renal function after 1 and 3 months, respectively, and they were not in need of dialytic treatment.

Two patients died (a 79-year-old female with severe cardiac failure and a 66-year-old diabetic female who died suddenly).

Five patients remain on CAPD.

TABLE 1.

Follow-up of 26 Patients — 105.5 Patient-Months

17	Transferred to hemodialysis	5	Catheter blockage
2	Improved renal function	2	No compliance with the treatment
2	Died	1	Hydrocele
5	Remained on CAPD	9	Peritonitis

When the 17 patients were transferred to hemodialysis treatment, the mean serum urea and creatinine levels were 160 mg%, S.D. = ±75, and 8.9 mg%, S.D. ±2.8, respectively.

In the nine patients who stopped the CAPD treatment and who were transferred to hemodialysis due to peritoneal infection, the bacterial culture showed the following organisms: *Pseudomonas putrefaciens*, 8; *Alcaligenes faecalis*, 5; *Pseudomonas aeruginosa*, 5; *Klebsiella pneumoniae*, 3; *Citrobacter* 1.

Six of the 26 patients underwent CAPD with three daily exchanges for more than 8 months. Their residual GFR was $\bar{X}$ = 1.58, S.D. = ±1.86, ml/minute and individual data are shown in Table 2.

Several mean laboratory values of six patients with a mean residual GFR of 1.58, S.D. = ±1.86, ml/minute who received CAPD more than 8 months (8 to 13) are shown in Table 3.

The previous results (pre-CAPD) are those obtained when CAPD was started after treatment with acute peritoneal dialysis (mean 18 hours).

Hematocrit. A slight rise (not significant) was found with a mean value of 30.3, S.D. = ±9.1, vol%.

Serum urea and creatinine. The serum urea and creatinine levels stabilized at 136, S.D. = ±39, mg/dl and 8.3, S.D. = ±2.8, mg/dl, respectively. The mean of serum urea was lower than predialysis values ($p < 0.001$, whereas the serum creatinine level fall was significantly lower ($p < 0.02$).

Serum uric acid. A mean of 8.1, S.D. = ±2.2 mg/dl was found, without changes in respect to predialysis values.

Serum electrolytes. The serum electrolytes generally remained normal in all the patients. Two patients developed hypokalemia (2.8 mEq/liter) without clinical symptomatology. Remission occurred after 3 weeks without clinical treatment.

Serum calcium and phosphorus. The serum calcium remained in normal values with a mean of 9.4, S.D. = ±0.65, mEq/liter. Serum phosphate showed a significant ($p < 0.05$) fall to normal values.

Serum cholesterol, lipids, and triglycerides. The serum cholesterol and lipids remained in normal values. A slight rise in the triglyceride level was found.

Glycemia. Glycemia remained slightly above normal values.

TABLE 2.
Clinical Data of Six Patients

Patients	Sex	Age	Kr[a] (ml/minute)	Etiology
M.H.	M	50	0.2	Polycystic K
S.R.	F	36	0.2	Chronic glomerulonephritis
B.P.	M	57	5.3	Interstitial nephritis
R.D.	F	66	2.2	Diabetic nephropathy
M.O.	M	52	0.5	Nephrosclerosis
S.C.	F	61	3.9	Chronic glomerulonephritis

[a] Kr: 1.58 ± 1.86 ml/minute.

TABLE 3.
Mean Values of Six Patients Undergoing CAPD (3 exchanges) for More Than 8 Months (8-13)

	Pre-CAPD[a]	n	CAPD[a]	n	Statistical Study
Hematocrit	27.0 ± 9	12	30.3 ± 9.1	97	N.S.
Serum urea	208 ± 74	20	136 ± 39	159	$p < 0.001$
Creatinine	10.0 ± 1.4	19	8.3 ± 2.8	171	$p < 0.002$
Uric acid	9.0 ± 3.0	12	8.1 ± 2.2	62	N.S.
Sodium	136 ± 2.0	21	138 ± 3.1	113	N.S.
Potassium	4.6 ± 0.1	30	4.5 ± 0.6	113	N.S.
Glycemia	110 ± 10	6	121 ± 36	72	N.S.
Cholesterol	185 ± 30	6	206 ± 42	62	N.S.
Triglycerides	170 ± 15	6	187 ± 37	17	N.S.
Total lipid	625 ± 45	6	595 ± 87	23	N.S.
Albumin	3.36 ± 0.70	6	3.04 ± 0.57	51	N.S.
Total protein	6.08 ± 1.00	6	5.72 ± 0.71	51	N.S.
Calcium	9.5 ± 0.3	6	9.4 ± 0.65	51	N.S.
Phosphorus	5.9 ± 2.9	6	4.6 ± 1.0	51	$p < 0.05$
Motor nerve conduction velocity	40.5 ± 9 / 40.08 ± 8.4	6	44.7 ± 10 / 41.5 ± 4.6	20	N.S.
Blood pressure					
Systolic	145 ± 23	45	138.5 ± 19.5	259	N.S.
Diastolic	88 ± 15	45	85.7 ± 9.5	259	N.S.

[a] Kr GFR: 1.58 ± 1.86 ml/minute.

Protein. The serum albumin stabilized in 3.04 g/dl.

Motor nerve conduction velocity. The bioelectrical studies of the patients did not show significant modifications on their nerve conduction studies.

Blood pressure. The blood pressure was 138.5, S.D. = ±19.5, and 85.7, S.D. = ±9.5, mm Hg. Ten of the 26 patients were hypertensive at the initiation of CAPD. Only one required antihypertensive medication.

Body weight. Mean predialysis body weight was 67.8 kg and rose to 69.2 kg at 8 months of CAPD treatment.

Table 4 shows the comparative data of two patients who received hemodialysis prior to CAPD.

Hematocrit level rose significantly ($p < 0.001$).

Serum urea level increased with low significance ($p < 0.2$).

The fall of serum phosphate level was significantly moderated ($p < 0.05$) not reaching the normal level.

The other controls were not significant.

After a period of more than 6 months when metabolic acidosis was found (bicarbonate levels less than 20 mEq/liter), sodium bicarbonate (10 to 25 g daily) was given to the patients with a rapid and significant rise of bicarbonate serum levels to normal values.

Peritoneal access. The 26 patients required 35 Tenckhoff catheters. In 18 only the initial access was required, whereas seven patients required two and one patient required three catheters.

Peritonitis occurred in 26 cases during the follow-up period (1 each 16.2 patient-weeks). In 85% the cultures were positive and in 15% they were negative. In 62% we found gram-negative bacteria: *Pseudomonas,* 13; *Kleb-*

TABLE 4.
Hemodialysis Versus CAPD. Mean Values Last 6 Months of Treatment
(Two Patients)

	Hemodialysis 16.5 hours/week — A = 1.36 m2		CAPD (3 exchanges/day)		Statistical Study
Hematocrit	27.4 ± 4.6	n = 15	37.9 ± 11.5	n = 11	$p < 0.001$
Serum urea	127.6 ± 14	n = 14	140.6 ± 15.5	n = 11	$p < 0.02$
Creatinine	9.7 ± 0.4	n = 15	11.0 ± 1.7	n = 12	N.S.
Uric acid	7.1 ± 0.1	n = 10	7.5 ± 1.6	n = 10	N.S.
Calcium	9.3 ± 0.4	n = 4	9.9 ± 1.0	n = 10	N.S.
Phosphorus	8.8 ± 1.7	n = 3	5.9 ± 1.8	n = 6	$p < 0.05$
Albumin	3.60 ± 0.70	n = 4	3.43 ± 0.17	n = 7	N.S.
Motor nerve conduction velocity	42.7 ± 9.5/43.5 ± 6.3	n = 4	43.2 ± 5.3/42.7 ± 4.8	n = 4	N.S.
Total protein	6.70 ± 0.14	n = 4	6.14 ± 0.39	n = 7	N.S.
Sodium	138 ± 1.4	n = 11	138 ± 3.6	n = 14	N.S.
Potassium	4.9 ± 0.4	n = 16	5.0 ± 0.1	n = 14	N.S.

[a] Kr: 0.2 ml/minute ± 0.15.

siella, 4; *Citrobacter*, 2; *Alcaligenes*, 5, *Enterobacter*, 1; *Acinobacter calcoaceticum*, 1. Gram-positive bacterial were found in 38% of the cases: *Staphylococcus aureus*, 4; *Staphylococcus epidermidis*, 3; *Streptococcus hemolyticus*, 1.

The main causes of the high percentage of peritonitis were related to incorrect technique and to the quality of the equipment used until March 1980.

DISCUSSION

The aim of this study was to determine if three daily CAPD exchanges could be an acceptable treatment in patients with ESRD regardless of the residual renal function.[5,11]

The data of Nolph *et al.*[15] regarding the relationship between the equilibrium of substances in dialysate solution and plasma and the dwell time of the dialysate were also considered for modification of the usual number of exchanges on CAPD.

With three daily exchanges, it is possible to obtain a weekly drain volume of 49 liters. When we use the clearance peritoneal formula, $D/P \times V/P$, and if we consider the D/P values of Nolph at 8 hours dwell time (urea 0.98, creatinine 0.9, uric acid 0.78, and inulin 0.48) the theoretical clearances could be as given in Table 5.

The weekly clearance of vitamin B_{12} with three daily exchanges is similar to that obtained with 15 hours weekly of hemodialysis[3,8] and it is related with adequate removal.[16,17]

Similarly the weekly clearance of inulin with three daily exchanges is nearly five times that obtained with 15 hours of weekly hemodialysis.[3,8]

The "clearance like kidney" concept[12,17,18] would indicate that the patients undergoing CAPD with five daily exchanges[3,4,8] are underdialyzed.

TABLE 5.
Theoretical Clearances

Substance	M.W.	Clearance (ml/minute)	Clearance (liter/week)
Urea	64	4.7	48
Creatinine	114	4.3	44
Uric acid	168	3.8	38
Vitamin B_{12}	1,350	2.9	30
Inulin	5,200	2.3	23

$$\text{"Clearance like kidney"} = \frac{\text{Kur. membrane (peritoneum)} + \text{Kur. residual}}{\text{body water}}$$

(Kur. membrane and Kur. residual in ml/week and body water in liters.)

Optimally it should be 2,500–3,000 ml/week/liter. The patients undergoing five daily CAPD exchanges,[3,4,8] if the Kur. residual were 0, have a "clearance like kidney" of 2,000 ml/week/liter. However, the average blood urea nitrogen (BUN) with five daily exchanges is 59 mg/dl,[8] which is adequate by current standards.[13,19] Theoretically with three daily CAPD exchanges the "clearance like kidney" goes down to 1,150 ml/week/liter but the BUN would be 90 mg/dl, which is quite acceptable.[13,19]

The mean serum creatinine and serum urea values in these six patients undergoing three CAPD exchanges during more than 8 months were 8.3 mg/dl and 136 mg/dl, respectively (residual GFR: $\bar{X} = 1.58$, S.D. $= \pm 1.86$, ml/minute).

These values are quite adequate according to the data of Sargent and Gotch[13,19] and Kjellstrand et al.[14] showing an adequate removal of small molecules.

Similarly the absence of pericarditis, deteriorating motor nerve conduction velocity or audiogram, and a steady hematocrit could be related with an adequate middle molecule clearance with three daily exchanges.

The degree of rehabilitation, increase in body weight, and feeling of well-being with three daily exchanges was similar to that other authors[1-6,8] obtained with CAPD utilizing more exchanges.

Consequently these preliminary data are encouraging and justify additional studies to confirm the utility of three daily CAPD exchanges.

References

1. Popovich, R. P., Moncrief, J. W., et al.: The definition of a novel portable-wearable equilibrium peritoneal dialysis technique. *Am Soc Artif Intern Organs* **5**: 64, 1976.
2. Locatelli, A., De Benedetti, L., et al.: Dialisis peritoneal continua ambulatoria. Fourth Congreso Latino Americano de Nefrologia, Perú, 1979, p. 45.
3. Moncrief, J. W., Nolph, K. D., et al.: Additional experience with continuous ambulatory peritoneal dialysis. *Trans Am Soc Intern Organs* **24**: 476–483, 1978.
4. Oreopulus, D. G., Robson, M., et al.: A simple and safe technique for continuous ambulatory peritoneal dialysis. *Trans Am Soc Artif Intern Organs* **24**: 484–487, 1978.

5. Oreopulus, D. G., Clayton, S., et al.: Experience with continuous ambulatory peritoneal dialysis. *Kidney Int* **16**: 234, 1979.
6. Popovich, R. P., Moncrief, J. W., et al.: Clinical development of the low dialysis clearance hypothesis via equilibrium peritoneal dialysis. *Proc Ann Contractor's Conf Artif Kidney* **10**: 123–126, 1977.
7. Popovich, R. P., Pyle, W. K., et al.: Preliminary verification of the low dialysis clearance hypothesis via a novel equilibrium peritoneal dialysis technique. *Trans Austr Conf Heat Mass Transfer* **2**: 217–220, 1977.
8. Popovich, R. P., Moncrief, J. W., et al.: Continuous ambulatory peritoneal dialysis. *Ann Intern Med* **88**: 449–459, 1978.
9. Cantarovich, F., Perez Loredo, J., et al.: Three daily exchanges on CAPD. Unpublished.
10. Tenckhoff, H.: Home peritoneal dialysis. In *Clinical aspects of Uremia and Dialysis,* Massrey Sellers, Ed. Charles C Thomas, Springfield, Ill., 1976.
11. Boun, S.: Discussion of manuscripts. *Trans Am Soc Artif Intern Organs* **24**: 488, 1978.
12. Ginn, H. E., Teschan, P. E., et al.: Neurobehavioral and clinical to hemodialysis. *Trans Am Soc Artif Intern Organs* **24**: 376–379, 1978.
13. Gotch, F. A., and Sargent, J. A.: Clinical results of intermittent dialysis therapy (ITD) guided by ongoing kinetic analysis of urea metabolism. *Trans Am Soc Artif Intern Organs* **22**: 175–188, 1976.
14. Kjellstrand, C. M., and Evans, R. L.: The unphysiology of dialysis. A major cause of dialysis side effects. *Kidney Int (Suppl)* **7**: 30–34, 1975.
15. Nolph, K. D., Twardowski, Z. J., et al.: Equilibration of peritoneal dialysis solutions during long-dwell exchanges. *J Lab Clin Med* **93**: 246–256, 1979.
16. Babb, A. L., Strand, M. J., et al.: Quantitative description of dialysis treatment. A dialysis index. *Kidney Int (Suppl)* **7**: 23–29, 1975.
17. Teschan, P. E., and Ginn, H. E.: Neurobehavioral responses to "middle molecule" in dialysis and transplantation. *Trans Am Soc Artif Intern Organs* **22**: 190–193, 1976.
18. Teschan, P. E.: Electroencephalographic and other neurophysiological abnormalities in uremia. *Kidney Int (Suppl)* **7**: 210–216, 1975.
19. Sargent, J. A., and Gotch, F. A.: The analysis of concentration dependence of uremic lesions in clinical studies. *Kidney Int (Suppl)* **7**: 35–44, 1975.

CHAPTER NINETEEN

The Initiation of a CAPD Program

DISA K. TAUNTON, R.N.

THE CONTINUOUS AMBULATORY PERITONEAL DIALYSIS (CAPD) home training program at Ochsner Foundation Hospital was incorporated into the existing home training program in April 1979. We felt CAPD would be a feasible alternative for some of our home dialysis learners by allowing more independence. A training program was organized to include policies, procedures, patient selection criteria, and a peritonitis protocol. The nursing staff was trained in all aspects of CAPD by a special workshop. Patients in existing hemodialysis and intermittent peritoneal dialysis programs were offered CAPD as an alternative mode of therapy. Others came to the program as referrals from nearby dialysis centers. Information on CAPD was given to all new patients during their initial interview.

The training program is extensive, and consistency in teaching is most important. Every effort is made to ensure consistency through a series of learning modules. The instructor's manual contains each module with a list of objectives, the teaching plan, and materials, including audiovisual aids, lecture content, demonstrations, or practice materials. Utilizing learning modules enables the course to be paced according to the learners' needs. Although the course is designed to cover 2 full weeks, learners have been able to complete it in as little as 1 week, whereas others have taken as much as 3 weeks. The modules include: 1) Sterile Technique; 2) Complications of CAPD; 3) Vital Signs; 4) Principles of Peritoneal Dialysis; 5) Medications; 6) Record Keeping; 7) Normal Kidney Function/Kidney Failure; and 8) Ordering Supplies/Supply Inventory.

The most important lesson for the learner to master is aseptic technique. therefore sterile technique is reinforced by presenting the information in numerous ways. Lectures on the basic theory are given and then applied to situations while teaching the exchange procedure. Filmstrips, flip charts, and discussions also prove to be valuable teaching aids. A practice apron was devised to enable the learner to simulate procedures without danger of contamination. Learners can be videotaped during practice sessions and

---

Ochsner Foundation Hospital, New Orleans, Louisiana

mistakes identified by the learner when played back. Posters decorating the walls of the training room also provide much information in that they use simple word and picture associations. Learning materials are kept short and relatively simple since lengthy or complex methods are difficult to retain. Frequent breaks must also be given and learners are encouraged to leave the room for their breaks.

Evaluation of learning is obtained through testing and return demonstrations. A comprehensive written pretest is given prior to the initiation of training. Following each learning module, short quizzes evaluate learning. In order to graduate, the learner must successfully complete a written comprehensive examination and return demonstrations of the exchange procedure, catheter care, and, if applicable, tubing change. Thereafter, learners are evaluated monthly. At these sessions, the learners have blood drawn, physician appointments, and demonstrate the tubing change procedure. If needed, a refresher course will be scheduled.

Eighteen learners have enrolled in the CAPD classes, with 16 of these completing the course. Two voluntarily withdrew from training and returned to in-center hemodialysis, stating that the responsibility of the meticulous, routine daily exchange procedure proved to be too much of a burden. Two others were removed from the program for noncompliance and repeated episodes of peritonitis.

In summary, the initiation of a CAPD training program requires:
1. A method to obtain patients.
2. A dedicated, enthusiastic nursing staff trained in peritoneal dialysis.
3. A set of policies, procedures, and manuals.
4. An organized, consistent teaching program, utilizing the principles of adult education.
5. A method of patient evaluation and follow-up.

CHAPTER TWENTY

The Quality of Life of the CAPD Patient

"P" A. J. SORRELS, R.N.

C. MULLINS-BLACKSON, R.N.

J. W. MONCRIEF, M.D.

R. P. POPOVICH, Ph.D.

DURING THE PAST 3 YEARS, there has been a great deal of discussion concerning the advantages of continuous ambulatory peritoneal dialysis (CAPD). A few of these advantages are: steady-state blood chemistries, minimum dietary restrictions, decrease in cost, and an enhanced sense of well-being, energy, and appetite. One subject that has not been addressed, however, is whether the patient's quality of life has improved or degenerated. At the Austin Diagnostic Clinic, Acorn Research Laboratory, a definite improvement in the quality of life has been manifested and expressed by a majority of the CAPD patients on several specific levels.

PHYSICAL CHANGES

After becoming established on a CAPD regimen, patients express surprise, and often shock, at the change in their general health. Some patients state, "I never thought I'd feel this good again." They note an improvement of sleeping habits; they fall asleep easily and usually are able to sleep through the night without the aid of medication. Most patients, who were previously on hemodialysis, report the loss of that "up and down" feeling experienced on intermittent dialysis.

With no dietary restrictions, patients feel very encouraged, since they are able to eat what they want. Appetites improve, and most patients note that food tastes better. Some patients who were accustomed to a salt-free diet have

---

The Austin Diagnostic Clinic, Acorn Research Laboratory, Austin, Texas

to be encouraged to add salt to their food and increase fluid intake; however, this usually disappears after the first 6 months of CAPD.

Changes in skin color and texture have been quite obvious in most patients transferred from hemodialysis. One patient who previously had calcinosis cutis on her face, arms, and back experienced complete sluffing of the skin in those areas with no subsequent recurrence of the condition. Most patients lose the chloasmalike grayish-yellow undertone that is present in many hemodialysis patients. Interestingly, one patient who had substantial amounts of hair loss from the armpits, scalp, and arms experienced regrowth of that hair; this is thought to be due to hormonal stimulation.

SEXUAL DIFFERENCES

Many male patients express an increase in libido after establishment on CAPD. However, a few sexually active males require testosterone for prolongation of erection.

Some female patients in the menarchal age range experienced menostasis while on hemodialysis. After 6 months on CAPD, two of these patients began to menstruate again. During menstruation, these patients often drain slightly bloody effluent; gram stains and cultures are negative with a white count of no more than 0–2. There have been no data obtained to ascertain if ovulation occurs in these patients.

Peritoneal catheters placed in a midline incision often cause both physical and emotional discomfort during sexual intercourse. Discussion with the surgeon has produced a lateral placement technique that removes the catheter from the common sexual activity area. Most patients have noted more ease of intercourse as well as less difficulty encountered by the sexual partner.

SOCIAL LIFE

Because there are minimal dietary restrictions, the CAPD patient may eat most types of food and is therefore able to go to restaurants with friends and family. The patient is also able to drink a limited amount of alcoholic beverages, which enhances a feeling of social freedom.

The concealment of the peritoneal catheter maintains self-image in many patients. During dwell times, when the empty bag is placed out of sight under the clothing, CAPD patients are indistinguishable from healthy people; in fact, many lay people are surprised to learn that dialysis is ongoing in these patients. Often, professionals visiting the Acorn Research Laboratory from other dialysis facilities comment that they cannot distinguish patients from staff members.

The ability to travel has been recognized by patients as a major plus for CAPD. Supplies are compact and can be stored in the trunk of an automobile or can be transported by air as "life support." The availability of CAPD back-up units throughout the country has also enhanced patient travel. There is no need for scheduling of back-up dialysis, but patients can make arrangements to replenish supplies or to be seen for complications on a transient basis.

FAMILIAL ACCEPTANCE

The Acorn staff encourages family involvement and education in the patient's dialysis therapy and disease. Most family members note the absence of chronic illness or invalidism in the CAPD patients. The patients are able to spend time in family activities and are able to be involved in family chores and responsibilities.

Most families express total acceptance of CAPD and state that patients are more "well" than expected or previously experienced with intermittent forms of dialysis. They view the home environment as healthier and relationships within the family as stronger and closer.

CONCLUSION

As seen at the Acorn Research Laboratory, quality of life may be the singularly most important factor in the future of CAPD patients. Patients have the opportunity to control their own lives and, for the most part, the treatment of their disease. They maintain a considerable amount of independence as well as the ability to pursue personal and professional goals that may have otherwise been futile.

References

1. Prowant, B. F., and Fruto, L.V.: Continuous ambulatory peritoneal dialysis. *Nephrol Nurse* 8–14, 1980.
2. Sorrels, A. J.: Continuous ambulatory peritoneal dialysis. *Am J Nurs* **79**: 1400–1401, 1979.
3. Moncrief, J. W., and Popovich, R. P.: Peritoneal dialysis for a greater number of patients. *Controv Nephrol* **1**: 35–45, 1979.
4. Moncrief, J. W., and Popovich, R. P.: Continuous ambulatory peritoneal dialysis: Today's art of peritoneal dialysis. *Contrib Nephrol* **17**: 139–145, 1979.
5. Popovich, R. P., Moncrief, J. W., Nolph, K. D., Ghods, A. J., Twardowski, Z. J., and Pyle, W. K.: Continuous ambulatory peritoneal dialysis *Ann Intern Med* **88**(4): 449, 1978.
6. Nolph, K. D., Popovich, R. P., and Moncrief, J. W.: Theoretical and practical implications of continuous peritoneal dialysis *Nephron* **21**: 117–122, 1978.

CHAPTER TWENTY-ONE

Peritoneal Catheter Complications in CAPD Patients

CHRISTINE LACKE, P.A.(C)

S. MARIE KOZAK, R.N.

HARRY O. SENEKJIAN, M.D.

THOMAS F. KNIGHT, M.D.

EDWARD J. WEINMAN, M.D.

THE DEVELOPMENT OF THE CHRONIC in-dwelling peritoneal catheter by Palmer, modification by Tenckhoff and Schecter,[1] and the more recent introduction of the 2-liter plastic bag[2] (Baxter-Dianeal) have resulted in an increase in the number of patients with end-stage renal disease (ESRD) who are maintained on continuous ambulatory peritoneal dialysis (CAPD).

With increasing experience with CAPD, it has become apparent that a number of complications occur in such patients. Of these complications, peritonitis remains the single most common problem encountered, particularly in the initial stages of a CAPD program. However, a number of other catheter-related problems are also noted to occur in CAPD patients. Table 1 illustrates the major complications of the permanent peritoneal catheter.

CATHETER MALFUNCTION

Catheter malfunction may be the consequence of malposition, encasement, or obstruction. With the exception of encasement, catheter malfunction usually occurs shortly after placement and is a rare occurrence in catheters that have been functional for a 10–14-day period. The most common cause of malfunction is malposition secondary to migration of the catheter. This in turn is the result of a failure to direct the catheter in a caudal direction, the failure to create a subcutaneous arch for the catheter, or entanglement of the catheter

Medical and Nursing Services, Veterans Administration Medical Center and the Department of Medicine, Baylor College of Medicine, Houston, Texas

TABLE 1.
Permanent Peritoneal Catheter Complications

1. Catheter malfunction
   Malposition
   Obstruction
   Encasement
   Functional
2. Exit site infection
3. Sinus tract infection
4. Catheter cuff erosion
5. Leakage

tip with omental fat. Diagnostic tests include a flat plate of the abdomen. If nonopaque catheters are used, it is sometimes necessary to instill x-ray contrast material for adequate visualization.

The clinical manifestations of malposition include the inability to drain the peritoneal cavity, with little or no difficulty during inflow, and the development of abdominal pain when suction is applied to the catheter during irrigation. Occasionally, this pain may be referred to the shoulder, if the catheter lies near the diaphragm. Treatment of catheter malposition usually requires replacement of the catheter, although repositioning of the catheter is occasionally successful.

Another frequent cause of catheter malfunction is obstruction of the catheter with blood or fibrin clots or incarceration with tissue. Blood and fibrin clots appear to occur shortly after catheter placement, and fibrin clots also occur during episodes of peritonitis, occasionally after the "off day" in patients dialyzing 6 days per week. The diagnosis is suggested by the presence of a bloody effluent or effluent containing large amounts of fibrin strands. Treatment by forceful irrigation of the catheter with a heparin-containing solution is usually successful. The addition of heparin to the dialysis solution during episodes of peritonitis and immediately after placement of the catheter is recommended as prophylaxis against this complication. Tissue incarceration occurs when omental tissue is drawn into the catheter tip during outflow. It is usually diagnosed by failure of the obstruction to be relieved by forceful irrigation. Repositioning or replacement of the catheter is required.

Encasement is the result of the formation of a fibrous sheath around the catheter and may be a consequence of recurrent or occasional asymptomatic peritonitis. The initial finding is frequently the inability to drain the abdomen of dialysate. Abdominal x-ray films reveal that, although the catheter is in the correct position, there is poor diffusion of x-ray contrast media into the peritoneal space. The contrast media can be seen to track or sheath along the catheter tract. Catheter replacement at another abdominal site is required to correct this complication.

Another important and frequent form of catheter malfunction is a functional and reversible problem, usually occurring in patients with constipation. Work-ups for other types of catheter malfunction are negative. Treatment includes enemas, laxatives, and stool softeners. Regular exercise and dietary manipulation to increase stool bulk should be included as a regular part of the

CAPD protocol. If the complication is recognized early, extensive diagnostic work-up can be avoided.

EXIT-SITE INFECTION

An exit-site infection is a potentially serious complication and one that can be difficult to manage. These infections may also lead to or occur in association with subcutaneous tunnel infections. Exit-site infections occur as a consequence of inadequate catheter care and are frequently seen in patients with poor personal hygiene. It may also be the result of traction on the catheter. The clinical manifestations include erythema, swelling, and tenderness at the exit site. Purulent drainage may also occur. Culture and sensitivity of the drainage is recommended. To date, the most common organisms have been *Staphylococcus aureus* or *epidermidis,* but infection with *Pseudomonas* and *Serratia* have also been encountered. Treatment includes an increase in daily local catheter care with a Betadine solution and oral antibiotics for 4 weeks. If the infection is not resolved in 4 weeks, replacement of the catheter is recommended. In addition, all patients are advised periodically to change the position of the external portion of the peritoneal catheter so as to prevent local irritation and reduce traction.

SINUS TRACT INFECTION

Sinus tract infections are a serious catheter-related problem and may develop as a secondary consequence of an exit-site infection or infection of the catheter cuff. The patient may be asymptomatic, with the only clinical manifestation being a persistently cloudy dialysis effluent. Occasionally, drainage around the exit site is noted. Often the first clue to a sinus tract infection is the failure of appropriate antibiotics to clear the dialysate, and the presence of persistently positive bacterial cultures. Overt and recurrent episodes of peritonitis may ensue if a sinus tract infection is not adequately treated. In general, it is difficult, if not impossible, to treat sinus tract infections with antibiotics alone. It is recommended that the catheter be removed and either a new catheter placed at a site remote from the sinus tract or placement of the new catheter delayed until the sinus tract heals. In the latter circumstance, the patient is maintained on hemodialysis during the interim period.

CATHETER CUFF EROSION

Catheter cuff erosion occurs as a consequence of a failure to create a sufficiently long subcutaneous tunnel during initial catheter placement. It usually becomes clinically evident within the first few weeks after catheter placement. The probable cause is pressure necrosis at the catheter exit site. Infection may or may not be noted in association with cuff erosion, but when it does occur, it is usually a late complication. Centers using double-cuff catheters have reported that it is possible to trim off the superficial Dacron cuff when a cuff erosion occurs, and to continue to use the catheter. However, when a cuff erosion occurs in a patient with a single-cuff catheter, the catheter must be replaced.

LEAKAGE

Leakage of dialysis fluid around the catheter usually occurs within the first few days after placement of the catheter and is due to failure of tissue to grow into the cuff. Occasionally, the dialysis fluid may dissect into tissue planes and result in scrotal or labial edema. The incidence of leakage appears to be increased in patients in whom initially large volumes of dialysate are used, in patients undertaking strenuous exercise before tissue growth into the cuff takes place, and in patients with poor abdominal musculature. Leakage is usually easily treated by stopping the dialysis for 3–4 days, placing the patient at bed rest, and using smaller fluid volumes when dialysis is resumed. Dressings should be changed frequently and the exit site kept as dry as possible to prevent the development of an exit-site infection.

SUMMARY

The clinical experience in a number of centers has demonstrated CAPD to be an effective alternative treatment modality for individuals with end-stage renal disease.[2-4] The development of new equipment and techniques that facilitate the exchange procedure has contributed to the decreasing incidence of both peritonitis and catheter-related complications. In our early experience, CAPD patients have required rehospitalization with peritonitis or catheter-related problems on an average of one every 4–6 months.[4,5] Of these rehospitalizations, approximatly 50% are due to the catheter-related problems with or without co-existent peritonitis. It seems likely that placement of the catheters by a single or only a few individuals, the assignment of personnel directly to the CAPD program, and a mechanism for easy access by the patient to the medical facility can reduce the high incidence of catheter-related complications. This becomes critically important in maintaining the patient's enthusiasm for and adherence to the CAPD regimen.

References

1. Tenckhoff, H., and Schecter, H.: A bacteriologically safe peritoneal access device. *Trans Am Soc Artif Internal Organs* **14:** 181, 1968.
2. Oreopoulos, D. G., Robson, M., Faller, B., *et al.:* Continuous ambulatory peritoneal dialysis: A new era in the treatment of chronic renal failure. *Clin Nephrol* **2:** 125, 1979.
3. Popovich, R. P., Moncrief, J. W., Knolph, K. D., *et al.:* Continuous ambulatory peritoneal dialysis. *Ann Intern Med* **88:** 449, 1978.
4. Lacke, C., Senekjian, H. O., Knight, T. F., Hatlelid, R., Frazier, M., Baker, P., and Weinman, E. J.: Twelve months' experience with continuous ambulatory and intermittent peritoneal dialysis. *Arch Intern Med* **141:** 187–190, 1981.
5. Weinman, E. J., Lacke, C., Kozak, S. M., Frazier, M., Senekjian, H. O., and Knight, T. F.: Continuous ambulatory peritoneal dialysis: Initial experience as a home-training and an in-hospital procedure. *Dial Transplant* **9:** 749–750, 1980.

CHAPTER TWENTY-TWO

Hypertriglyceridemia, Diabetes Mellitus, and Insulin Administration in Patients Undergoing Continuous Ambulatory Peritoneal Dialysis

J. W. MONCRIEF, M.D.

W. K. PYLE, Ph.D.

P. SIMON, R.N.

R. P. POPOVICH, Ph.D.

DERANGEMENT OF LIPID METABOLISM is a common accompaniment of end-stage renal disease.[1-3] Hypertriglyceridemia, hypercholesterolemia, and abnormal concentrations of lipoprotein subfractions have been described. Carbohydrate and insulin metabolism are also abnormal.[4] Similar abnormalities in carbohydrate, insulin, and lipid metabolism have been demonstrated in patients undergoing chronic dialytic therapy.[5]

Accelerated atherosclerosis is a major complication and a leading cause of death in patients with abnormal insulin-glucose metabolism (diabetes mellitus) and in patients undergoing chronic dialytic therapy.[6] The early reports of hypertriglyceridemia in patients undergoing continuous ambulatory peritoneal dialysis (CAPD) have been confirmed.[7] Severe hypertriglyceridemia has become a major concern in some of these patients.

Since October of 1978, when dialysate in collapsible plastic containers became available in the United States, 36 patients have been trained to perform CAPD at the Austin Diagnostic Clinic, Acorn Research Laboratory. After training, seven patients were transferred to other CAPD units. Five patients were subsequently transferred to intermittent hemodialysis. Two patients died from cardiac failure. Twenty-two patients are currently being

---

Acorn Research Laboratory, Austin, Texas

144   CAPD Update

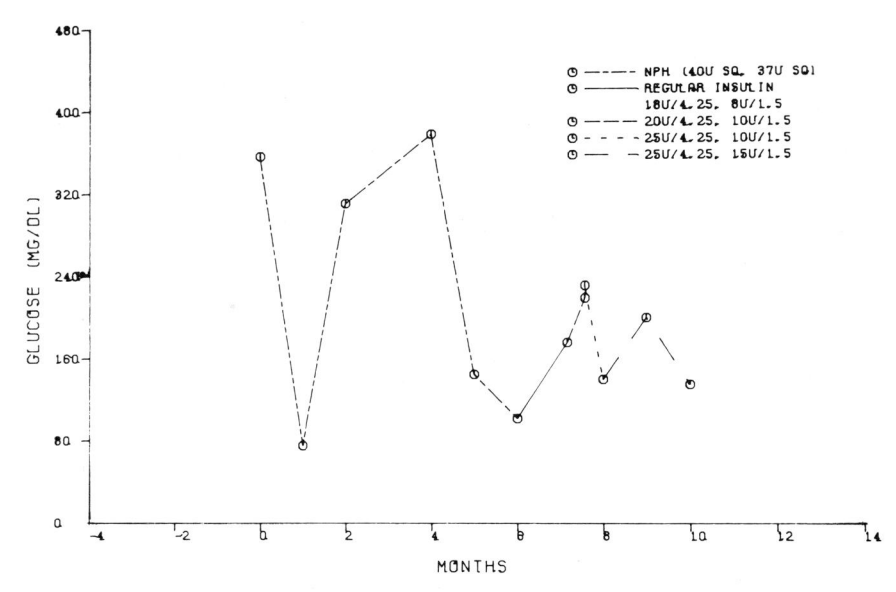

Figure 1. Random fasting glucose: patient 1.

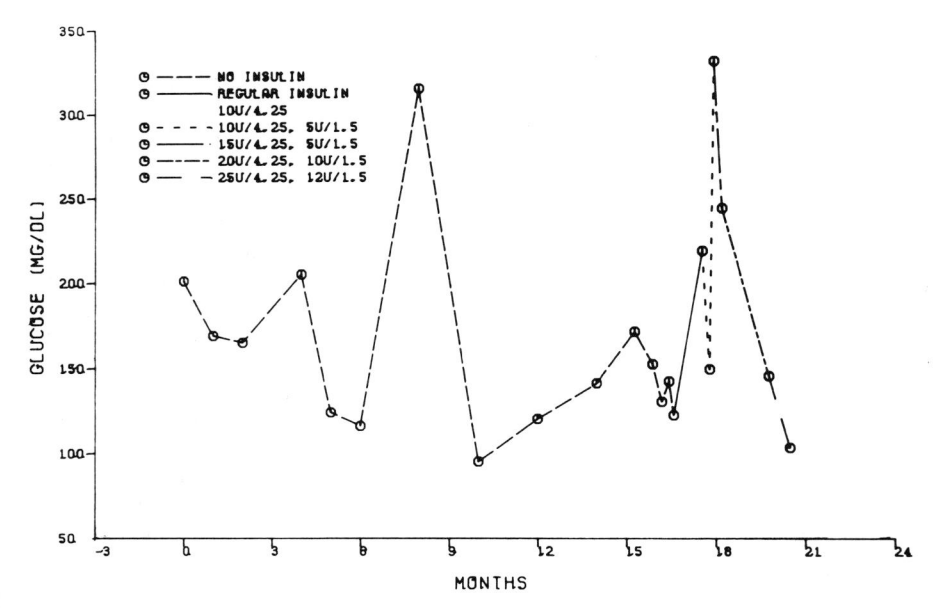

Figure 2. Random fasting glucose: patient 2.

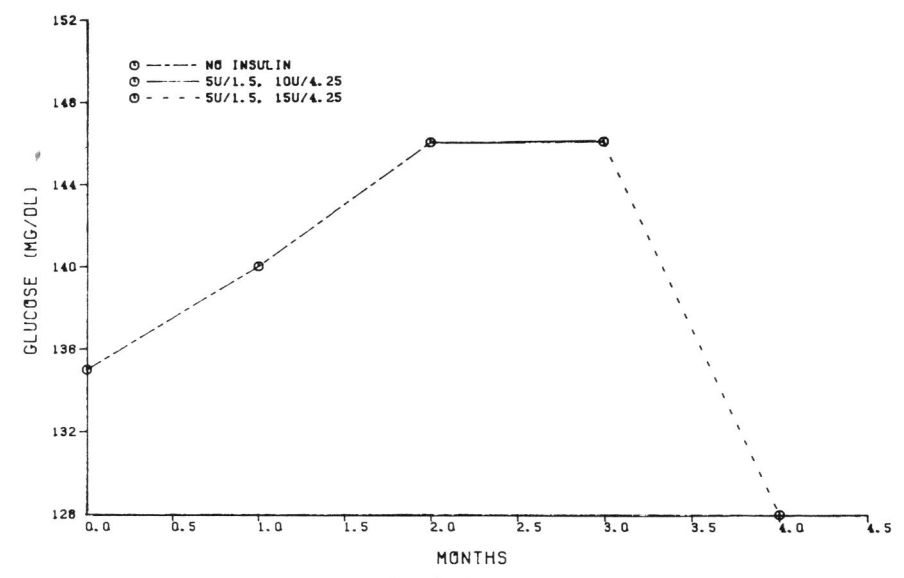

Figure 3. Random fasting glucose: patient 3.

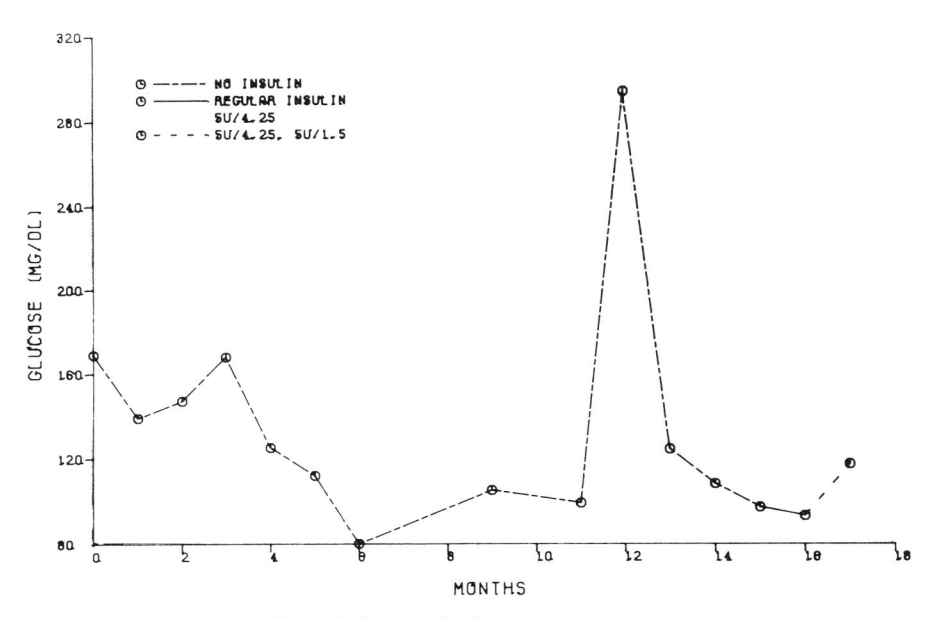

Figure 4. Random fasting glucose: patient 4.

146   CAPD Update

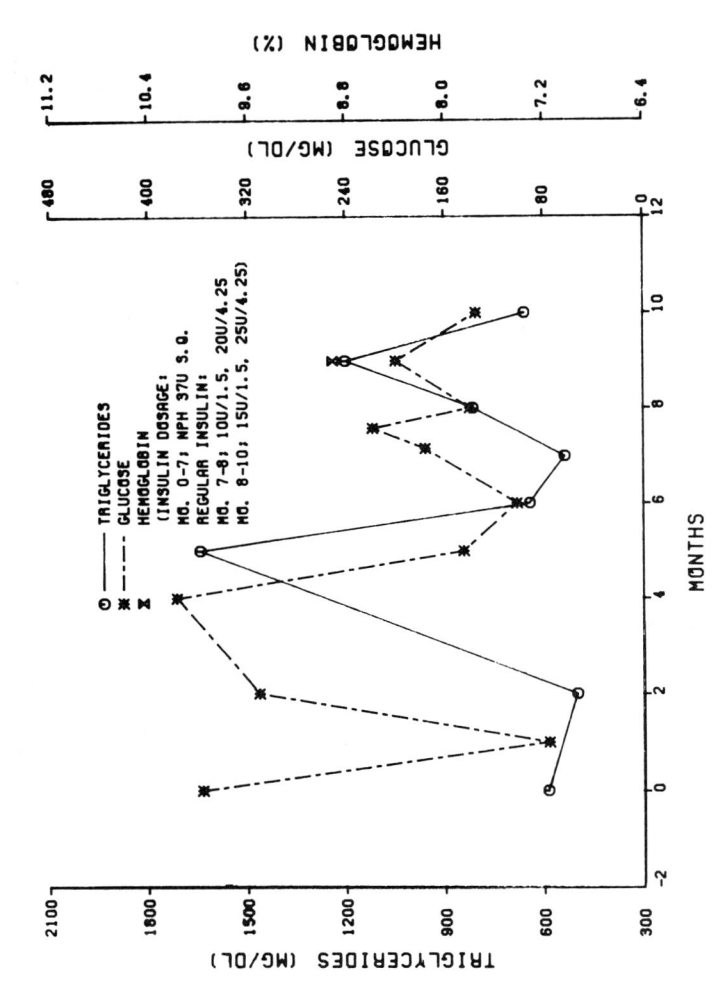

Figure 5. Triglycerides, glucose, and hemoglobin beta-1: patient 1. (Normal: female, over 60 years, T.G. < 146 mg/dl, Hb < 8.5.)

Patients Undergoing Continuous Ambulatory Peritoneal Dialysis 147

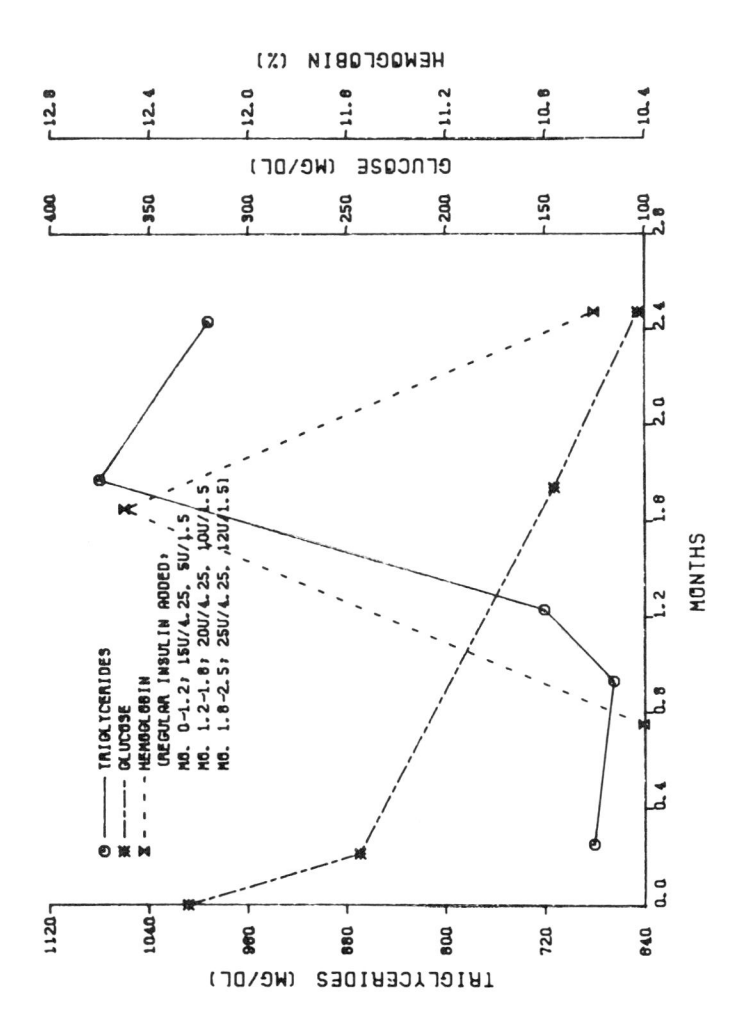

Figure 6. Triglycerides, glucose, and hemoglobin beta-1: patient 2. (Normal: male, 50–59 years, T.G. < 197 mg/dl, Hb < 8.5%.)

followed at the Austin Diagnostic Clinic who have been undergoing CAPD for 2–22 months, a mean of 10 months. In this population, the mean serum triglyceride level is 210 ± 84 mg%, above normal when compared with the general population but in the same range as patients undergoing intermittent hemodialysis.[5] Four of these patients have developed modest to severe hypertriglyceridemia (greater than 300 mg%), and two of these patients have developed extremely high levels of serum triglycerides (greater than 1,500 mg%). Three of the four patients with triglyceride levels greater than 300 mg% had diabetes mellitus. Only one patient required subcutaneous insulin for blood sugar control (patient 1). Blood sugar was monitored by random fasting (Fig. 1–4) and by glycosylated hemoglobin levels (Fig. 5–8 and Table 1) and considered to be well controlled. Glucose tolerance curves were performed in the patients with triglyceride levels greater than 300 mg% who did not have overt diabetes mellitus and are depicted in Figures 9 and 10. All patients with serum triglycerides greater than 200 mg% were instructed in a prescribed exercise program[8] after undergoing cardiorespiratory evaluation with pulmonary function studies, bicycle ergometry, and electrocardiographic evaluation. Patients with triglyceride levels greater than 300 mg% were placed on a restricted carbohydrate diet and efforts were made to reduce the number of hypertonic 4.25% glucose exchanges. No patient was administered oral lipolytic medication, and androgens were administered in only one patient (patient 4). Despite this program, progressive evaluation of serum triglycerides occurred, and in two patients the levels exceeded 1,500 mg%.

Continuous insulin infusion has been demonstrated to produce extremely "tight" glucose control in diabetic patients, and a reduction in the serum triglyceride level to normal has been demonstrated in some of these patients.[9–11] Excellent control of blood sugar in patients undergoing CAPD by the administration of regular insulin into the peritoneal cavity with the dialysate solution was reported by Flynn and Nanson.[12] These authors did not find the erratic insulin absorption previously suggested by others.[13,14]

Because of the severe hypertriglyceridemia, insulin was added to the dialysis solution and infused into the patient in an attempt to achieve better glucose control.

CASE REPORTS

Patient 1

Patient 1 had insulin requiring diabetes mellitus and took 37 units of NPH insulin subcutaneously each morning. CAPD was initiated in May of 1979. In

TABLE 1.
Glycosylated Hemoglobin (Hb $\beta - 1$) Normal <8.5%

February	4.3	8.8	7.4	6.9	10.7[a]	10.7[a]	10.4[a]		8.9[a]			
March			7.4		8.3[a]	9.7[a]	12.5[a]	7.1	7.6		8.8	6.9	7.3
April	4.1	7.8			6.7[a]	9.7[a]	10.6[a]	8.0		7.0	9.5

[a] Patients with hypertriglyceridemia.

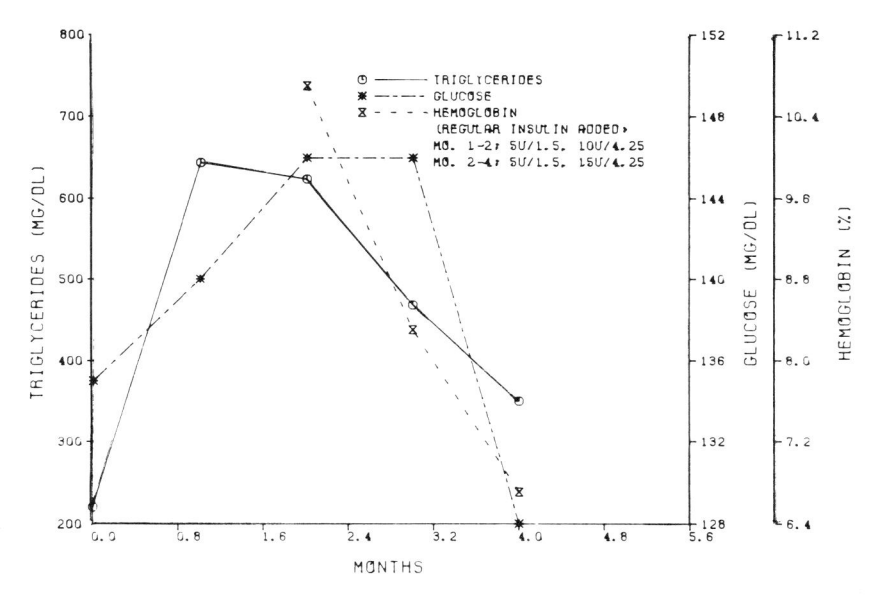

Figure 7. Triglycerides, glucose, and hemoglobin beta-1: patient 3.

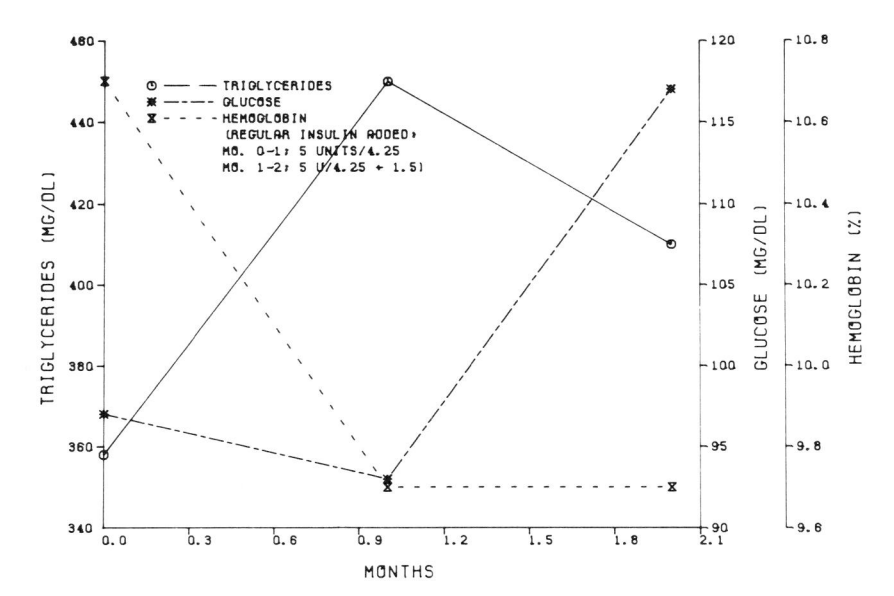

Figure 8. Triglycerides, glucose, and hemoglobin beta-1: patient 4. (Normal: male, 40–49 years, T.G. < 193 mg/dl, Hb < 8.5%.)

150   CAPD Update

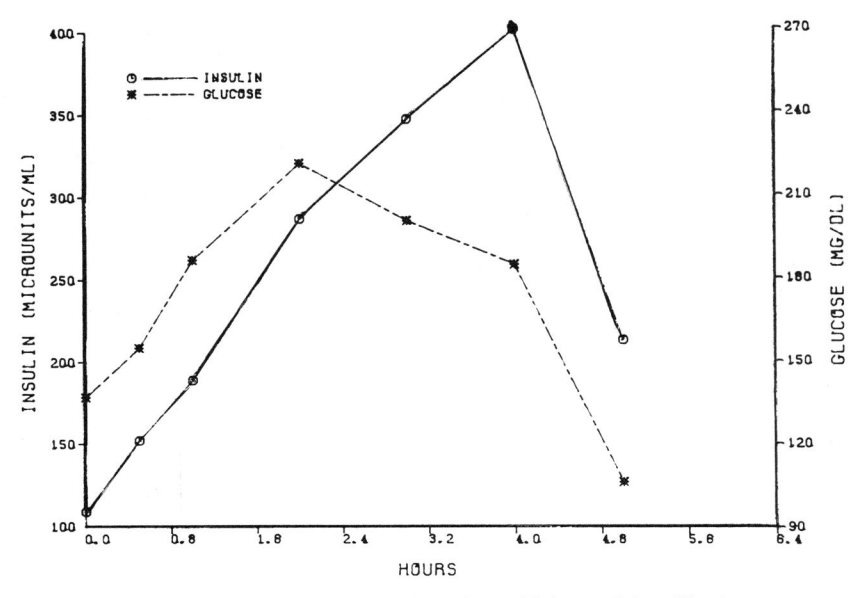

Figure 9. Glucose tolerance test in patient with hypertriglyceridemia.

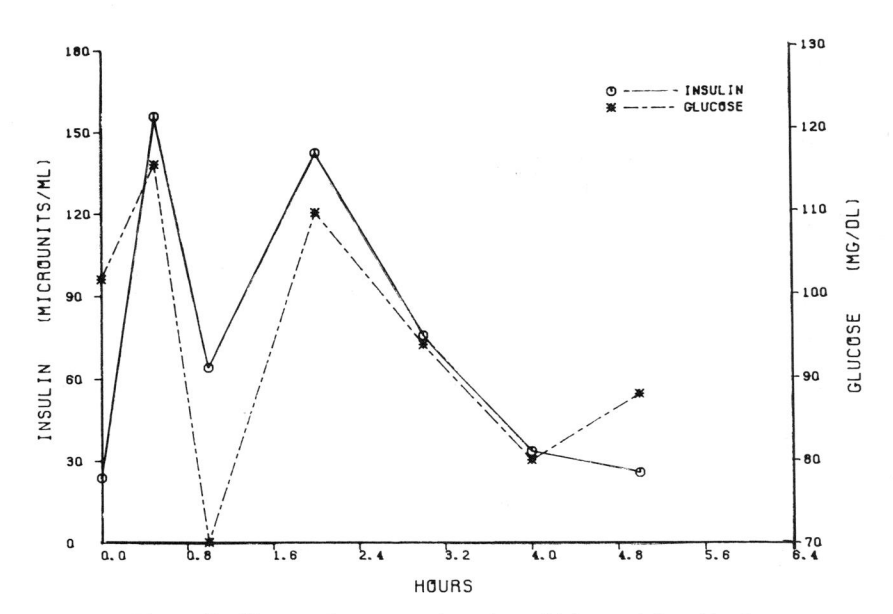

Figure 10. Glucose tolerance test in patient with hypertriglyceridemia.

July of 1979 the patient had a serum triglyceride level of 497 mg%. During the next 3 months, the serum triglyceride level rose to 1,643 mg% in spite of acceptable blood sugar control (Fig. 11). In October of 1979 insulin was added to the dialysate solution prior to infusion. Subcutaneous insulin was discontinued. Eighteen units of regular insulin was added to each 4.25% glucose exchange, and 8 units of regular insulin to each 1.25% glucose exchange. Within 1 month, the serum triglyceride level had fallen to 640 mg% and by December 1979 the triglyceride level had fallen to 534 mg%. Insulin levels were slightly increased in December of 1979. Twenty units was added in each 4.25% glucose exchange and 10 units to each 1.25% glucose exchange. During the following 3 months, the serum triglyceride level again rose to a high of 1200 mg% by February 1980, and the insulin in the solution was increased to 25 units in each 4.25% glucose exchange and 15 units in each 1.25% glucose exchange. In the following month the serum triglyceride level fell again to 654 mg%.

Patient 2

Patient 2 began on CAPD in August of 1978, and although he had random blood sugars slightly above normal during the following year, he did well and required no insulin for blood sugar control. His random blood sugars improved slightly in the following 6 months, August 1979 through December

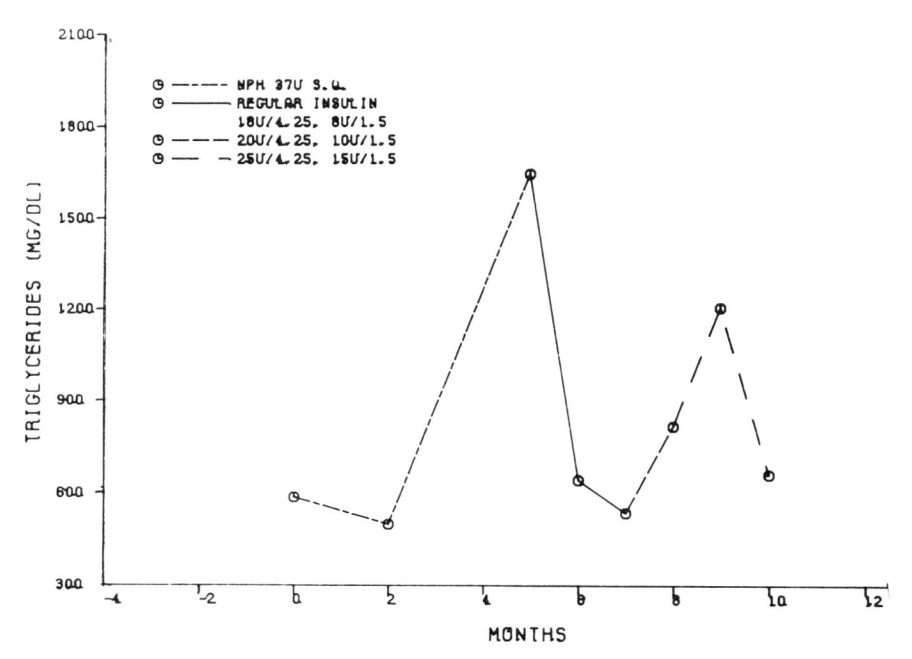

Figure 11. Effect of insulin in dialysate on triglyceride levels: patient 1. (Normal: female, over 60 years, <146 mg/dl.)

1979 (Fig. 2). During this time, he gained 21 kg in body weight. In December of 1978, his serum triglyceride level was 377 mg% (Fig. 12) and, with slight fluctuation, it remained in this range until June of 1979. Between June of 1979 and November of 1979, his serum triglyceride levels rose precipitously from 445 mg% to 1,931 mg%. During this same period, his random fasting blood sugar ranged from 95 to 171. In November 1979, his random blood sugar was 152 mg% and small doses of insulin were begun in his dialysate solution in an attempt to control the serum triglyceride level. Five units of regular insulin was added to each exchange. The patient at that time was using two exchanges of 4.25% dextrose solution and two 1.25% dextrose solutions. A rapid fall in the serum triglyceride level occurred, and by December 24, 1979, the serum triglyceride level had fallen to 1,152. In January 1980 the triglyceride level had fallen to 952, and at that time the insulin in the dialysate solutions was increased to 10 units of regular insulin in each 4.25% dextrose solution and 5 units in each 1.5% dextrose solution. A continued gradual fall occurred during the following month reaching 804 mg% by the end of January. At that time, the insulin was again increased to 15 units of regular insulin for each 4.25% dextrose solution and 5 units for each 1.5% dextrose solution. By early February 1980, the patient's serum triglyceride had fallen to 680 mg%. During the period of the addition of larger doses of insulin to the dialysis solution, there appears to have been a deterioration of the control of blood sugars as evaluated by random blood sugars, and a secondary rise in the serum triglyceride occurred. Increased

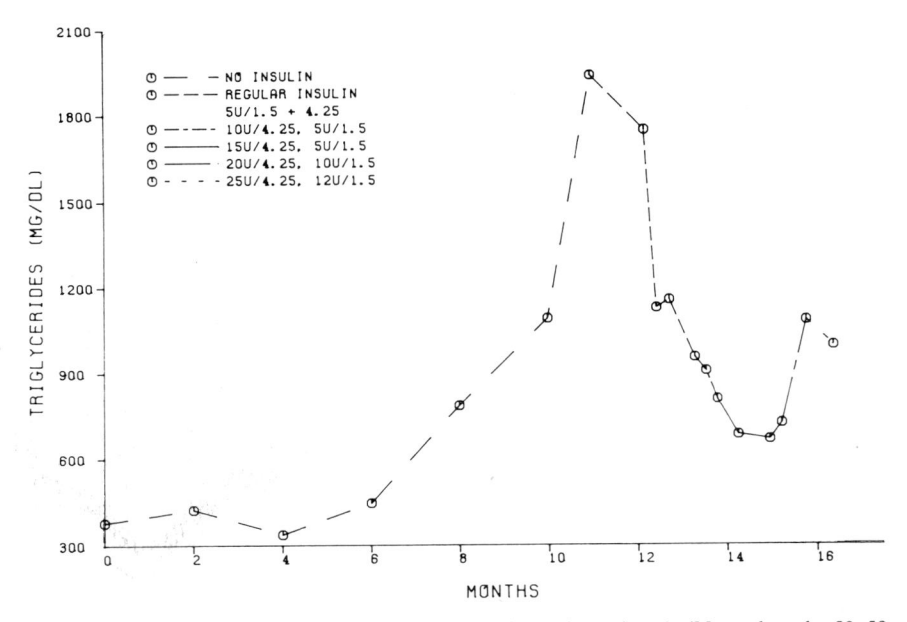

Figure 12. Effect of insulin in dialysate on triglyceride levels: patient 2. (Normal: male, 50–59 years, <197 mg/dl.)

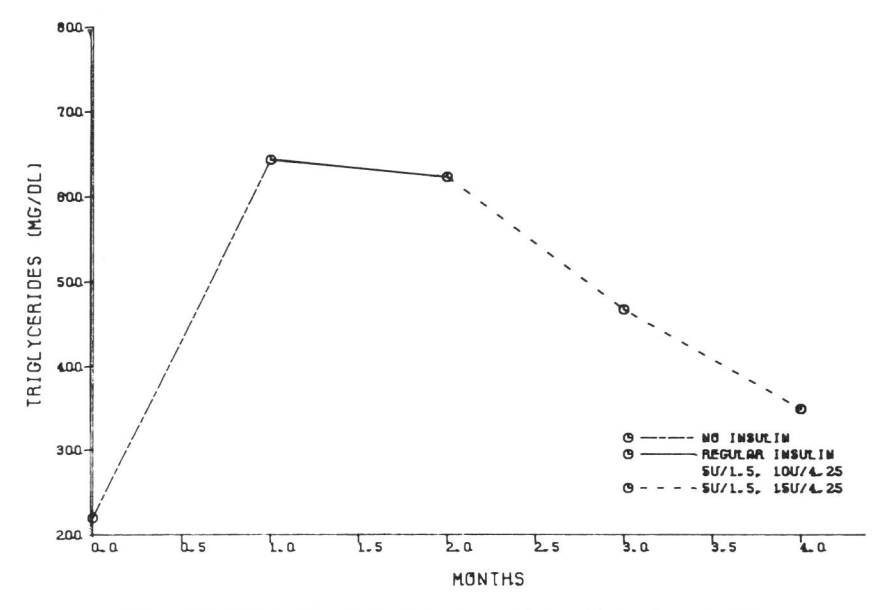

Figure 13. Effect of insulin in dialysate on triglyceride levels: patient 3.

insulin in the dialysate caused a control of the blood sugar and a fall in the triglyceride level to 565 mg% by March of 1980.

Patient 3

Patient 3 was not known to have diabetes and had normal random blood sugars. With initiation of CAPD in December of 1979, the serum triglyceride level rose rapidly from a value of 220 mg% and by January 1980 reached 640 mg% (Fig. 13). A 5-hour glucose tolerance curve (Fig. 9) demonstrated only a slight abnormality with a peak blood sugar of 222 mg% 2 hours after glucose loading and a gradual fall to baseline levels of 106 at the end of 5 hours. There was, however, a delay in insulin release and absence of an early insulin peak following glucose loading. A late peak occurred at 4 hours after glucose loading followed by a rapid fall in serum insulin levels at 5 hours. Even at that time, however, serum insulin levels were twice baseline levels. In January of 1980, insulin was added to the dialysis solution (Fig. 13), a dose of 5 units for each 1.25% exchange and 10 units for each 4.25% glucose exchange (subsequently increased to 15 units/4.25% exchange), and a fall in serum triglyceride levels had occurred. The last serum triglyceride level measured in April of 1980 was 350 mg%.

Patient 4

Patient 4 had CAPD initiated in November of 1978. A gradual rise in the serum triglyceride level occurred during the next 10 months from a level of

154   CAPD Update

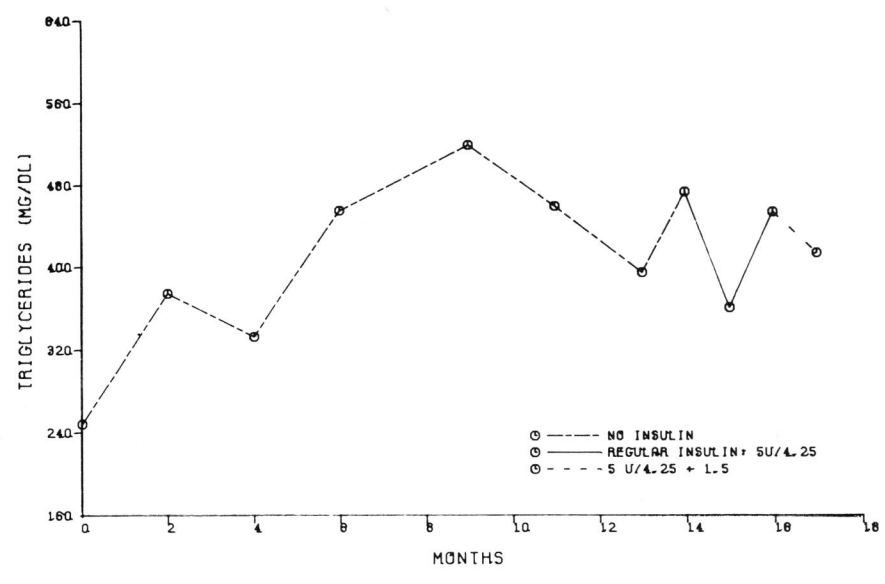

Figure 14. Effect of insulin in dialysate on triglyceride levels: patient 4. (Normal: males 40–49 years, <193 mg/dl.)

248 mg% in November 1978 to a peak of 517 mg% in August of 1979 (Fig. 14). During this time, testosterone enanthate 200 mg% each 2 weeks was given for hemopostic and androgen effect. Glucose tolerance curve was performed (Fig. 10), and this was completely normal with a fasting blood sugar of 102 mg%, a peak at ½ hour of 116 mg% returning to baseline levels of 88 mg% at 5 hours. A rapid rise in serum insulin levels occurred with glucose loading within ½ hour. A rapid fall occurred in serum insulin level as a decreased blood sugar occurred, and a second serum insulin peak occurred at 2 hours with a secondary slight rise in the blood sugar level. The serum insulin level had fallen to normal baseline levels at 5 hours. Because of the hypertriglyceridemia (Fig. 14), insulin was added to the dialysate solution in a dose of 5 units of regular insulin for each exchange. No significant fall in the triglyceride level has been demonstrated at this time.

INSULIN AND ULTRAFILTRATION

With the addition of insulin to the dialysis solution, each patient noticed and reported an increase in the drain volume. This occurred with both the 4.25% glucose solution and the 1.5% glucose solution. Two patients who had previously had stable blood pressure and stable weight developed intervascular volume depletion, weight loss, and orthostatic hypotension. Both patients reduced the number of 4.25% glucose exchanges.

To determine the ultrafiltration effect of the addition of insulin to the dialysis solution, water transport studies were performed on two patients, *the protocol for which is in the appendix*. These were performed with 1.5% dextrose solutions. Without insulin, the ultrafiltration volume in patient 4 was 242 ml ± 102 ml. Addition of insulin caused an ultrafiltration volume of 432 ml. This volume is greater than the 95% probability maximum of 394 ml in this patient. The reabsorption rate was −0.82 ml/minute and was not significantly different from controlled values. In this patient, no change in the mass area transfer coefficients for urea creatinine, uric acid, and glucose was demonstrated by the addition of insulin. Patient 2 had severe hypertriglyceridemia (1,100 mg%), and no change in ultrafiltration volume could be demonstrated with the addition of insulin.

LIPOPROTEIN SUBFRACTIONS

Patients undergoing CAPD had been reported to have decreased levels of high-density lipoprotein (HLD) cholesterol concentrations.[7] This was present in our patients. Two of our patients with extremely high triglyceride levels demonstrated low normal to below normal levels, 120 ± 6. These levels did tend to change opposite to the triglyceride levels with the addition of insulin to the dialysate solution. After initiation of CAPD, a gradual rise in the level of the very low-density lipoprotein (VLDL) cholesterol concentrations was observed, and this lipoprotein fraction declined approximately parallel to the

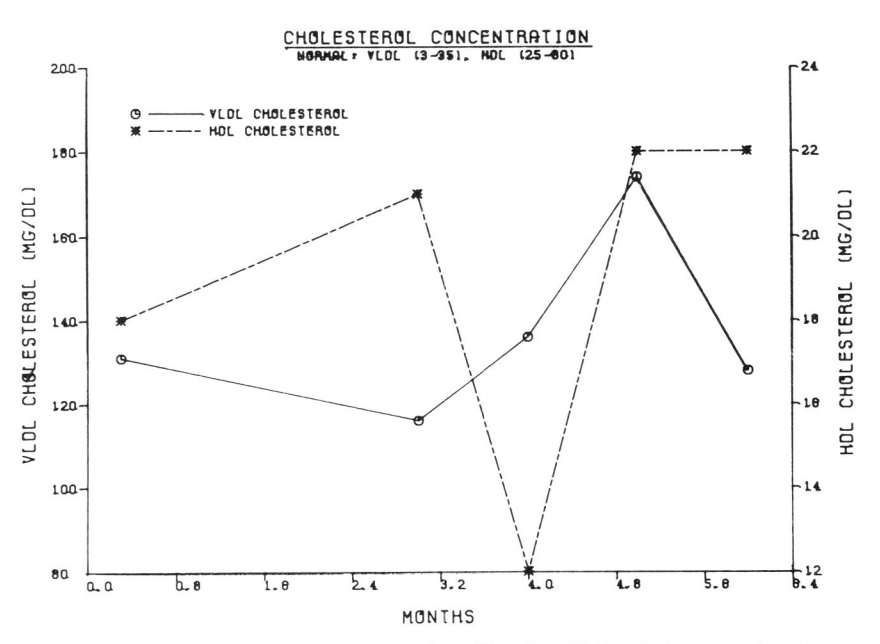

Figure 15. Lipoprotein subfractions. Effect of insulin added to dialysate: patient 1.

156 CAPD Update

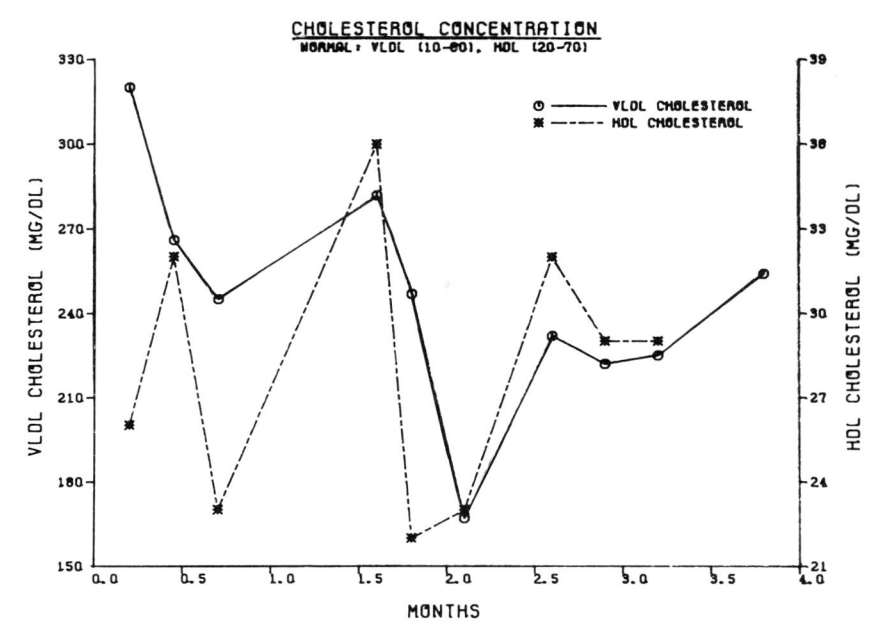

Figure 16. Lipoprotein subfractions. Effect of insulin added to dialysate: patient 2.

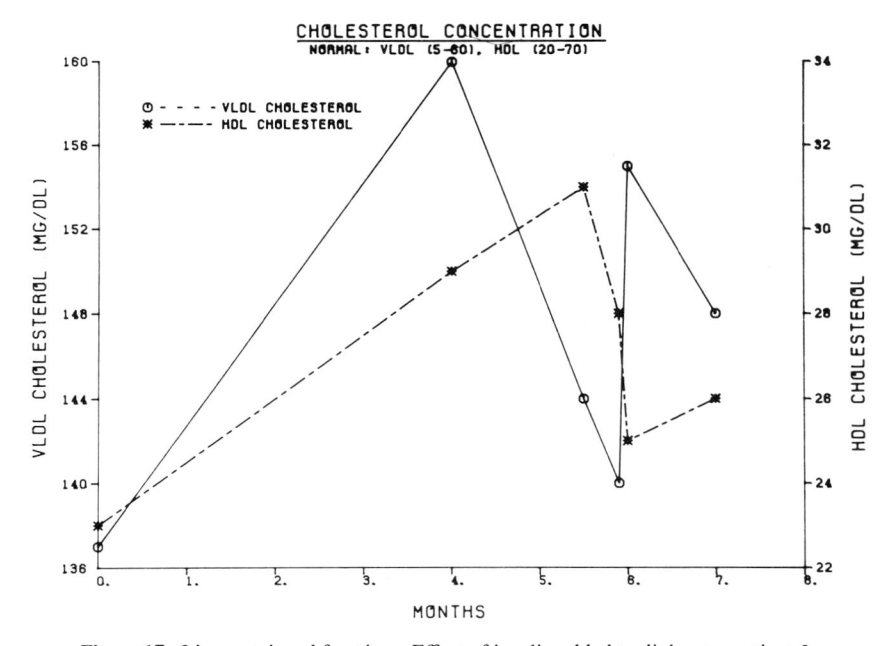

Figure 17. Lipoprotein subfractions. Effect of insulin added to dialysate: patient 3.

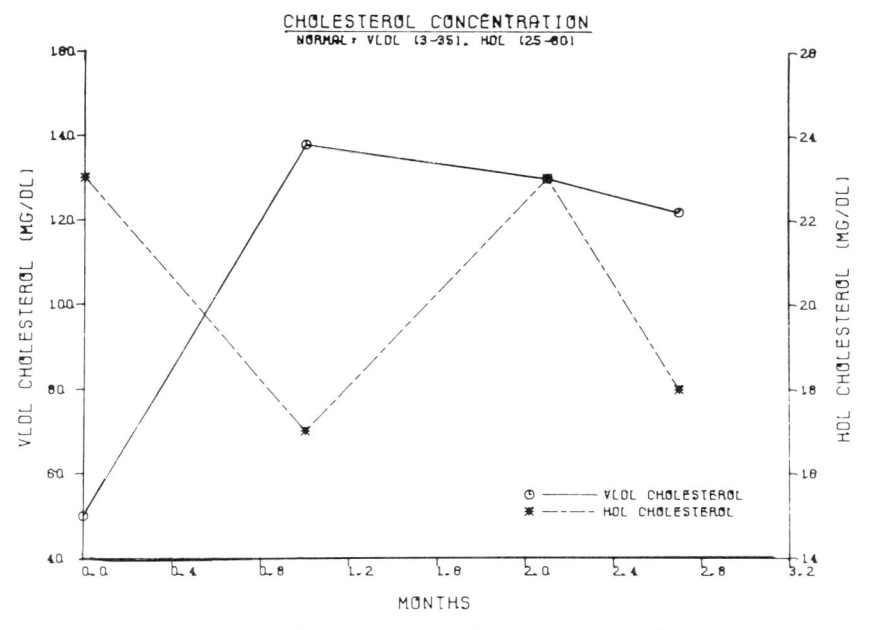

Figure 18. Lipoprotein subfractions. Effect of insulin added to dialysate: patient 4.

fall in serum triglyceride levels when insulin was added to the dialysis solution (Figs. 15–18).

A gradual rise occurred in the total serum cholesterol level with a mean serum cholesterol of 340 mg% in these patients. This is similar to levels found in patients undergoing other forms of dialysis.[15,16] These levels were unaffected by the addition of insulin to the dialysis solution (Figs. 19–22).

Discussion

Twenty percent of the patients followed in our program for longer than 2 months experienced a rise in the serum triglyceride level to above 300 mg%. Nine percent of the patients (2 of 22) developed hypertriglyceridemia with levels above 1,500 mg%. These extremely high triglyceride levels have been reported by other investigators and are considered an important complication and a potentially limiting factor in the treatment of patients with CAPD.[17] Hyperglycemia in patients with juvenile onset diabetes has been observed to increase the fasting levels of cholesterol triglyceride and VLDL subfractions[18,19] and to lower the HDL subfractions. These changes have been related to accelerated atherosclerosis in this patient population.[20,21]

Long-term follow-up in patients undergoing CAPD is unavailable at this time, but there is concern that these levels of severe hypertriglyceridemia may manifest themselves as accelerated atherosclerosis. Control of hyperglycemia in patients undergoing diabetic therapy is difficult. Continuous infu-

158   CAPD Update

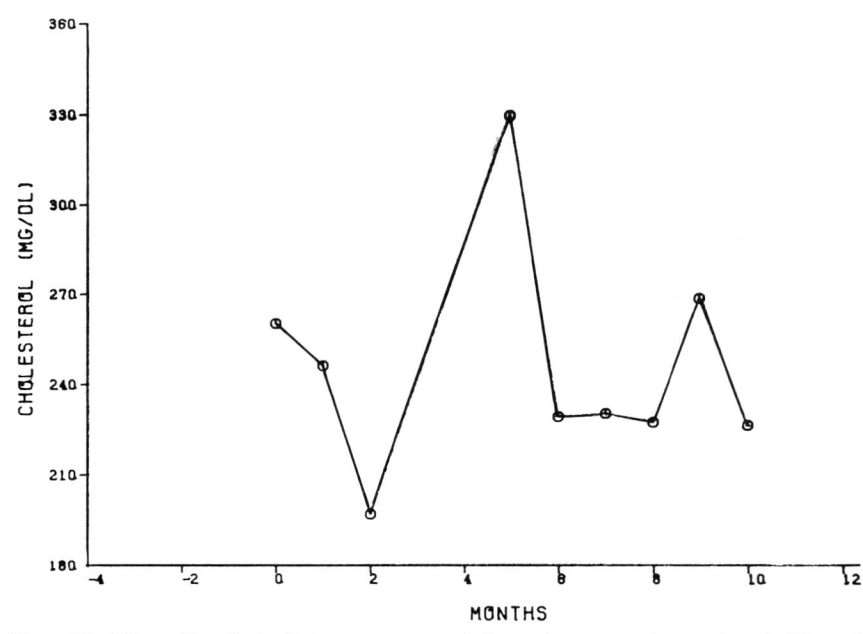

Figure 19. Effect of insulin in dialysate on serum cholesterol concentration: patient 1. (Normal: 160–330 mg/dl.)

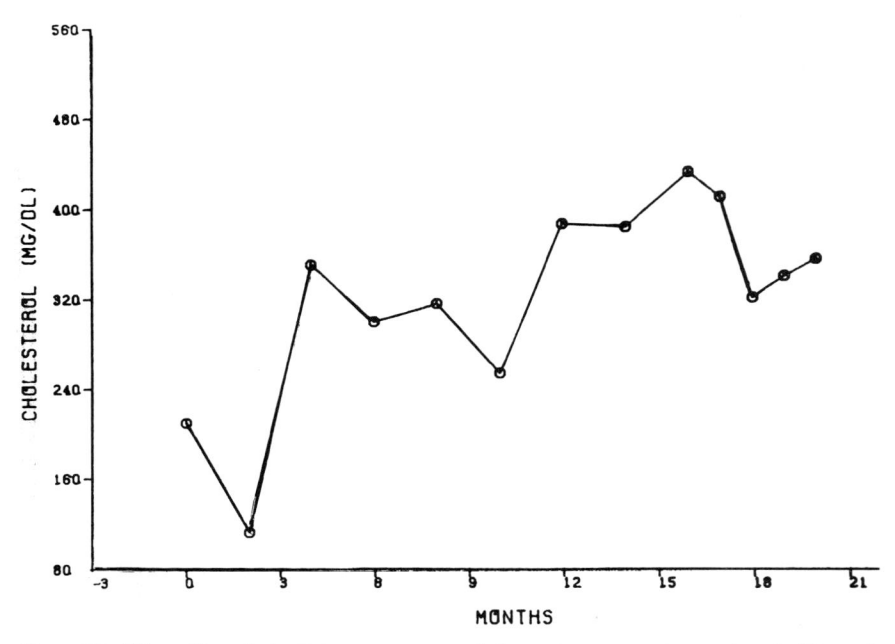

Figure 20. Effect of insulin in dialysate on serum cholesterol concentration: patient 2. (Normal: 160–330 mg/dl.)

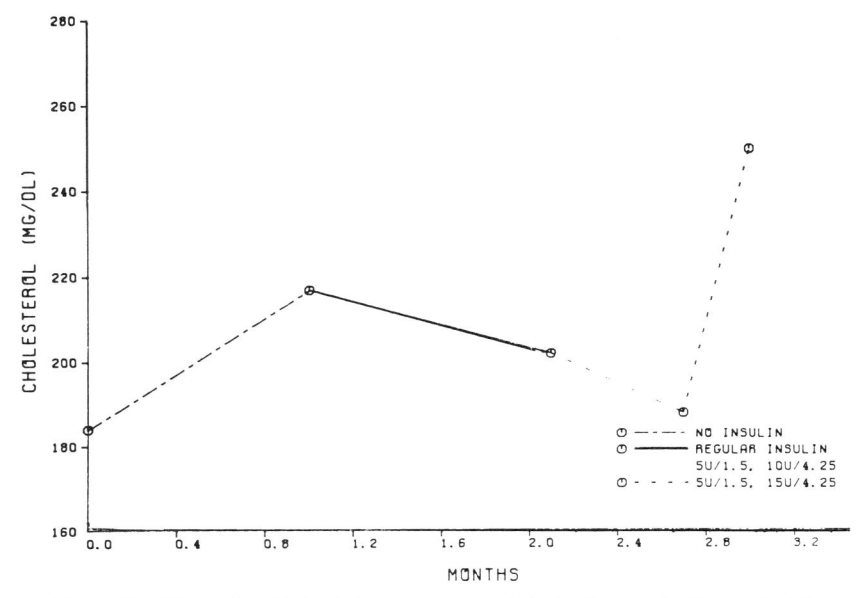

Figure 21. Effect of insulin in dialysate on serum cholesterol concentration: patient 3.

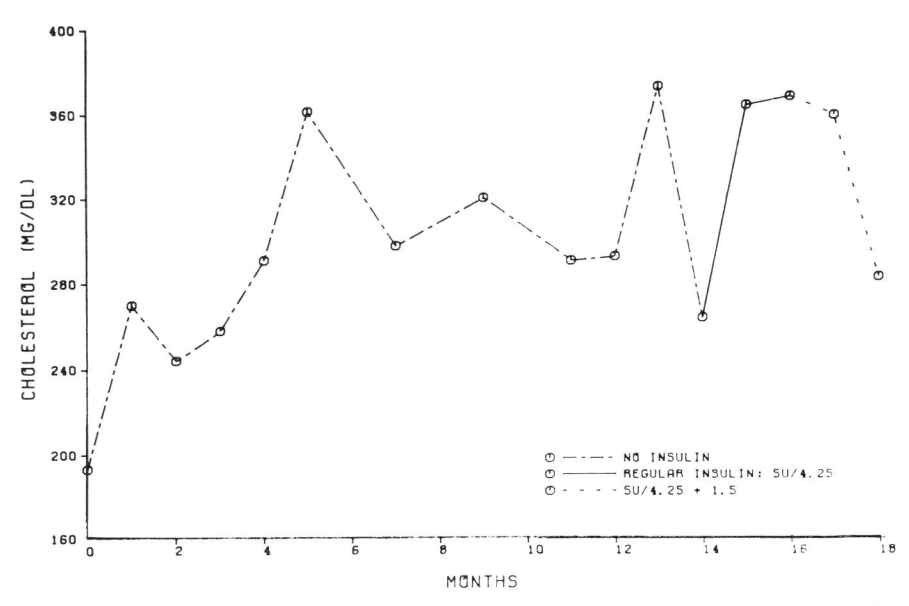

Figure 22. Effect of insulin in dialysate on serum cholesterol concentration: patient 4. (Normal: 160–330 mg/dl.)

sion of insulin may, however, produce basal normoglycemia, which in most patients is associated with a reduction in the serum triglyceride level to normal. Continuous insulin infusion can be achieved by addition of regular insulin to the dialysis solution in patients undergoing CAPD. Hypertriglyceridemia associated with either an abnormal glucose tolerance curve or late insulin release suggestive of insulin-glucose metabolic abnormality (diabetes mellitus) has been lowered by addition of insulin to the dialysis solution in three patients. Total cholesterol levels have been unaffected. A fall in the VLDL cholesterol concentration and a rise in the HDL cholesterol levels also occurred, but the small number of patients make definite interpretation difficult.

Felig and Wahren[22] have suggested that the liver is the primary target organ whereby glucose homeostasis is achieved with small increments of insulin. Improvement in the glucose metabolism was documented by random blood sugars to correlate directly with the serum triglyceride. These levels fall with the addition of insulin to the dialysis solution.

A theoretical analysis of the infusion rate of insulin was done in our laboratory and suggests that less insulin absorption should occur with a 4.25% glucose solution than with a 1.5% glucose solution (Fig. 23). We are evaluating insulin transport in patients at this time (related to the volume changes due to ultrafiltration). Figure 24 indicates that infusion of 10 units of regular insulin in a 4.25% glucose solution with a dwell time of 5 hours should produce an absorption of 6 to 7 units of insulin, 1.4 units of insulin absorbed per hour. The infusion of 2 liters of 1.5% glucose solution with 20 units of regular insulin and a dwell time of 5 hours should produce an absorption of 10 to 11 units of insulin, 2 to 2.2 units per hour. Clinical measurement of insulin concentrations in drain dialysate volume was carried out in one patient, and further investigation of the absorption rates of insulin is under way.

Conclusion

Partial control of the severe hypertriglyceridemia associated with insulin-glucose intolerance and large glucose loads in patients undergoing CAPD has been achieved by the addition of insulin to the dialysis solution. Mild hypercholesterolemia was observed and was unaffected by the addition of insulin to the dialysis solution. Increase in drain volumes was reported by the patients upon addition of the insulin to the dialysis solution. This was confirmed by transfer studies in one patient.

Hypertriglyceridemia unassociated with glucose-insulin metabolism abnormalities was unaffected by the addition of insulin to the dialysis solution. The addition of insulin to the dialysis solution in patients with severe hypertriglyceridemia undergoing CAPD appears indicated at this time. The present technique requires injection of the insulin into the sterile bag and has the potential risk of secondary contamination of the dialysis solution. No episode of peritonitis has occurred in any patient during the period of addition of insulin to the dialysis solution. The long-term effects of hypertriglyceridemia, mild hypercholesterolemia, decreased levels of HDL cholesterol fractions, and elevated levels of VLDL cholesterol fractions are unknown at this time.

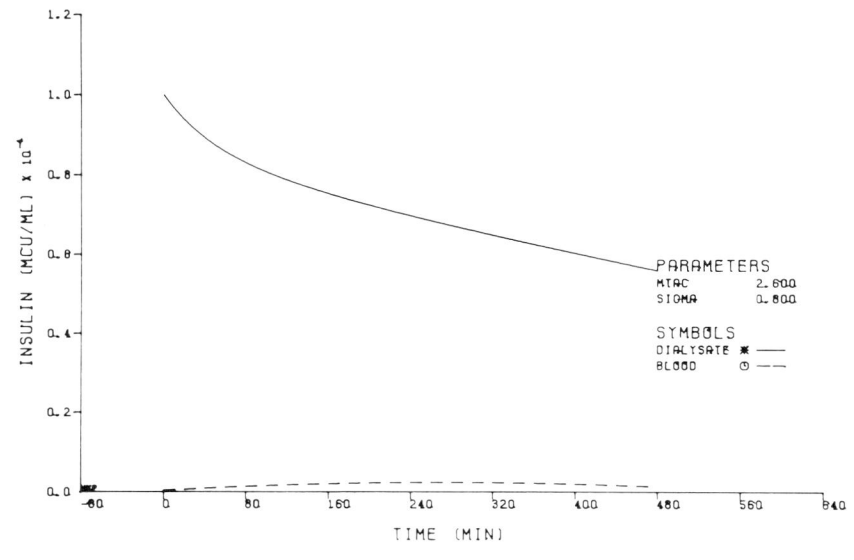

Figure 23. Theoretical mass transfer determination: Insulin–insulin transfer study: 1.5%.

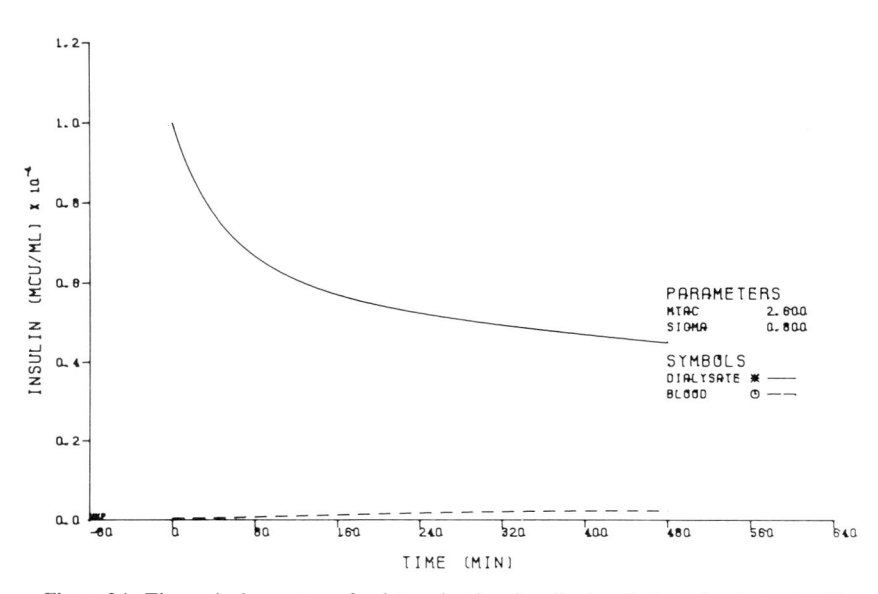

Figure 24. Theoretical mass transfer determination: Insulin–insulin transfer study: 4.25%.

ACKNOWLEDGMENT

This work was supported in part by NIH contract No. NOI-AM-9-2208.

APPENDIX: MASS TRANSFER EVALUATION

Background

Although CAPD is a relatively simple procedure for the trained patient to perform, the events that occur within the patient are quite complex. Following is a brief description of these processes and a study protocol designed to evaluate them.

The process of mass transfer in peritoneal dialysis is comprised of two major categories: solute transport and fluid transport. In fact, solute and fluid transport are so closely interrelated that it is impossible to discuss one fully without mentioning the other. In solute transport, two mechanisms exist to move a dissolved substance between the dialysate and plasma. The first and best-understood mechanism is diffusion. Whenever a difference in concentration of a solute exists between the dialysate and plasma, that solute will tend to move or diffuse across the peritoneum into the fluid where the lower concentration exists. This mechanism will therefore tend to equalize the concentrations. Small (low molecular weight) solutes tend to diffuse rapidly, whereas larger solutes move more slowly. That is, the rate of solute diffusion is inversely proportional to the solute molecular weight. This rate of diffusion across the peritoneum for a given solute is characterized by the mass transfer area coefficient (MTAC). The MTAC may be determined by mathematically evaluating the variations of plasma and dialysate concentrations with time.

Second, solutes may be transported as a result of fluid transport. Whenever fluid moves between the dialysate and plasma, the substances dissolved in that fluid will be dragged along (sometimes referred to as "solvent drag"). Solvent drag may either add to or counter the effects of diffusional solute transport. Since fluid transport may cause the dialysate volume to vary by more than 1,000 ml as well as altering solute transfer, fluid transport must be considered to characterize solute transport adequately.

In peritoneal dialysis, hypertonic dialysis solution is used to remove excess fluid from the patient. Fluid movement between the dialysate and plasma is the result of the difference in tonicity or osmolality of these two fluids. The plasma osmolality is relatively constant due to the body's regulatory mechanisms and is maintained by the presence of various salts. Dialysate osmolality is the result of salts in essentially plasma concentrations (to eliminate most diffusion) and of very high glucose (dextrose) concentrations. As a result of the substantial difference in osmolality, fluid will move by osmosis between the dialysate and plasma. The rate of fluid transport is termed the ultrafiltration rate (UFR). Here, solute transport considerations are once again of importance, since the glucose in the dialysate will diffuse or be pulled into the plasma. This will change the dialysate osmolality, which changes the UFR, which changes the rate of solvent drag.

In order to determine the UFR accurately, some means of measuring the dialysate volume in the patient's abdominal cavity is needed. The most accurate method suitable for use in human beings is to determine the dilution of a known amount of some large molecular weight radioisotope, such as carbon-14 tagged dextran-70 (molecular weight, 70,000). By measuring the dialysate dextran concentration as it changes with time in the dialysate and plasma, the dialysate volume and UFR may be calculated. Untagged solutes, such as inulin, for which an assay is available, may be substituted for the radioisotope if necessary. However, the accuracy of the procedure will not be as high in this case.

The study protocol that follows will result in a sufficient amount of information to allow quantitation of the processes described. The study will require that the subject patient be available for about 7–8 hours per exchange studied. It is important not to shorten the study unless unavoidable, since this will limit the information that may be derived from the experiment. Primarily, the study consists of obtaining dialysate and plasma samples according to the indicated schedule and having them analyzed for desired solutes. At a minimum, samples should be analyzed for blood urea nitrogen (BUN), glucose, albumin, dextran (or inulin), and osmolality. Other endogenous solutes, such as creatinine or uric acid, may be included, if desired. Unqualified informed consent must be obtained from the patient or guardian prior to the study and administration of the exogenous material. It may also be necessary to obtain the approval of a Human Subjects Review Committee if your institution has one.

If any questions arise, please contact: Keith Pyle (512-471-1216) or Robert Popovich (512-471-5080): Biomedical Engineering Department, ENS 621, University of Texas, Austin, TX 78712.

Protocol

The purpose of this procedure is to obtain timed blood and dialysate samples and to measure the concentration levels of selected substances in these samples. These data will be analyzed to determine peritoneal mass transfer parameters.

Prior to exchange of interest

1. Obtain informed consent (in writing) from patient or guardian.
2. Complete the general information section of the attached data report form or otherwise record this information.
3. Place bag of fresh solution on work area and apply port wrapping: place Betadine-soaked gauze pad around injection port, wrap with a sterile 4×4 gauze pad and tape in place.

Exchange procedure

1. Dialysate in the peritoneal cavity should be drained as completely as possible.
2. Any exogenous solutes to be added to the dialysis solution should be

carefully measured and aseptically added to the fresh dialysate bag. The solution should be mixed well by repeated inversion of the bag.
3. The fresh solution bag should be connected to the patient and infusion initiated. Note the time required for infusion. No solution should remain in the bag.
4. Approximately 2 minutes *before* completion of infusion, an initial blood sample sufficient for analysis must be taken. The time should be carefully recorded.
5. As soon as infusion of the fresh solution is complete, the initial dialysate sample (D1) should be taken in the manner to be described. The elapsed time from the completion of infusion must be recorded (*actual time,* not necessarily the ideal time indicated). The volume of the samples should be kept to the minimum necessary for accurate analysis.
6. Additional dialysate samples should be obtained and noted as above at 30, 60, 90, 120, 180, 240, 360, and 480 minutes (measured from the completion of infusion).
7. Additional blood samples should be obtained and the time recorded at 180 minutes and immediately after initiation of drainage.
8. Record the drained volume.

Dialysate sampling procedure

1. Unroll the dialysate bag and place in the drain position.
2. Release the tubing clamp and allow approximately 50 ml of dialysate to flow into the bag. Close the tubing clamp. Record the time that the clamp is closed as the "actual sample time."
3. Place the bag on a suitable surface and remove the injection port wrapping.
4. Aseptically withdraw a sufficient volume of dialysate for analysis from the bag via the injection port.
5. Raise the bag and reinfuse any dialysate remaining in the bag into the patient.
6. Wrap the injection port with a fresh wrapping as already described.
7. Transfer the sample to a clean, suitably labeled container.

Blood sampling procedure

Blood samples are obtained in the normal manner. Note and record the sample time when about half of the blood sample has been collected. Label the container appropriately.

Completing the evaluation

1. Submit all samples for analysis.
2. Send the completed data forms, results of all analyses (*not* the samples), and a copy of the signed and witnessed consent form to Keith Pyle or Robert Popovich.

References

1. Bagdade, J. D., Porte, D. Jr., and Bierman, E. L.: Hypertriglyceridemia: A metabolic consequence of chronic renal failure. *N Engl J Med* **269**: 181–185, 1968.
2. Bagdade, J. D.: Uremic lipemia. *Arch Intern Med* **126**: 875–881, 1970.
3. Bagdade, J. D.: Disorders of carbohydrate and lipid metabolism in uremia. *Nephron* **14**: 153–162, 1975.
4. Samar, R. E.: Hyperthiglyceridemia in chronic uremia and hypertriglyceridemia response to mega vitamin therapy. Doctoral dissertation, University of Texas at Austin, May, 1976.
5. Klein, K. L., and Kurokawa, K.: Metabolic and endocrine alterations in end-stage renal failure. *Postgrad Med* **64**: 99–108, November 1978.
6. Rapoport, J., Aviram, M., Chaimovitz, C., and Brook, J. G.: Defective high density lipoprotein composition in patients on chronic hemodialysis. *N Engl J Med* **299**: 1326–1329, 1978.
7. Moncrief, J. W., Popovich, R. P., Nolph, K. D., Rubin, J., Robson, M., Dombros, N., deVeber, G. A., and Oreopoulos, D. G.: Clinical experience with continuous ambulatory peritoneal dialysis. *Am Soc Artif Intern Organs* (3), 1979.
8. Cooper, K. H.: *Aerobics*. Bantam Book, New York, 1979.
9. Holman, R. R., and Turner, R. C.: Diabetes: The quest for basal normoglycemia. *Lancet* 469–474, 1977.
10. Turner, R. C., McCarthy, S. T., Holman, R. R., and Harris, E.: Beta-cell function improved by supplementing basal insulin secretion in mild diabetes. *Br Med J* **1**: 1252–1254, 1976.
11. Streja, D., Steiner, G., and Kwiterovich, P. O., Jr.: Plasma high-density lipoproteins and ischemic heart disease. *Ann Intern Med* **89**(6): 871–880, 1978.
12. Holman, R. R., and Turner, R. C.: Maintenance of basal plasma glucose and insulin concentrations in maturity-onset diabetes. *Diabetes* **28**: 227-230, 1979.
13. Flynn, C. T., and Nanson, J. A.: Intraperitoneal insulin with CAPD—An artificial pancreas. *Trans Am Soc Artif Intern Organs* **25**: 114–116, 1979.
14. Personal communication.
15. Ponticelli, C., Barbi, G., Cantaluppi, A., Donati, C., Annoni, G., and Bramacaccio, D.: Lipid abnormalities in maintainance dialysis and renal transplant recipients. *Kidney Int* **13**(Suppl 8): 5-72–5-78, 1978.
16. Levine, J., Falk, B., Henriquez, M., Raja, R. M., Kramer, M. S., and Rosenbaum, J. L.: High-density lipoproteins–correlation with cardiovascular disease in hemodialysis patients. *Trans Am Soc Artif Intern Organs* **24**: 43–49, 1978.
17. Popovich, R. P., Moncrief, J. W., Nolph, K. D., Ghods, A. J., Twardowski, Z. J., and Pyle, W. K.: Continuous ambulatory peritoneal dialysis. *Ann Intern Med* **88**(4): 449, 1978.
18. Reaven, G. M.: Effects of different in amount and kind of dietary carbohydrate on plasma glucose and insulin response in man. *Am J Clin Nutr* **32**: 2568–2578, 1979.
19. Turner, R. C., Mann, J. I., Simpson, R. D., et al.: Plasma glucose, insulin and triglyceride changes in response to a standard breakfast on an oral glucose tolerance test in normal obese and diabetic subjects. *Clin Endocrinol* **6**: 253–254,
20. Sosenko, J. M., Breslow, J. L., Miettinen, O. S., and Gabbay, K. H.: Hyperglycemia and plasma lipid levels. *N Engl J Med* **302**: 650–654, 1980.
21. Tamborlane, W. V., Sherwin, R. S., Genel, M., and Felig, P.: Restoration of normal lipid and aminoacid metabolism in diabetic patients treated with a portable insulin-infusion pump. *Lancet* **1**: 1258–1261, 1979.
22. Felig, P., and Wahren, J.: Influence of exogenous insulin secretion on splanchnic glucose and amino-acid metabolism in man. *J Clin Invest* **50**: 1702–1711, 1971.

CHAPTER TWENTY-THREE

New Materials

"P" A. J. SORRELS, R.N.

V. KRUGER, R.M.A.

J. W. MONCRIEF, M.D.

R. P. POPOVICH, Ph.D.

AS CONTINUOUS AMBULATORY PERITONEAL DIALYSIS (CAPD) has gained recognition in the dialysis community, it has become apparent that the development of specifically designed materials is necessary for the success of such a dialytic therapy. Baxter Travenol Laboratories has been the frontrunner in the development of these materials and has developed an entire line of CAPD products. Interest from other companies is rapidly growing; however, the availability of materials has not been forthcoming.

TITANIUM ADAPTOR

Titanium is a lightweight, semiprecious metal with which a peritoneal catheter adapter has been made. The adapter weighs little more than the plastic adapters previously used, and it allows for a leur-locking system to prevent disconnection from the transfer tubing, which was a major problem with previously utilized materials. The titanium adapter may be used for extended periods with no cracking, which often occurs with plastic adapters. The adapter produces a double-locking seal with the tubing, which prevents leakage of fluid from the catheter. Some patients have developed skin irritation due to the ridges on the adapter, but this problem has been alleviated by placing a simple gauze dressing around the connection site.

The Austin Diagnostic Clinic, Acorn Research Laboratory, Austin, Texas

TRANSFER TUBING SET

The transfer tubing was developed to be utilized with the titanium adapter and to make connection to and disconnection from the bag easier for the patient. The proximal end of the tubing is again a leur-locking system to prevent disconnection from the catheter. The distal end of tubing consists of a key-grip spike that allows the patient to maintain a firm grasp when making a bag change. The ease with which the spike is removed from the used bag and inserted into the new bag makes CAPD a much easier procedure. There has been no cracking of the key-grip spike, which, too, was a major difficulty noted with previously utilized equipment.

GRIPPER CLAMP

The gripper clamp is made of plastic and was designed to prevent the flow of solution during an exchange and therefore to alleviate the use of a hemostat, which often crushes the spike. The round disc on the clamp is a finger guard, and when used properly it alleviates the risk of contamination by fingers slipping onto the outlet port of the bag or the spike during a bag change. If the gripper clamp is used improperly, however, the risk of contamination is increased by placement of fingers under the outlet port. Therefore there is only one way to use the gripper clamp, which may be a disadvantage for some patients with manual dexterity difficulties.

CAPD PREP KIT

Previously, exchange supplies were shipped to the patient in bulk form and required a large area for storage. The development of the CAPD prep kit has alleviated this problem because it is small and consolidates the materials needed for an exchange. There are 30 kits per case, and depending upon the number of exchanges per day, the patient receives that number of cases per month.

TUBING CHANGE KIT

With the development of the titanium adapter and transfer set, the technique for changing the tubing has been modified to encompass a 5-minute Betadine soak of the adapter-tubing connection and another 5-minute soak of the adapter itself prior to the connection of a new transfer set. With this new technique, it has become painfully obvious that some form of tubing change tray would be most beneficial.

Several companies have displayed interest in the development of such a tray, and a few have actually presented a prototype. The Tri-state Hospital Supply Company has designed a small, compact tray that allows for proper Betadine immersion techniques without unnecessary waste. The Clinipad

CAPD CYCLER

American Medical Products has developed a CAPD "cycler" with a timing device that has been modified for a dwell time up to 10 hours and a volume selector to monitor the amount of fluid infused. This allows the patient to have a prolonged dwell time during the day and connect to the cycler at bedtime with shorter dwell times overnight. We, at the Austin Diagnostic Clinic, Acorn Research Laboratory, consider that this is not in adherence to the philosophy of CAPD, but we see it as a possible advantage to those patients who do not want to cope with an exchange during an active day and can perform the aseptic techniques required for connections to and disconnections from a machine.

CONCLUSION

The development of new and more sophisticated materials is important to the future of CAPD and is currently of utmost priority. The results seen with the materials now available indicate that peritonitis will not remain the major complication of CAPD and that it will, in fact, be almost alleviated with future advancement in techniques and equipment. Materials developed to make the techniques of CAPD easier will increase the future availability to the dialysis patient population and enhance the well-being of patients currently being treated with this modality.

References

1. Popovich, R. P., Moncrief, J. W., Decherd, J. F., Bomar, J. B., and Pyle, W. K.: The definition of a novel portable/wearable equilibrium peritoneal dialysis technique. *Trans Am Soc Artif Intern Organs* **5:** 64, 1976.
2. Popovich, R. P., Moncrief, J. W., Nolph, K. D., Ghods, A. J., Twahdowksi, Z. J., and Pyle, W. K.: Continuous ambulatory peritoneal dialysis. *Ann Intern Med* **88:** 449, 1978.
3. Oreopoulos, D. G., Robson, M., Izatt, S., Clayton, S. L., and deVeber, G. A.: A simple and safe technique for continuous ambulatory peritoneal dialysis (CAPD). *Trans Am Soc Artif Intern Organs* 1978.
4. Moncrief, J. W., and Popovich, R. P., Continuous Ambulatory Peritoneal Dialysis, today's art of peritoneal dialysis. *Contrib Nephrol* **17:** 139–145, 1979.
5. *Going Home with Confidence,* Procedure for Continuous Ambulatory Peritoneal Dialysis, Patient Program, Baxter-Travenol Laboratories, 1979.
6. Moncrief, J. W., Rutherford, C. E., Sorrels, A. J., Bailey, A., and Popovich, R. P. Technical aspects of CAPD, new connection devices developed by Baxter Travenol Laboratories, 1979. Excerpta Medica (in press).

CHAPTER TWENTY-FOUR

A Comparison of CAPD and Hemodialysis in Adaptation to Home Dialysis

R. M. LINDSAY,* M.D., F.R.C.P.(C)

D. G. OREOPOULOS,† M.D., Ph.D., F.R.C.P.(C)

H. BURTON,‡ M.Sc., M.S.W.

J. CONLEY,‡ Ph.D.

G. WELLS,‡ M.Sc.

INTRODUCTION

FEWER ADVENTS IN THE HISTORY of nephrology have carried greater impact than the first description of continuous ambulatory peritoneal dialysis (CAPD) given in 1978.[1] Since then, the growth of CAPD has been enormous and currently in Ontario, Canada, approximately 55% of all patients placed on home dialysis are being treated by this therapy mode (unpublished survey data). There is no question that the CAPD works and already there are several publications describing the biochemical and physical status of patients at home on such therapy.[2] It is believed by most to be cost-effective; Robson and Oreopoulos[3] have suggested that the patient on CAPD will create costs of approximately $5,000 per year and Fenton and his colleagues[4] suggest that it is at least as cost effective as hemodialysis (HD). However, these quoted figures have not completely considered the question of hospital admission

---

*Victoria Hospital, London, Ontario, Canada and The University of Western Ontario, London, Ontario, Canada
†Toronto Western Hospital, Toronto, Ontario, Canada and The University of Toronto, Toronto, Ontario, Canada
‡Health Care Research Unit, The University of Western Ontario, London, Ontario, Canada

rates, which obviously have implication for cost effectiveness, nor do any studies so far published address themselves to determining the quality of life experienced and to assessing which patients are best treated by CAPD and which by HD.

As part of a major study on the factors that might influence successful adaptation to home dialysis, we have had the opportunity to examine information pertaining to the physical and psychosocial well-being of a large group of patients undergoing home dialysis in the province of Ontario, and have, thus, set out to compare the influence of the treatment modality (CAPD versus HD) on these parameters. This paper presents additional information to that already given to the first International Symposium on CAPD in Paris in 1979.[5]

PATIENTS AND METHODS

Adaptation to home dialysis*

The objectives of the study are: 1) to evaluate the influence that physiological, psychological, social, and economic functioning and the training and support received by the dialysis patients have on their ability to adapt to a program of home dialysis; 2) to analyze those factors that facilitate the adaptation of the home dialysis patients so that more accurate predictions in patient selection may be made; 3) to analyze the influence of treatment methods used on the adaptation of the dialysis patient. It is hoped that the realization of these objectives may lead to successful home dialysis adaptation in a higher percentage of patients with end-stage renal disease. The study design incorporates two stages; a retrospective study to explore adaptation in persons who commenced a home dialysis training program between June 1, 1975, and June 1, 1978; and a prospective study to follow patients from commencement of home dialysis training through their first and second years of adjustment to home dialysis.

Data collection involves the patient and his partner being questioned by trained interviewers who obtain data on psychological, physical, social, and economic functioning, and sources of social support. From chart abstraction and renal unit records, data are obtained to assess physiological and physical functioning. Finally, the parent renal unit is asked to assess each patient to give an evaluation of the patient's adaptation level. The questionnaires contain established tools used by psychologists, sociologists, and behavioral scientists to enable assessments to be made on such conditions as anxiety, denial, and depression, and to recognize stresses. Indeed, stresses are not merely identified, but the degree to which stress is experienced is indicated on a score from 0 to 5. All the information so obtained is coded and computer stored, which will allow the interrelationship between any factors to be assessed. The nature of data collection and the potential for mathematical scoring might eventually make it possible to apply numerical weightings to each factor so that "a coefficient for adaptation" can be created. At present, the retrospective study is completed and the data so obtained are being subjected to statistical analysis and the prospective study is under way.

Patients

The retrospective sample contains 260 home dialysis patients from 16 renal centers throughout the province of Ontario. Of these patients, 150 were treated by HD and 89 by CAPD. Another 21 patients were at home being treated by intermittent peritoneal dialysis; these will not be considered here. Of the 260, 59% were male, but there were more male patients undergoing HD (67%) than CAPD (54%) ($p < 0.01$). The mean age of the HD patients at the time they commenced their home dialysis training was 41.06 ± 13.49 years (M $\pm$ S.D.). The CAPD patients were significantly ($p < 0.01$) older at 49.83 ± 13.23 years. The duration of home dialysis at the time of data collection was 20.08 ± 11.96 months for the HD population and 7.42 ± 5.86 months for those undergoing CAPD. This difference is statistically different ($p < 0.01$).

Statistical analyses

All information was subjected to chi-square analysis or to Student's t-test where appropriate. Interrelationships between variables were examined by regression analysis or by Pearson coefficients. In the text mean values are presented ± 1 S.D.

AREAS OF COMPARISONS AND RESULTS

Training time

This was significantly less for the CAPD patients at 2.9 ± 1.9 weeks as compared with 6.7 ± 3.4 weeks for HD ($p < 0.0001$).

Physiological data

Significant differences in physiological parameters as found at 6 months after the commencement of home dialysis on a particular treatment modality and again at 1 year are shown in Table 1. Not all patients had experienced 6 months or 1 year treatment and therefore the number of patients suitable for analysis is indicated on that table. It can be seen that any differences found are unlikely to have any clinical significance.

Hospital admission rates

Hospital admissions were significantly higher in those treated by CAPD ($p < 0.007$). The respective mean rates were 0.326 ± 0.483 per patient-month (CAPD) and 0.133 ± 0.197 (HD). In spite of this, there was no significant difference in the days per patient-month spent in the hospital between the two groups (2.1 ± 2.8, CAPD; 1.25 ± 2.5, HD).

Reasons for hospital admissions

In total, 66 separate reasons for hospital admission were found, but in only one area was there a significant difference that could be related to the

TABLE 1.
Physiological Data at 6 Months and 1 Year

	6 Months[a] CAPD	6 Months[a] HD[b]	1 Year[a] CAPD	1 Year[a] HD[b]
	(M ± S.D.)	(M ± S.D.)	(M ± S.D.)	(M ± S.D.)
Total proteins (g%)	6.3 ± 0.9 (34)	6.9 ± 0.6 (90)	6.4 ± 0.9 (8)	7.0 ± 0.6 (66)
	$p < 0.0001$		NS	
Albumin (g%)	3.5 ± 0.6 (34)	4.1 ± 0.5 (88)	3.6 ± 0.7 (8)	4.2 ± 0.5 (64)
	$p < 0.0001$		$p < 0.05$	
Calcium (mg%)	9.1 ± 0.9 (45)	9.5 ± 0.9 (118)	9.1 ± 0.8 (9)	9.8 ± 0.8 (85)
	$p < 0.006$		$p < 0.008$	
Phosphorus (mg%)	5.0 ± 1.8 (45)	5.2 ± 1.7 (118)	4.7 ± 1.5 (9)	5.4 ± 1.5 (85)
	NS		NS	
Alkaline phosphatase (mU/ml)	110.7 ± 52.0 (41)	104.4 ± 54.1 (114)	149.3 ± 143.3 (9)	118.7 ± 101.3 (82)
	NS		NS	
Blood urea nitrogen (mg%)	55.1 ± 18.5 (31)	65.9 ± 20.8 (120)	54.6 ± 18.9 (7)	66.1 ± 21.6 (87)
	$p < 0.01$		NS	
Creatinine (mg%)	11.0 ± 3.4 (33)	11.6 ± 3.6 (124)	11.5 ± 2.4 (7)	11.5 ± 3.2 (90)
	NS		NS	
Potassium (mEq/liter)	4.1 ± 0.8 (33)	4.9 ± 0.8 (124)	3.8 ± 0.2 (7)	4.8 ± 0.7 (89)
	$p < 0.0001$		$p < 0.001$	
Hemoglobin (g%)	9.0 ± 2.2 (43)	8.2 ± 2.0 (126)	8.5 ± 2.9 (9)	8.3 ± 2.2 (91)
	$p < 0.02$		NS	

[a] Numbers in parentheses indicate number of observations.
[b] All data for HD are predialysis values.

treatment modality. This was with peritonitis in the CAPD population ($p < 0.0001$). The most common other causes for hospital admission were access revision (shunt, fistula, peritoneal catheter), diabetic complication, transplantation, infection, fluid overload, pericarditis, and nephrectomy.

Employment

To examine the effect of treatment upon employment an Employment Adaptation Index (EAI) was created. This was based on the responses to three questions:

Comparison of CAPD and Hemodialysis   175

1. Were you able to continue with your type of employment after commencement of dialysis?
   Ai —Yes (same job)
   Aii —Yes (different job)
   Aiii—No
2. Did your renal failure and its treatment force this change?
   Bi —Yes
   Bii—No
3. Did you become unemployed, retired, or laid off because of your renal failure?
   Ci —Yes
   Cii—No

It was assumed that the best EAI was obtained with a patient who continues in the same type of employment, with no job change due to renal failure or dialysis, and who has remained employed. The worst EAI would be with an individual not able to continue his line of work, for whom renal failure or dialysis forced the change, and who has become unemployed. Ten combinations of answers are possible and thus an ordinal scale from 1 (best) to 10 (worst) was made, the number obtained for any given individual being his or her EAI. The EAI was obtained for 117 HD and 35 CAPD patients, that is, for those who held a job (as classified by Canadian Manpower) before dialysis therapy was required. The mean EAI for HD patients was 5.7 ± 4.1, which was significantly ($p < 0.02$) lower, that is, better, than the 7.6 ± 3.4 for CAPD patients. When corrected for sex, it was found that HD scored better for males ($p < 0.005$), but there was no difference related to treatment modality in the female population. When examined by age, it was found that CAPD consistently had a detrimental effect, that is, a higher score on the EAI, but this only became significant in the older age group (>60). There was no correlation between the EAI and the duration of HD. An EAI was also created for housewives based on four questions relating to the theme, "Does dialysis interfere with housework?" in a manner similar to that described above. Again, HD scored better than CAPD and a special significance was noted in the older than 60 age group ($p < 0.003$).

Treatment modality as a stress factor in relationship to work

Patients being treated by CAPD indicated significantly more stress when asked the question, "Does your treatment modality interfere with your work?" ($p < 0.001$). Similarly, the female patients indicated that CAPD caused more stress when asked, "Does your treatment modality interfere with your household duties?" ($p < 0.01$).

Dialysis procedure as a stress factor

When patients were asked the question, "Does your dialysis procedure cause you stress or concern?" it was found that CAPD was associated with significantly less stress ($p < 0.003$).

TABLE 2.
CAPD Versus HD

A. Sexual Functioning as a Stress Factor by Modality and Sex of Patient

	None or Mild				Moderate or Severe			
	Male		Female		Male		Female	
	N	%	N	%	N	%	N	%
Home hemodialysis	58	64	31	71	33	36	18	30
CAPD	18	72	13	82	7	28	4	18
Total	76	66%	44	74%	40	34%	22	26%

B. Sexual Functioning as a Stress Factor by Modality and Age

	None or Mild						Moderate or Severe					
	<45		46–59		>60		<45		46–59		>60	
Home hemodialysis	50	71	19	44	21	95	20	29	24	59	1	5
CAPD	12	80	14	67	10	90	3	20	7	39	1	10
Total	62	73%	33	52%	31	94%	23	27%	31	48%	2	6%

Sexual functioning

Of all patients, 69% indicated that the degree of stress encountered by their level of sexual function was "none or mild" (0–1 on questionnaire scale) and 31% indicated that it was of "moderate or severe intensity" (4–5 on questionnaire). As shown in Table 2, treatment modality had no influence on sexual functioning as a stress factor analyzed by both sex and age of patients. Furthermore, when the stress factors as defined by decreased sexual ability, level of sexual satisfaction (interspousal), change of sexual satisfaction, and degree of difficulty experienced with any change in sexual satisfaction were analyzed by modality, age, and sex, no significant differences were found.

Stress and concerns

The frequency of identifiable stresses (relating to illness or dialysis, such as fear of blood clotting) and concerns (relating to life, such as marriage strain) were analyzed by age, sex, and treatment modality. Stress counts were scaled 0 → 14, concerns 0 → 8. The mean values for these counts are shown in Table 3, where significant differences are indicated. It is interesting that as patients get older they experience far less stress from their treatment modality. Also it was observed that there was no correlation between stress and concern counts with time on dialysis.

Internality–externality scale

Rotter has developed a numerical score based upon questions designed to define the degree of internality or externality or locus of control that is part of an individual personality.[6] An individual who scores strongly as an "internal"

TABLE 3.
Stresses and Concerns (Mean Counts)

	HD	CAPD	p
1. All			
Stress	7.4	6.1	<0.02
Concern	3.6	2.4	<0.001
2. Males			
Stress	7.2	6.2	NS
Concern	3.7	2.6	<0.02
3. Females			
Stress	8.0	5.9	<0.01
Concern	3.5	2.3	<0.02
4. Effect of Age: ↑ Age ↓ Counts			
e.g. Females <49:			
Stress	9.2	6.7	<0.05
Concern	4.0	2.3	<0.05
Females >60:			
Stress	5.8	5.5	NS
Concern	2.1	2.5	NS
5. No correlation with time on dialysis			

is generally one who believes that he is in control of his own destiny and can cope with external stresses. The individual who scores as an "external" tends to believe that everything that happens is determined by chance or fate and is very much influenced by important events. This scale is a widely used tool of behavioral scientists and its uses are well reviewed by MacDonald.[7] The score for any individual may not be constant and, indeed, may change with dramatic events and may be influenced by the degree of exposure to a powerful external stress.[7] When this scale was applied to our home dialysis population, no significant difference between the population scores was found between the CAPD and the HD patients. Furthermore, in the HD group when the score was analyzed in relationship to the duration of hemodialysis therapy, no such correlation existed.

TABLE 4.
BPI Numerical Scores (Mean ± S.D.)

	HD	CAPD	Normal (n = 210)
Depression	5.1 ± 4.4	5.1 ± 4.2	2.3 ± 3.2
Denial	8.5 ± 3.6	9.5 ± 2.8	6.9 ± 3.4
Anxiety	7.5 ± 4.4	7.4 ± 5.1	5.2 ± 3.6
Self-depreciation	3.2 ± 2.7	3.1 ± 3.0	2.0 ± 2.5
Social introversion	4.9 ± 3.2	5.1 ± 4.2	3.3 ± 3.2

NS

Basic Personality Inventory scale

The Basic Personality Inventory (BPI) scale is a tool, developed from the work of Jackson and Carlson,[8] which gives indications of the degree of depression, denial, anxiety, self-deprecation, and social introversion found in an individual. In Table 4 the mean scores for these five aspects of personality are presented for the HD and CAPD populations and can be compared with those scores found in 210 normal persons (male and female) interviewed in Southwestern Ontario. It can be seen that there are no significant differences between the two treatment groups but patients on dialysis do score higher in all aspects when compared with the normal population. When the five components of the BPI scale were analyzed in relationship to the appreciation of stresses and concerns, it was found that there was a strong positive correlation between (individually) depression, anxiety, self-deprecation, and social introversion with (individually) stresses and concerns ($p < 0.02 \rightarrow p < 0.001$); there was a strong negative correlation between denial and the appreciation of stresses and concerns ($p < 0.001$). There was also a positive correlation between self-deprecation and a high (externality) Rotter score.

DISCUSSION

This retrospective study gives some insight into the problems experienced by patients on home dialysis. Furthermore, where the treatment modality appears to influence these problems the information obtained may lead to the appropriate selection of a treatment modality for a given patient. It would appear that CAPD requires a shorter training time than hemodialysis, which is obviously beneficial in a cost-effective sense. On the other hand, CAPD patients have a higher hospital admission rate because of peritonitis and this, in spite of the fact that there is no difference in bed occupancy rates, is still likely to be cost ineffective. There is no doubt that those patients who are working find that CAPD interferes with both job and housework. Furthermore, there is strong evidence that the use of CAPD as a treatment modality will hamper the individual patient's return to work, especially if he is male or of the older age group. On the other hand, the frequency and degree of stresses and concerns are much more relevant to those patients treated by HD, especially so in the younger age groups. Furthermore, the experience of stress and concern is directly related to the degree of depression, anxiety, self-deprecation, and social introversion that the individual patient has as part of his basic personality make-up (BPI). Thus, it can be assumed that a patient who demonstrates high levels of depression, anxiety, self-deprecation, or social introversion will find home HD a stressful form of therapy; a patient who demonstrates a high denial score, on the other hand, may well easily cope with that treatment modality. The results of this study were obtained by a greater in-depth analysis of the retrospective data than the preliminary information presented at the Paris meeting.[5] These results strongly suggest that a life-style profile of the patient could be conducted and this might be the major factor in assigning that patient to CAPD or HD as his treatment modality. It seems clear that a male patient who is strongly motivated to continue working, especially if he is of an older age group, would best be treated by HD; the young female patient with a family and not working, however, will likely prefer CAPD, a treatment modality associated with less concern in regard to her marriage and the problems of vacations with her family, and this preference would be enhanced if her BPI shows increased scores for depression, anxiety, self-deprecation, or social introversion. A trial of such an approach is logical, since there are no important differences in the physiological effects (at least in the short term) of the treatment modalities (Table 1). These observations will be tested in a longitudinal manner with the prospective study, and a further report will be subsequently given.

ACKNOWLEDGMENTS

This study was supported by a grant from the Ministry of Health of Ontario (No. DM338). The principal investigators in this study are Mr. Howard Burton, Dr. Lino Canzona, Dr. Robert Lindsay, and Mrs. Sally Palmer. The participating nephrologists are listed herewith and their help is acknowledged: Doctors R. W. Johnson, R. Manning, P. Morrin, B. Haberstroh, T. Liu, W. Cameron, W. P. Fay, C. Cameron, G. A. Posen, R. Couture, D. Page, C. J. Barnes, B. Hall, E. Kinsey-Smith, J. Lien, A. G. Shimizu, P. E. Cordy, D. C. Cattron, S. S. A. Fenton, C. S. O. Saiphoo, C. C. Williams, D. Oreopoulos, and R. Uldall.

References

1. Popovich, R. P., Moncrief, J. W., Nolph, K. D., Ghods, A. J., Twardowski, Z. J., and Pyle, W. K.: Continuous ambulatory peritoneal dialysis. *Ann Intern Med* **88**: 449, 1978.
2. Oreopoulos, D. G., Clayton, S., Dombros, N., Zellerman, G., and Katirtzoglou, A.: Nineteen months' experience with continuous ambulatory peritoneal dialysis. *Proc Eur Dial and Transplant Assoc,* **16**: *178, 1979.*
3. Robson, M. D., and Oreopoulos, D. G.: A revolution in the treatment of chronic renal failure. *Dial Transplant* **7**: 999, 1978.
4. Fenton, S. S. A., Cattran, D. C., Allen, A. F., Rutledge, P., Ampil, M., Dadson, J., Locking, H., Smith, S. D., and Wilson, D. R.: Initial experiences with continuous ambulatory peritoneal dialysis. *Artif Organs* 3(3): 206, 1979.
5. Lindsay, R. M., Oreoupolos, D., Burton, H., Conley, J., Wells, G., and Fenton, S.: Adaptation to home dialysis; a comparison of CAPD and hemodialysis. *CAPD: Proceedings of an International Symposium,* M. Legrain, Ed. Excerpta Medica, Amsterdam, 1980.
6. Rotter, J. B.: Generalized expectancies for internal versus external control of reinforcement. *Psychol Monogr* **80**: 1, 1966.
7. MacDonald, A. P.: Internal-external locus of control. In *Measures of Social Psychological Attitudes,* Robinson, J. P., and Shaver, P. R., Eds. Institute of Social Research, University of Michigan, Ann Arbor, Chap. 4, p. 169.
8. Jackson, D. N., and Carlson, K. A.: Convergant and discriminant validation of the differential personality inventory. *J Clin Psychol* **29**(2): 214, 1973.

CHAPTER TWENTY-FIVE

Chronic Intermittent and Continuous Ambulatory Peritoneal Dialysis: A Comparison

WADI N. SUKI, M.D.

BRIGID JAYNES, R.N.

SHERRY BARLOW-SNEAD, R.D.

JEANNE LOVELL, R.N.

CRAIG G. PRICE, P.A.

THE DEVELOPMENT OF PERMANENT IN-DWELLING PERITONEAL CATHETERS, and the design of equipment for the automatic mixing and/or cycling of dialysate, have made it possible for patients suffering from end-stage renal disease to undergo chronic peritoneal dialysis. For the past 3 years, we have been engaged in the training of patients in chronic intermittent peritoneal dialysis (CIPD) for use in the home.

The recent innovation of continuous ambulatory peritoneal dialysis (CAPD) is another advance that offers several theoretical and practical advantages but also has some distinct limitations. Over the past year, we have trained 21 patients in CAPD. Thirteen of these had been treated with CIPD, six with chronic maintenance hemodialysis, and the remaining two patients were begun on CAPD *de novo*. The change to CAPD from the established treatment modalities of CIPD and hemodialysis has permitted us to compare these three approaches to the management of patients with chronic renal failure.

A comparison of the laboratory results of 13 patients first treated by CIPD and then changed to CAPD is depicted in Table 1. There was no significant change in the values for hemoglobin, hematocrit, creatinine, total serum proteins, serum albumin, calcium, and phosphate. However, in spite of the liberalization of the diet, both the blood urea nitrogen (BUN) and the serum

Department of Medicine, Baylor College of Medicine and The Methodist Hospital, Houston, Texas

TABLE 1.
Laboratory Results in Patients Changing from CIPD to CAPD

	Hemoglobin		Hematocrit		Blood Urea Nitrogen		Creatinine		Total Proteins		Albumin		Potassium		Calcium		Phosphate	
	I[a]	A[b]	I	A	I	A	I	A	I	A	I	A	I	A	I	A	I	A
Mean	8.7	8.9	26	27	81	71	15.0	13.6	7.0	6.7	4.5	4.3	4.6	3.9	9.5	9.6	6.1	5.6
S.E.M.	0.4	0.5	1.1	1.5	5.6	5.4	1.8	1.4	0.2	0.1	0.2	0.1	0.2	0.2	0.2	0.2	0.2	0.5
p	NS		NS		<0.05		NS		NS		NS		<0.02		NS		NS	

[a] I is CIPD.
[b] A is CAPD.

TABLE 2.
Laboratory Results in Patients Changing from Hemodialysis to CAPD

	Hemoglobin		Hematocrit		Blood Urea Nitrogen		Creatinine		Total Proteins		Albumin		Potassium		Calcium		Phosphate	
	H[a]	A[b]	H	A	H	A	H	A	H	A	H	A	H	A	H	A	H	A
Mean	8.8	8.7	26	27	83	60	12.3	11.2	6.6	6.6	4.1	4.2	4.7	4.0	8.6	9.2	5.4	5.0
S.E.M.	1.3	0.5	2.2	1.5	6.9	6.4	1.6	1.1	0.4	0.3	0.3	0.3	0.4	0.3	0.5	0.3	0.3	0.5
p	NS		NS		<0.05		NS		NS		NS		NS		<0.10		NS	

[a] H is hemodialysis.
[b] A is CAPD.

potassium fell significantly. These results indicate that CAPD is equal or superior to CIPD in maintaining hematological and biochemical balance in these patients. Specifically, there was no evidence for increased loss of serum proteins during CAPD.

The laboratory results in six patients changed from chronic maintenance hemodialysis (H) to CAPD are compared in Table 2. The hemoglobin, hematocrit, creatinine, total serum proteins, serum albumin, calcium, and phosphate during CAPD were not significantly different from those during hemodialysis. However, BUN again was significantly lower during CAPD, and the serum calcium was higher, although the difference just missed statistical significance ($0.1 > p > 0.05$). Thus, CAPD appears to be equal or superior to hemodialysis in maintaining hematological and biochemical balance in these patients.

An important consideration in evaluating CAPD as a treatment modality is patient acceptance. To assess this, we devised a grading system wherein 3+ means the patient liked the treatment extremely well and better than any previous form of dialysis, and offered no significant complaints; 2+ means the patient liked the treatment very well and offered some minor complaints; 1+ means the patient accepted the treatment but offered a number of complaints; and unacceptable means the patient could not tolerate the treatment and/or had major complaints. Following this scoring system, 16 patients found CAPD acceptable; the acceptance was 1+ in 2, 2+ in 2, and 3+ in 12 (Table 3). Five patients found the treatment unacceptable and had to be withdrawn and returned to alternate forms of dialysis. Of those who found the treatment acceptable, two additional patients had to be withdrawn. The reasons for withdrawal in the two groups are depicted in Table 4. Of the patients in the high acceptance group, one was withdrawn because of return of function and the second because of recurrent peritonitis. In the low acceptance group, however, the reasons for withdrawal consisted of intolerable abdominal distension in three, eye to hand incoordination in two, hypotension in two, dehydration in one, and uncontrollable anxiety and/or depression in three. CAPD therefore was highly acceptable to 70% or more of patients so treated.

Aside from the 21 patients trained in CAPD, we have trained an additional 34 patients in CIPD over a 3-year period (Table 5). During this time the patients developed 36 episodes of peritonitis, 20 episodes among the CIPD

TABLE 3.
Acceptance of CAPD

			Total Number
Acceptable	1+	2	
	2+	2	
	3+	12	
			16
Unacceptable			5
Total			21

TABLE 4.
Reasons for Discontinuing CAPD

High Acceptance Group (2 Patients)	
Return of function	1
Recurrent peritonitis	1
Low Acceptance Group (5 Patients)	
Abdominal distension	3
Eye to hand incoordination	2
Hypotension	2
Dehydration	1
Anxiety/depression	3

patients and 16 among the CAPD patients. No organism could be identified in 9 (25%) of these; of the remaining 27, *Staphylococcus* accounted for 14, *Pseudomonas* and *Streptococcus* for 4 each, *Escherichia coli* for 2, and *Acetobacter, proteus,* and *Candida* accounted for 1 each.

It is important to note that the majority of our patients had no peritonitis at all. Fifty-nine percent of CIPD patients (20/34) and 67% of CAPD patients (14/21) had no peritonitis; 29% of CIPD patients (10/34) and 14% of CAPD patients (3/21) had only one episode (Fig. 1). Thus, 38% of the patients accounted for 100% of the peritonitis episodes and 9% accounted for 44% of peritonitis episodes. Also, the occurrence of peritonitis did not correlate with the duration of treatment either with CIPD or with CAPD. There are

TABLE 5.
Peritonitis in Peritoneal Dialysis

Number of Patients		
CIPD	34	
CAPD	21	
Total		55
Number of Episodes		
CIPD	20 (3 years)	
CAPD	16 (1 year)	
Total		36
Cause		
No Growth		9
Known Growth		
Staphylococcus epidermidis	6	
Staphylococcus aureus	8	
Pseudomonas	4	
Gamma *Streptococcus*	3	
E. coli	2	
Alpha *Streptococcus*	1	
Acetobacter	1	
Proteus	1	
Candida	1	
Total		27

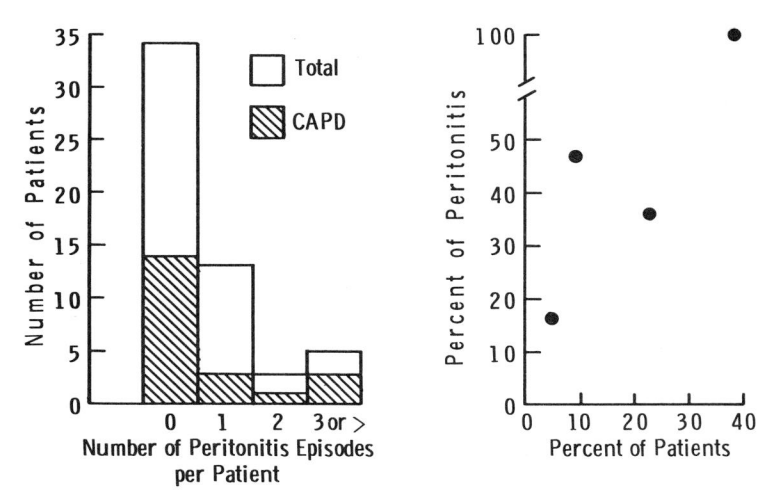

Figure 1. Numbers of patients with 0, 1, 2, or 3 or more episodes of peritonitis (left), and the percentage of patients responsible for different percentage of peritonitis episodes (right).

patients who have had no peritonitis after 23 months on CIPD, whereas others had two or more episodes of peritonitis in 10–15 months of therapy (Figs. 2 and 3). The frequency or incidence of peritonitis, however, was higher in CAPD, being one episode per 4.6 patient-months in contrast to one episode per 22 patient-months in CIPD. Another difference between CIPD and

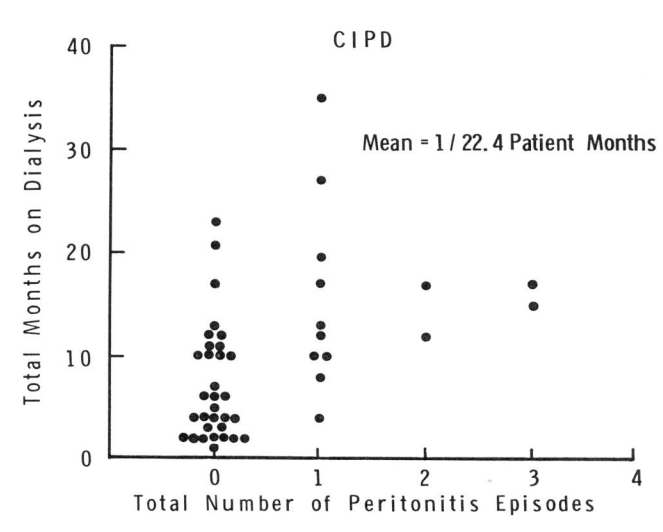

Figure 2. Duration of dialysis in CIPD patients who have had 0, 1, 2, 3, or 4 episodes of peritonitis.

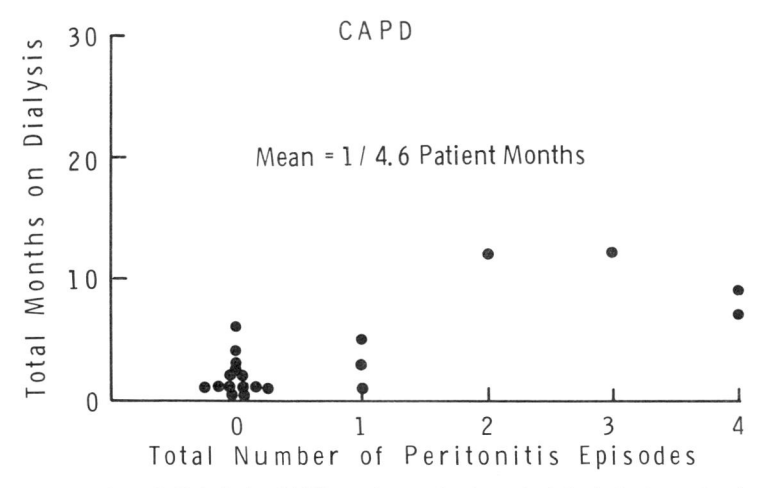

Figure 3. Duration of dialysis in CAPD patients who have had 0, 1, 2, 3, or 4 episodes of peritonitis.

CAPD has to do with the interval after commencing dialysis at which peritonitis was first noted (Fig. 4). In CIPD the first episode of peritonitis occurred after variable intervals that could number many months. Second and third episodes also followed at variable intervals. By contrast, in patients treated with CAPD five of the seven first episodes of peritonitis occurred

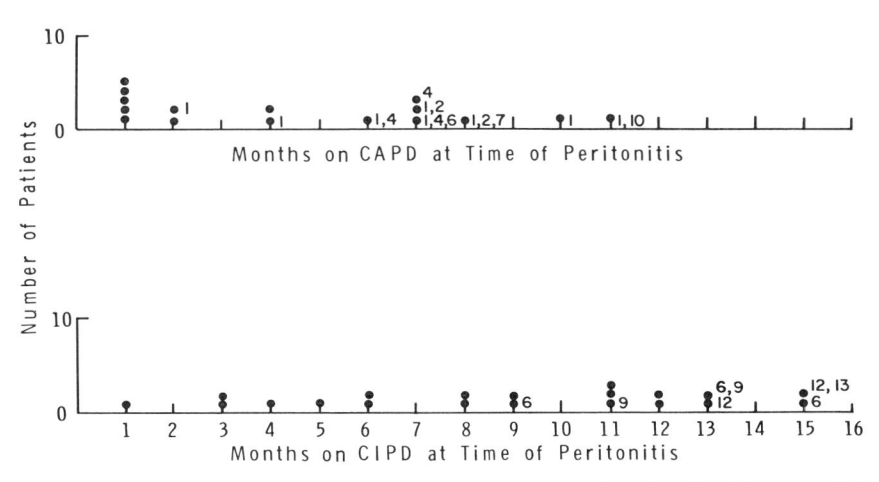

Figure 4. Time on dialysis at which first or subsequent episodes of peritonitis occurred in individual patients undergoing CAPD (top) or CIPD (bottom). First episodes of peritonitis are indicated by closed circles alone; closed circles followed by numbers indicate repeat peritonitis episodes. The number next to a closed circle indicates the month during which the repeat episode occurred.

TABLE 6.

Laboratory Results in Patients Changing from CIPD to PDPD

	Blood Urea Nitrogen		Creatinine		Total Protein		Albumin		Potassium		Calcium		Phosphate	
	I[a]	PD[b]	I	PD	I	PD	I	PD	I	PD	I	PD	I	PD
Mean	76	75	15.4	14.6	6.4	6.2	3.5	3.3	3.9	4.3	9.5	9.1	4.9	4.6
S.E.M.	17	4.9	1.6	1.7	0.2	0.3	0.2	0.3	0.6	0.4	0.2	0.2	0.7	0.6
p	NS		NS		NS		NS		NS		NS		NS	

[a] I is CIPD.
[b] PD is PDPD.

within the first 4 weeks of commencing treatment, and 60% of these went on to develop second, third, or fourth episodes of peritonitis.

Although the reasons for these differences are not understood, it does not seem unreasonable to propose that patients selected for CAPD who develop episode of peritonitis within the first month be removed from the program in an effort to reduce the high incidence of peritonitis in what is otherwise an extremely effective and highly accepted approach.

Finally, we wish to draw attention to a subset of patients for whom CAPD may not be practicable because of impaired vision or manual dexterity, and where a mate or assistant may not be able to effect all four or five exchanges. In a group of four such patients we have been able to prolong the dwell time on the AMP cycler to 3–4 hours for the first three exchanges. The fourth exchange is then instilled and the patient disconnected until the time of the next day's dialysis. We have labeled this form of dialysis, automated prolonged-dwell peritoneal dialysis (PDPD). The laboratory results on four patients during this form of dialysis are compared to the results during treatment with CIPD in Table 6. There were no specific differences between the results during either treatment modality. PDPD is therefore an effective alternative to CIPD in patients not eligible for CAPD.

In summary, CAPD is equal or superior to hemodialysis and CIPD in effecting metabolic control in patients with end-stage renal disease requiring dialysis. It is also highly accepted and preferred to other forms of dialysis. CAPD, however, is associated with high incidence of peritonitis. This may possibly be improved upon by withdrawing the small percent of patients who are responsible for most episodes of peritonitis. Finally, a modification of CAPD may be applicable to patients previously considered ineligible.

CHAPTER TWENTY-SIX

Cost and Social Benefits of CAPD in a Pediatric Population

JAMES SHMERLING, M.S.

EDWARD KOHAUT, M.D.

STEPHEN PERRY, M.S.

RECENTLY A NUMBER OF AUTHORS have demonstrated that adults with end-stage renal failure could be successfully and easily managed at home with continuous ambulatory peritoneal dialysis (CAPD).[1-5] Since the current management of end-stage renal failure in children is less than optimal, a CAPD program was initiated on a trial basis at The Children's Hospital in Birmingham, Alabama (TCH). Most children with end-stage renal failure are poor home dialysis candidates. This is due to many factors, most of which are related to their instability during dialysis. Since CAPD does not cause rapid shifts of fluid and solute,[1,2] it was our feeling that this might be an ideal method of home dialysis for young patients. Since most children do require in-center dialysis, the cost of maintenance dialysis in the pediatric population is high. The purpose of this chapter is to compare the cost of in-center hemodialysis with that of CAPD in the pediatric population and to relate this to patient acceptability and other social benefits.

METHODOLOGY

Although seven patients were entered into the program, four children aged 6–18 years are currently maintained on CAPD at TCH. Total costs of these patients were analyzed. Costs have been broken down into three categories. First, direct costs include expenses directly attributable to the services and supplies provided during dialysis therapy. Second, indirect costs include all expenses incurred while procuring those services. Third, direct patient costs

The Children's Hospital of Birmingham, Birmingham, Alabama

are those that must be borne directly by the family. These costs were compared with costs incurred in in-center hemodialysis. The direct costs were determined by several methods. This included interviews with the dialysis team members, who compiled a list of supplies used weekly by the patients undergoing both hemodialysis and CAPD. The cost of these supplies was then computed using the hospital supply cost schedule. The costs of labor were taken from the hospital's 1979 Medicare cost report. In that report the percentage of time spent by each team member providing dialysis treatment was applied to the total salary. This computation allocated the appropriate amount of the salary to the cost of providing dialysis therapy. Indirect costs were taken from the hospital's 1979 Medicare report form. Direct patient costs incurred as a consequence of dialysis therapy were computed after interviews with the patient and family members.

An attempt was also made to determine patient acceptability and social benefit of therapy. The major benefit, of course, would be an improved quality of life; therefore a questionnaire was developed to analyze subjective impressions of the pediatric patients undergoing CAPD who had previously undergone hemodialysis. The questionnaire was not intended to be a definitive test for determining the psychological impact of dialysis; rather it was intended to reflect the attitudes of several patients regarding both dialysis modalities.

RESULTS

Detailed costs are shown in Table 1. The first item identified in the table is supply cost. This category is comprised of supplies obtained from the central

TABLE 1.
Comparison of Total Costs of CAPD and In-Center Hemodialysis

	Hemodialysis Annual	CAPD Annual	Projected CAPD Annual
Direct Costs			
Supplies, general	$13,965.14	$ 1,763.84	$ 1,763.84
Pharmacy	235.79	13,635.96	8,400.00
Total supplies	$14,200.93	$15,399.80	$10,163.84
Laboratory	2,374.29	558.48	558.48
Labor	11,394.22	7,123.65	2,606.33
Miscellaneous	813.28	372.32	372.32
Total direct	$29,623.04	$23,454.25	$13,700.97
Indirect Costs			
General overhead	$ 3,857.19	0.00	0.00
Other indirect	2,240.16	447.27	447.27
Total indirect costs	6,097.35	447.27	447.27
Total Direct and Indirect Costs	$35,720.39	$23,901.52	$14,148.24

supply department and pharmacy. Although the general supply costs from central supply appear to be less for CAPD than for hemodialysis, CAPD supplies became 20% more expensive once the pharmacy costs were added. This would appear to be contrary to previous studies, which indicated the need for fewer supplies at less expense for CAPD patients.[1-7] A more detailed analysis of the pharmacy supply costs follows. Ninety percent of the total supply cost originated in the pharmacy. Of the $296.00 weekly cost of CAPD, pharmacy costs comprised approximately $186.00 that was attributed to the dialysis fluid. The total cost of labor was $7,123.65 per year for CAPD compared with $11,394.22 per year for hemodialysis. This 37% difference is attributed to the additional man-hours required to maintain pediatric patients on hemodialysis. Previously, it had been documented that pediatric patients require more supervision while on hemodialysis than do adults.[8] Pediatric patients managed on CAPD spend a minimum amount of time in the hospital, consequently utilizing fewer personnel. The social workers' and dietitians' salaries remained the same because there was no correlation between their daily patient activities and the amount of time each patient spent in the hospital for routine treatment. Therefore analysis for direct cost revealed that CAPD was 20% less than hemodialysis. Indirect cost for general overhead such as building depreciation, housekeeping, and plant operations were not incurred by the CAPD patients since they spent the majority of time at home. According to the Medicare cost report $3,857.19 was spent per patient undergoing treatment on hemodialysis. Other indirect costs include business office, communication, purchasing, employee health and welfare, central supply, and medical records utilized by CAPD patients. However this indirect cost was only $8.60 per week, or 90% less than for the hemodialysis patient. Corresponding costs for each of these areas are shown in Table 1. Indirect costs incurred by patients, of course, vary greatly. However, the average patient spent three times as much in travel costs getting back and forth from hemodialysis. The patient suffering from chronic renal failure who is on hemodialysis incurred a total yearly cost of $35,720.00; however, those managed on CAPD incurred an annual expense of only $23,902.00. This represents a 33% over-all saving for the patient treated with CAPD.

Total costs for CAPD and hemodialysis are also demonstrated in Table 1 as well as the projected cost of CAPD when two very important variables are changed. First, currently we have an increased pharmacy cost since fluid is only available in 2-liter bags and our pharmacy must transfer these into smaller bags. Second, the current figures are based on a patient to nurse ratio of 4 to 1. It is our aim to have approximately an 8 to 1 nurse-to-patient ratio. It is therefore projected that once the CAPD program becomes fully operational costs will fall further.

The social and psychological benefits as determined by the response to our questionnaire were found to include patient's adaptability in respect to social life, peer relationship, mood, effect, activity levels, school performance, behavioral changes, and his/her feelings and fantasies regarding dialysis therapy. Hemodialysis was cited by all four patients as an impediment to their social life, recreational activities, and school performance. All of the children in school who were on hemodialysis expressed discontent with the arrangements made for them to continue their schooling while receiving hemodialysis therapy. These arrangements usually were home-bound teachers. They stated that since they were on CAPD and could attend school regularly they were getting a much wider educational experience as well as feeling much more content because of increased peer contact. Only one of the patients expressed a degree of psychological discomfort regarding the CAPD catheter protruding from his abdomen. The wearing of the appliance seemed to arouse fear of being stigmatized by his peers. However, one question posed to that same patient concerning his social life suggested that in actuality this had improved since being placed on CAPD. No mention of stigmatization was made by any of the other patients.

When the patients were asked what they liked and disliked most about CAPD and hemodialysis the responses were very similar. All the patients indicated that the freedom of time and movement were the most advantageous aspects of CAPD. Two patients also cited their ability to manage their own therapy and therefore control of their own life as being a significant advantage that hemodialysis had not permitted. The only displeasure for CAPD was expressed by one of the patients who again did not like wearing the external appliance. The final question required each of the patients to rate hemodialysis and CAPD on a scale of 1 to 10; one representing the least amount of satisfaction and 10 representing the most. The over-all rating reflected a significant and more favorable attitude for CAPD than for hemodialysis.

DISCUSSION

From both a cost and patient acceptance aspect, CAPD seems to be a viable alternative for the pediatric patient with end-stage renal failure. The costs even at this point in time are less than in-center hemodialysis. We would expect the cost to fall even further. The cost analysis done during this study was done at a time when only 2-liter bags were available. It is our understanding that shortly bags of varying size will be available, which will eliminate pharmacy labor costs.

Not included in this cost summary were hospitalizations for extraordinary events. This was not included since, although the incidence of peritonitis in our CAPD patients is significant, only two patients have required hospitalization. Most cases of peritonitis are treated at home with intraperitoneal antibiotics and therefore the cost is minimal. We feel that this is more than offset by cost of shunt revisions, which occur in our hemodialysis patients with a fair degree of regularity.

The direct family costs were not tabulated in exact figures since this study was done retrospectively and the families had not kept accurate records. All of the families suggested that CAPD was much less of a burden on them than in-center hemodialysis. In Alabama we deal with a rural population, many of our patients living 50 to 200 miles from the center. At current transportation costs if a patient lived 50 miles away, an $18.00 transportation fee for each round trip for hemodialysis would be incurred. We are currently seeing our CAPD patients every 2 weeks; therefore transportation costs are only 17% of in-center hemodialysis transportation costs. I suspect as our patient group stabilizes even further and we have the availability of bags of varying size that could be shipped directly to the patient's house, trips will become even less frequent.

Although this series was small, the response of our patients to CAPD was gratifying. As is typical of most children and adolescents, all of them showed initial fear of trying something different. This was especially true of the patients who had been doing reasonably well on hemodialysis. After a short period of time, however, all found that CAPD was a more acceptable form of therapy.

References

1. Popovich, R., Moncrief, J., Nolph, K., et al.: Continuous ambulatory peritoneal dialysis. *Ann Intern Med* **88**: 449–56, 1978.
2. Oreopoulos, D.: The coming of age of continuous ambulatory peritoneal dialysis (CAPD). *Dial Transplant* **8**: 460–1, 517, 1979.
3. Sorrels, A.: Continuous ambulatory peritoneal dialysis. *Am J Med* 1400–1401, 1979.
4. Moncrief, J., Nolph, K., Rubin, J., et al.: Additional experience with continuous ambulatory peritoneal dialysis (CAPD). *Trans Am Soc Artif Intern Organs* **24**: 476–482, 1978.
5. Nolph, K., Popovich, R., and Moncrief, J.: Theoretical and practical implications of continuous ambulatory peritoneal dialysis. *Nephron* **21**: 117–122, 1978.
6. Orepoulos, D., Robson, M., and Izatt, S.: A Simple and safe technique for continuous ambulatory peritoneal dialysis (CAPD). *Trans Am Soc Artif Intern Organs* **24**: 484–489, 1978.
7. Oreopoulos, D., Robson, M., Faller, B., et al.: Continuous ambulatory peritoneal dialysis: A new era in the treatment of chronic renal failure. *Clin Neph* **2**: 125–128, 1979.
8. Levy, N.: *Living or Dying; Adaption to Hemodialysis.* Charles C Thomas, Springfield, Ill., 1978.

CHAPTER TWENTY-SEVEN

Clinical Parameters in Continuous Ambulatory Peritoneal Dialysis for Infants and Children

STEVEN R. ALEXANDER,* M.D.

CLEVERT H. TSENG,* M.D.

KRISTINE A. MAKSYM,* R.N.

ROBERT A. CAMPBELL,* M.D.

Y. B. TALWALKAR,* M.D.

E. C. KOHAUT,† M.D.

WHEN POPOVICH AND MONCRIEF conceived the chronic dialysis technique now called continuous ambulatory peritoneal dialysis (CAPD) in 1975, they were not sure the method could be practically adapted for use in children.[1] The initial proposal predicting successful dialysis using the CAPD technique carefully noted that the analysis was based on daily dialysate volumes of 10 liters.[2] Joined by Nolph in further collaborative studies, their initial reports documenting effective dialysis using the CAPD technique continued to limit the practical application and implications of these early clinical trial results to use in the adult patient.[3,4] And with good reason. Forced to use heavy 2-liter bottles of dialysate, the Texas/Missouri original CAPD technique was inconvenient and unwieldy, even for some adults. The full peritoneal catheter connect/disconnect procedure required at each exchange and the design of the dialysate bottle's entry port also contributed to an unacceptable rate of peritonitis, which threatened continuation of the method, despite excellent results in control of uremia.

Fortunately, the same dialysate solution (Dianeal, Travenol) was available in Canada, but in 2-liter plastic bags. In Toronto, Oreopoulos enthusiastically embraced the concept of CAPD for his adult patients and devised the delivery method now used in most CAPD programs.[5] Use of plastic bags reduced the

---

*Division of Pediatric Nephrology, Department of Pediatrics, Doernbecher Memorial Hospital for Children, University of Oregon Health Sciences Center, Portland, Oregon

†Division of Pediatric Nephrology, University of Alabama in Birmingham, Birmingham, Alabama

incidence of peritonitis to one episode every 7.1 patient-months,[6] a tolerable, if not entirely acceptable, rate. By 1978, plastic bags of dialysate were finally available for use in the United States, leading to increased activity in evaluating CAPD in adult patients.[7]

Pediatric nephrologists followed these developments with interest, but they remained leery of CAPD. The availability of dialysate only in 2-liter bags versus the need for variable intraperitoneal volumes as low as 200 cc in their smaller patients created an immediate stumbling block. The peritonitis issue was also a strong deterrent for many pediatric nephrologists.[8]

The Pediatric Nephrology Division of the University of Oregon Health Sciences Center began a limited study of CAPD in a small child then being maintained on in-center chronic intermittent peritoneal dialysis (IPD) in October of 1978. Preliminary results were encouraging and led to the development of a Pediatric CAPD Program in February 1979.

During a 5-month period from February to June of 1979, three children, aged 9 months to 5 years, required definitive therapy for end-stage renal disease (ESRD) and were unacceptable candidates for renal transplantation. In-center dialysis was also a poor alternative, since all children lived 100–250 miles from the pediatric dialysis center. More importantly, each of these families was highly motivated to engage in home dialysis. A fourth child (aged 5.5 years) who had been on in-center intermittent peritoneal dialysis for the previous 2 years joined the CAPD program because of frequent catheter dysfunction and the desire of the family to dialyze the child at home.

This chapter primarily describes our clinical experience with CAPD in these four young children, all of whom have been maintained on CAPD for 12 ± 2 months. Data from three older children (10–20 years of age) who entered the Oregon CAPD program within the past 6 months are included where appropriate for comparison with the small children. Growth data on four children maintained on CAPD at the University of Alabama in Birmingham are also included.

This report must be considered preliminary, if for no other reason than the small number of patients involved. One of the purposes of such a report is to stimulate interest in the development of CAPD programs within other Pediatric Nephrology Divisions. We hope to achieve this by describing in sufficient detail those clinical parameters that have proved most helpful to us in the care of the young CAPD patient.

METHODS

Patient selection

All aspects of the Pediatric CAPD Program were first approved by the University of Oregon Health Sciences Center Committee for Research Involving Human Subjects.

Pediatric patients to be considered for CAPD must first meet the usual physiological criteria for ESRD of sufficient severity to mandate some form of chronic dialysis therapy. In our Center this usually also will imply that the child is not a suitable candidate for renal transplantation at the time dialysis is initiated. Age, size, previous transplant rejections, and high titers of preformed cytotoxic antibodies are some of the factors that prevent or delay renal transplantation. A child will also be considered for CAPD if he or she must begin dialysis while on the list awaiting a cadaveric renal transplant.

Second, there must be good indication that the child and parents are sufficiently motivated to learn and comply with a home dialysis program. Economic factors play a small role here in the case of the single working parent, but this has not proved a real obstacle to home CAPD when the dialysis schedule is designed around the parent's work schedule. Children younger than 16 years of age must have at least one parent willing to take primary responsibility for their CAPD. This parent (usually the mother) will receive the most intensive training. It is essential that a second adult receive training if the child is too young to do self-dialysis. Fathers or grandparents usually fulfill this back-up role.

Before acceptance for CAPD training, any other medically acceptable chronic dialysis techniques available in our center (in-center hemodialysis or intermittent peritoneal dialysis, home automated peritoneal dialysis) are presented in detail. Written informed consent is then obtained from parents and from the child if 8 years of age or older.

The training program

Details of the CAPD training program have been described elsewhere.[9] We have found a team approach essential to successful training. If medically possible, 2 weeks are devoted to education and preparation of the child and family, both for the operative catheter placement and the subsequent CAPD training course.

Peritoneal catheter placement

All catheters are placed surgically. It is of inestimable value to develop a close working relationship with a surgeon who is either experienced in this procedure or interested in developing expertise in surgical management of chronic peritoneal catheters. On the day prior to catheter placement, it is our practice to have the attending pediatric nephrologist and the surgeon see the child together to determine placement site and measure directly on the child the proposed tunnel course. This allows preparation of the catheter to suit the individual child by gluing each of the two Dacron velour cuffs at the appropriate sites on the catheter. The catheter is then allowed to cure overnight before resterilization preoperatively.

We use only "adult" size Tenckhoff catheters with two unattached cuffs. The length of the intraperitoneal portion is estimated to be a centimeter or so longer than the distance between symphysis and umbilicus. Infants and small children may need removal of up to 5.0 cm of the intraperitoneal portion to prevent coiling in the pelvis. At least 5 cm should remain between the peritoneum and the first catheter side hole.

Placement of the proximal cuff has been most successful when a "collar" of peritoneum is sutured in a purse-string fashion, which encloses 0.1–0.2 cm of the base of the cuff. This same suture is secured to the cuff at a single point through the substance of the cuff before tightening the purse string to form a collar (Fig. 1).

The subcutaneous tunnel should be short (4–6 cm) and straight, usually passing at a slight angle from the midline to an exit wound on the upper abdomen in infants and small children, more laterally in older children (Fig. 1). Adolescent patients may prefer a tunnel and entry site well away from the midline for cosmetic reasons. The catheter exit wound must be at least 0.5 cm from the distal edge of the superficial cuff to prevent skin erosion and infection at the exit site.

An exception to the use of the "adult" size Tenckhoff is the infant weighing less than 5 kg. It is hoped that a wider choice of pediatric catheters will become more readily available.

Catheter position is checked intraoperatively by x-ray before closure of the peritoneum. The use of a radio-opaque catheter facilitates this procedure. More important than the x-ray is successful institution of dialysis before skin closure.

We routinely use continuous low volume passes (15 cc/kg) to document

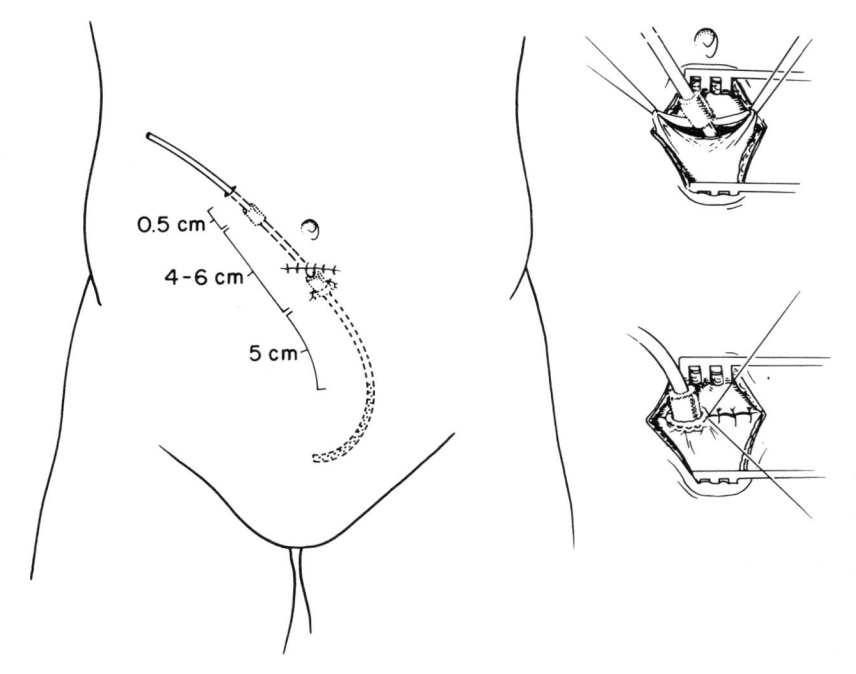

Figure 1. Schematic drawing of the technique of peritoneal catheter placement (see text for details).

catheter function and provide additional irrigation with a dialysis solution containing a cephalosporin at a concentration of 100 mg/liter.

Intraoperative peritoneogram and partial omentectomy have also been adopted as routine procedures and are described in detail elsewhere.[10]

Initiation of dialysis

Dialysis begins in the operating room and continues without interruption ideally until the patient is on a CAPD schedule 6–8 days later. For the first 6 hours postoperatively, an exchange volume of 15 cc/kg of 1.5% dialysate is used, to which has been added heparin: 500 U/liter. More hypertonic dialysate may be required if the child is clinically hypervolemic. Of concern at this point is prevention of catheter obstruction or migration. For the first 6 hours postoperatively, two exchanges per hour are used; drain times are limited to 5 or 10 minutes per exchange. After 6 hours, the exchanges are extended to 1 hour, again avoiding prolonged drains, which can engulf the catheter in omentum at a time when there is a greater risk of fibrin plugs becoming lodged within its lumen.

A single dialysate return sample is cultured daily for the first 4 to 7 days postoperatively. It is no longer our practice to use prophylactic intraperitoneal cephalosporin during this period in an attempt to slow emergence of cephalosporin-resistant strains in our unit.

In search of the "dry weight"

From the second postoperative day, standard 1-hour intermittent peritoneal dialysis is gradually converted to a CAPD regimen by sequential increases in dwell periods and dialysate volumes. This continuous process allows the gentle removal of excess body water to approach the patient's dry weight. Blood pressure control is maintained as long as necessary with antihypertensives, but our experience has shown an ability to reduce antihypertensive dosage beginning as soon as the first full week of CAPD. We routinely use a CAPD regimen consisting of five exchanges per day at a volume that is slowly increased to 28–30 cc/kg.

During this period, CAPD training begins in earnest and takes approximately 2 weeks. The second week may be accomplished as an outpatient in older children, but infants and young children will often require the full 2 weeks for stabilization in the hospital.

The home training program

Daily training sessions are required to instruct parents in the fundamental pediatric CAPD procedures: 1) the continuous peritoneal dialysis process; 2) methods required to apply the small volume bag technique; 3) safe dialysate bag exchanges; 4) meticulous exit site care; 5) sterile connecting tubing change; and 6) dialysate culture methods. Our patients are currently maintained on five exchanges per day, 7 days per week using exchange volumes of 20–35 cc/kg for each child. This yields actual exchange volumes of 200–400

TABLE 1.
Characteristics of Pediatric Patients at Initiation of CAPD; University of Oregon Health Sciences Center

Patient	Sex	Diagnosis	Date of CAPD Onset	Age	Weight (kg)/ Height (cm)	Distance (miles) of Home from CAPD Center
M.P.	Male	Focal glomerulosclerosis	2/16/79	17 months	9.92/75.8	245
M.W.	Female	Rapidly progressive glomerulonephritis	5/01/79	9 months	7.25/67.5	110
C.B.	Female	Left renal dysplasia Right renal aplasia	6/19/79	$5^{9}/_{12}$ years	10.82/86.4	15
J.H.	Male	Renal dysplasia Posterior urethral valves	6/20/79	$5^{11}/_{12}$ years	14.1/100.3	110
K.F.	Female	Systemic lupus erythematosis nephritis	2/7/80	20 years	49/152.8	200
D.H.	Male	Chronic glomerulonephritis Renal transplant rejection	3/05/80	15 years	24/115	177
A.S.	Male	Henoch-Schönlein nephritis	4/14/80	10 years	23.8/135	600

TABLE 2.
Characteristics of Pediatric Patients at Initiation of CAPD; University of Oregon Health Sciences Center

Patient	Age	Residual Creatinine Clearance (cc/minute/1.73 m^2)	Average Urine Output (cc/day)	Prior ESRD Therapy	Reasons for Selecting CAPD
M.P.	17 months	Anuric	Anuric	None	Size/age
M.W.	9.5 months	Anuric	Anuric	None	Size/age
C.B.	5^{9}/$_{12}$ years	2.5	650	In-center IPD for 14 months. Two cadaveric transplants Parathyroid autotransplant	Parent preference Highly sensitized
J.H.	5^{11}/$_{12}$ years	2.83	600	Two cadaveric transplants Parathyroid autotransplant	Parent preference Highly sensitized
K.F.	20 years	3.1	200 cc	None	Parent and patient preference Distance from CAPD center
D.H.	15 years	<1.0	100 cc	Three cadaveric transplants in-center HD (1½ years)	Parent and patient preference; status after 3 renal transplants
A.S.	10 years	<1.0	75 cc	In-center IPD (2 months); in-center HD (1 year)	Parent and patient preference

ml. (With only 2-liter plastic bags available, the small volume bag technique using 600–1000 cc transfer packs is still mandatory.) Parents learn, using strict aseptic techniques, how to add heparin and other medications to the 2-liter bags and then how to measure and transfer the appropriate exchange volume of dialysate solution from the 2-liter bag into 600 or 1000 ml capacity transfer packs. Since the CAPD locking tubing with titanium adapter became available, tubing changes are made monthly by the head CAPD nurse. Parents are still instructed in this technique so that in an emergency they can safely perform this procedure.

Parents are also taught a daily routine of brief but careful assessment and recording of their child's weight, blood pressure, the quality and quantity of the peritoneal fluid, and the condition of the skin at the exit site. This, plus teaching parents about the possible complications that can occur, enable the parents quickly to recognize and report problems to the pediatric nephrologist or lead CAPD nurse.

Process for follow-up

The child's home CAPD program is monitored closely after discharge by the pediatric nephrologist and the lead CAPD nurse. Methods used are: 1) home visits during the first month and at intervals thereafter; 2) biweekly telephone contact with the family; 3) reports from the child's local physician; and 4) monthly visits to the pediatric CAPD clinic. During these monthly visits, the child receives a thorough evaluation, the sterile tubing change is performed, and parents are given refresher minicourses on CAPD procedures and other aspects of the child's care as required. Group meetings involving all parents and medical support team members have been utilized to provide ongoing support and communication.

TABLE 3.

Average Biochemical Values Among Four Pediatric Patients on CAPD[a] for 10 Months

Serum creatinine	6.8 mg%
Blood urea nitrogen	66.0 mg%
Serum sodium	137.0 mEq/liter
Serum potassium	4.6 mEq/liter
Total CO$_2$	22.1 mEq/liter
Serum calcium	9.0 mg%
Serum phosphorus	5.3 mg%
Total protein	5.7 g%
Albumin	3.4 g%
Glucose	99.0 mg%
Cholesterol	190.0 mg%
Triglycerides	287.0 mg%
Hematocrit	25.8%
Hemoglobin	8.2 g%
Dialysate protein losses	2.7 g/24 hours

[a] Five exchanges/day; "2.5%" dialysate; exchange volume = 30 cc/kg.

PATIENT POPULATION

Tables 1 and 2 summarize descriptive data for each CAPD patient: age at onset of CAPD, sex, weight/height, diagnosis, residual creatinine clearance and average daily urine volume, prior ESRD therapy, reason for selecting CAPD over other forms of therapy, date CAPD was begun, and distance patient lives from dialysis center.

Table 3 gives average biochemical values of the four small children who have been maintained for 10 or more months on CAPD. By a slow but definite progression, dialysate glucose concentration has been increased in all to an average of 2.5 g% to give adequate ultrafiltration on an unlimited diet.

Figure 2 is a composite of the linear growth charts of the four small children in Oregon. Growth has corresponded directly to periods of adequate calorie intake in the absence of any complications, such as peritonitis or inguinal hernia.

Table 4 is a similar representation of linear growth of the four children in Alabama.

COMPLICATIONS

Table 5 lists complications encountered in six patients in Oregon on CAPD for at least 1 month. Peritonitis occurred in three children and is examined in more detail in Table 6. The severity of the infection was directly related to where the organism was acquired. All home-acquired episodes of peritonitis responded to intraperitoneal antibiotics alone in 7 days, usually without alteration in CAPD schedule. A more detailed description of this treatment plan is in preparation.

DISCUSSION

Infants and small children with ESRD present particularly difficult management problems using standard forms of chronic dialysis therapy. CAPD was considered for these patients as a new alternative. Although our experience remains limited, the over-all results are encouraging and prompt a brief comparison with other available methods.

TABLE 4.
Linear Growth of Children Maintained on CAPD in Alabama

Patient	Sex	Age at Onset CAPD (years)	Months on CAPD	Height at Onset CAPD (cm)	Present Height (cm)
S.W.	Male	16½	8	154.5	158
J.T.	Male	5½	6	103.5	105.0
S.W.	Female	15	9	142.0	144.5
S.J.	Male	19	5	164.5	165.5

204   CAPD Update

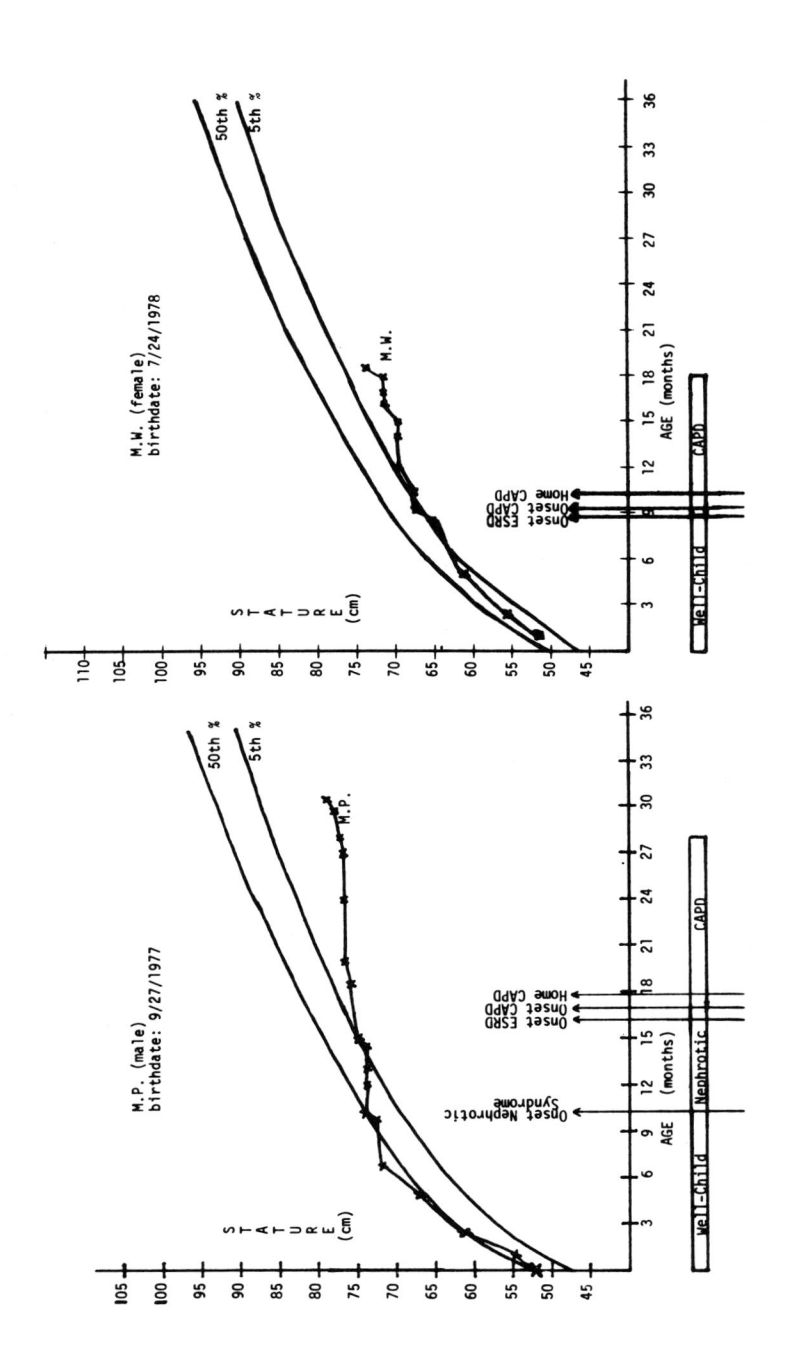

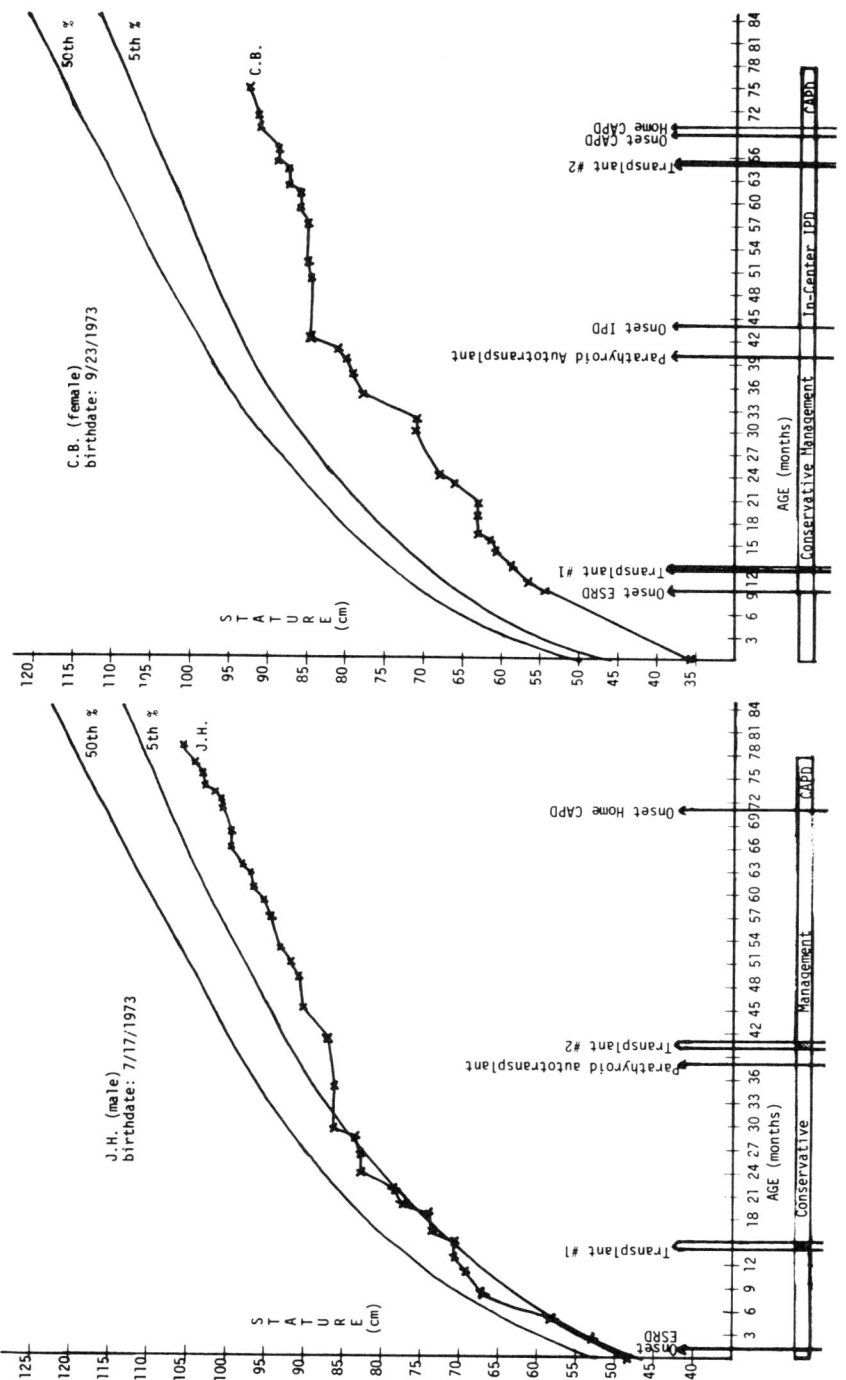

Clinical Parameters in CAPD for Infants and Children 205

Figure 2. Linear growth of the four youngest children in the Oregon CAPD program.

TABLE 5.
Complications Seen in Pediatric Patients on CAPD for More Than One Month

	$N = 6$
Peritonitis	3
Inadequate ultrafiltration, chronic mild hypervolemia, hypertension	3
Transient hypovolemia, vomiting, mild hypotension	3
Periods of poor feeding	3
Hypokalemia or hypophosphatemia early in CAPD course	2
Hyponatremia	1
Exit-site infection	1
Dialysate leakage from exit site lasting more than 7 days after post catheter placement	1
Tunnel trauma producing self-limited bloody dialysate	1
Incisional hernia	1
Inguinal hernia	2
"Parent fatigue"	4

TABLE 6.
Bacterial Peritonitis in Pediatric Patients on CAPD[a]

Patient	Months on CAPD	Number of Episodes	Causative Organisms		"Hospital Acquired"
M.W.	11	None	—		
M.P.	14½	7	*Staphylococcus* coagulase negative	(2)	(1)
			Streptococcus faecalis	(1)	(1)
			Staphylococcus epidermidis	(2)	
			Staphylococcus aureus		
C.B.	10	8	*Streptococcus viridans*	(2)	
			Staphylococcus, coagulase positive	(2)	
			Staphylococcus, coagulase negative	(2)	(1)
			Streptococcus faecalis	(1)	(1)
			Pseudomonas aeruginosa	(1)	(1)
J.H.	10	None	—		
K.F.	2	None	—		
D.H.	1	1	Actinobacter	(1)	(1)
A.S.	½	None	—		

[a] Compiled April 30, 1980.

Hemodialysis

Chronic hemodialysis is technically difficult in small children, although a few major centers have developed a truly remarkable expertise.[11-15] Problems of vascular access, poor patient/family acceptance as a home dialysis technique, distance from an experienced center, and over-all cost have made chronic hemodialysis unavailable for most small children with ESRD.[16,17]

Intermittent peritoneal dialysis

Increased interest in chronic intermittent peritoneal dialysis for children predated the appearance of CAPD and has enjoyed singular success as a home dialysis program in many centers.[18-20] The procedure is dependent upon expensive, somewhat temperamental machinery that, to date, has not been adapted to the child whose exchange volume is less than 500 cc. Frequent catheter dysfunction and the combination of inefficiency with immobility (40 or more hours per week attached to the machine) have also set limits on the acceptance of this form of therapy.[21]

Transplantation

A functioning kidney remains the goal of all forms of maintenance dialysis. Transplantation has not been successful in infants younger than 1 year of age and has had only limited success in children younger than 3 years of age.[22]

CONCLUSION

CAPD has filled an important gap in existing maintenance dialysis therapy by providing a method by which infants and small children may be maintained at home.

Our early experience suggests that CAPD is an effective, safe, and well-tolerated technique for the chronic maintenance dialysis of infants and small children with ESRD, pending transplantation. It is a home dialysis technique of relative simplicity; it is quickly learned and skillfully performed by parents and other committed adults. Home dialysis offers children and their families an opportunity for near-normal psychosocial development at a critical period in the life of the young child.

Bacterial peritonitis occurs with alarming frequency in some patients and is not seen in others despite similar CAPD methods, training programs, and extensive support services. Peritonitis that is acquired outside the hospital has been a mild infection in our patients, presenting as cloudy dialysate in a minimally symptomatic child. Treatment with intraperitoneal antibiotics alone or in combination with oral antibiotics for 5 to 7 days without altering the standard CAPD regimen has been successful.

Nutrition can theoretically be maximized in children on CAPD. Unlimited protein and augmented caloric intake using dietary supplements and considering glucose absorbed from the dialysate provides an advantage not seen in other forms of chronic dialysis therapy.

Careful attention to fluid balance is required to avoid insidious development of volume overload. Increased fluid intake can be offset by adjusting dialysate glucose concentration to increase ultrafiltration.

Early optimism regarding theoretical growth potential in children on CAPD has been only partially supported by limited experience to date. Truly "stable" CAPD conditions including maximal nutrition have only intermittently been achieved in all patients due to poor appetite or other complications. A more complete evaluation of the metabolic state of young children stabilized on CAPD is now in progress. However, a multicenter cooperative study of pediatric CAPD is needed to obtain statistically adequate data.

ACKNOWLEDGMENTS

This work was supported in part by a grant from the Medical Research Foundation of Oregon. The authors gratefully acknowledge the contributions of the pediatrics nursing and residency staffs of the Doernbecher Memorial Hospital for Children, University of Oregon Health Sciences Center. We are particularly indebted to the following pediatricians who have each provided comprehensive medical care in their home communities for one or more of the patients described in this report: William B. Kohn, M.D., Grants Pass, Oregon; Thomas Roe, M.D., Eugene, Oregon; and Max Stephenson, M.D., Springfield, Oregon.

References

1. Popovich, R.: Personal communication, September 1979.
2. Popovich, R. P., Moncrief, J. S., Decherd, J. B., et al.: The definition of a novel portable/wearable equilibrium peritoneal dialysis technique. *Abstr Am Soc Artif Intern Organs* **5**: 64, 1976.
3. Popovich, R. P., Moncrief, J. W., Nolph, K. D., et al. Continuous ambulatory peritoneal dialysis. *Ann Intern Med* **88**: 4, 1978.
4. Nolph, K. D., Popovich, R. P., and Moncrief, J. W.: Theoretical and practical implications of continuous ambulatory peritoneal dialysis. (Invited editorial.) *Nephron* **21**: 117–122, 1978.
5. Oreopoulos, D. G., Robson, M., Izatt, S., et al.: A simple and safe technique for continuous ambulatory peritoneal dialysis. *Trans Am Soc Artif Intern Organs* **22**: 484–487, 1978.
6. Robson, M. D., and Oreopoulos, D. G.: Continuous ambulatory peritoneal dialysis. *Dial Transplant* **7**: 999–1003, 1978.
7. Moncrief, J. W., Popovich, R. P., Nolph, K. D., et al.: Additional experience with continuous ambulatory peritoneal dialysis (CAPD). *Trans Am Soc Artif Intern Organs* **24**: 476–483, 1978.
8. McEnery, P. T.: Personal communication, October 1979.
9. Maksym, K. A.: A training program for parents of young children on home continuous ambulatory peritoneal dialysis (CAPD). *J Am Assoc Nephrol Nurses Tech* (in press).
10. Alexander, S. R., and Tank, E. S.: Surgical aspects of continuous ambulatory peritoneal dialysis in infants and children. *J Urol* (in press).
11. Mauer, S. M., and Lunch, R. E.: Hemodialysis techniques for infants and children. *Pediatr Clin North Am* **23**: 4, 1976.
12. Cameron, J. S.: The treatment of chronic renal failure in children by regular dialysis and transplantation. *Nephron* **11**: 221, 1973.
13. Potter, D.: Management of the child on chronic dialysis. In *Clinical Pediatric Nephrology*. E. Lieberman, Ed. J. B. Lippincott, Philadelphia, 1976, p. 439.

14. Fine, R. N., and Grushkin, C. M.: Hemodialysis and renal transplantation in children. *Clin Nephrol* **1**: 243, 1973.
15. Mauer, S. M.: Pediatric renal dialysis. In *Pediatric Kidney Disease.* C. M. Edelmann Jr., Ed. Little, Brown, Boston, 1978, pp. 487–502.
16. Potter, D. E.: Comparison of peritoneal dialysis and hemodialysis in children. *Dial Transplant* **7**: 8, 1978.
17. Potter, D.: Management of the child on chronic dialysis. In *Clinical Pediatric Nephrology.* E. Lieberman, Ed., J. B. Lippincott, Philadelphia, 1976, p. 449.
18. Baluarte, J. J., Grossman, M. B., Polinsky, M. S., *et al.:* Experience with intermittent home peritoneal dialysis in children (personal communication).
19. Counts, S., Hickman, R., Garbaccio, A., *et al.:* Chronic home peritoneal dialysis in children. *Trans Am Soc Artif Intern Organs* **19**: 157, 1973.
20. Brouhard, B. H., Berger, M., Travis, L. B., *et al.:* Chronic peritoneal dialysis in children. *Tex Med* **72**: 84, 1976.
21. Day, R., and White, R.: Peritoneal dialysis in children. *Arch Dis Child* **52**: 56, 1977.
22. Hodson, E. M., Najarian, J. S., Kjellstrand, C. M., *et al.:* Renal transplantation in children ages 1 to 5 years. *Pediatrics* **51**: 3, 1978.

CHAPTER TWENTY-EIGHT

An Assessment of Continuous Ambulatory Peritoneal Dialysis (CAPD) in Children

JOHN WILLIAMSON BALFE, M.D., F.R.C.P.(C)

MARGARET-ANN IRWIN, R.N., R.M.N., B.Sc.N., C.D.P.

DIMITRIOS G. OREOPOULOS, M.D., Ph.D., F.R.C.P.(C), F.A.C.P.

IN MANY COUNTRIES continuous ambulatory peritoneal dialysis (CAPD) has now become accepted as an important adjunct for the management of uremia for patients with end-stage renal failure.[1,2] With improved technique, it is relatively safe and easy to perform.[3] Peritonitis continues to be a problem but with technical improvements this should eventually become an infrequent complication.

Experience with children, especially the very young and thus small child, is still limited.[4] Older children have been shown to tolerate the procedure well. The younger patient presents new problems. The response of nutrition, growth, and bone development to CAPD is at present unanswerable. The assessment of children is difficult. Usually their stay on CAPD treatment is short since our current policy is to perform a renal transplant as soon as their condition is relatively stable and safe.

However, the future prospects for CAPD are encouraging and the purpose of this paper is to present our experience and to assess the effect of such therapy.

MATERIALS AND TECHNIQUES

We have admitted 16 patients to our CAPD program over the past 18 months, and Table 1 summarizes the characteristics of these patients. The first 15

Associate Professor of Pediatrics, University of Toronto, Toronto, Ontario, Canada
Head Nurse, Renal Unit, Hospital for Sick Children, Toronto, Ontario, Canada
Associate Professor of Medicine, University of Toronto, Toronto, Ontario, Canada

TABLE 1.
Pediatric CAPD Patients

Patient Number	Sex	Age (years)	Diagnosis	Reason for Choosing CAPD
1	M	15	Medullary cystic disease	No vascular sites High antibodies Two previous transplants
2	M	12	Reflux, pyelonephritis	No vascular sites High antibodies Two previous transplants
3	F	12	Reflux, pyelonephritis	No vascular sites High antibodies Two previous transplants
4	M	5	Triad syndrome	No vascular sites High antibodies Two previous transplants Parent's request
5	F	4	Wilm's tumor	Elective observation Small size
6	F	16	Focal glomerulosclerosis	No vascular sites High antibodies Two previous transplants
7	M	2.5	Congenital nephrosis	Small size High antibodies Distance from unit
8	M	1.5	Obstructive uropathy (urethral valves)	Small size
9	F	5	Focal glomerulosclerosis	Distance from unit Preference
10	F	0.5	Oxalosis	Small size Elective observation
11	F	1.9	Familial hemolytic uremic syndrome	Small size Distance from unit Physician request
12	M	7.9	Hemolytic uremic syndrome	Parent's request
13	M	1.5	Obstructive uropathy (urethral valves)	Small size Distance from unit
14	M	1.7	Obstructive uropathy (dysplastic kidneys)	Small size Distance from unit
15	F	6.8	Renal vein thrombosis Reflux uropathy	Small size Distance from unit
16	M	15.7	Glomerulonephritis	Distance from unit Small size

patients have been treated for 1 month or more, whereas patient 16 is new to the program and thus will have no follow-up data. There are nine males and seven females, with ages ranging from 0.5 to 16 years. The underlying renal disease was pyelonephritis in two, obstructive uropathy or reflux nephropathy

TABLE 2.
Indications for CAPD in Children

1. Very small patient with end-stage renal disease.
2. Very small patient with early renal failure with serious growth failure and/or bone disease.
3. Small patient who requires prolonged elective dialysis prior to renal transplant (for instance, patient with Wilms' tumor).
4. High titer of preformed cytotoxic antibodies.
5. No availability of home or center hemodialysis.
6. Preference of the patient or parent or referring physician.

in five, and glomerulonephritis in five. Medullary cystic disease, triad syndrome, congenital oxalosis, and Wilms' tumor were present in one patient each. The patient with Wilms' tumor was tumor free but was being observed electively for 2–3 years prior to receiving a renal transplant. Five children required CAPD because they had no remaining vascular access sites, a high titer of preformed cytotoxic antibodies, and had rejected two previous renal transplants. In six children their small size would have made hemodialysis extremely difficult, even in a children's dialysis center. Table 2 summarizes what we consider indications for CAPD.

We have found that CAPD in the older pediatric patient has presented no new problems than those already described in adult patients and thus they can be managed technically like an adult. However, for the small child with less than 20 kg body weight, the approach must be modified. Placement of the peritoneal catheter is critical for proper function. We have used various

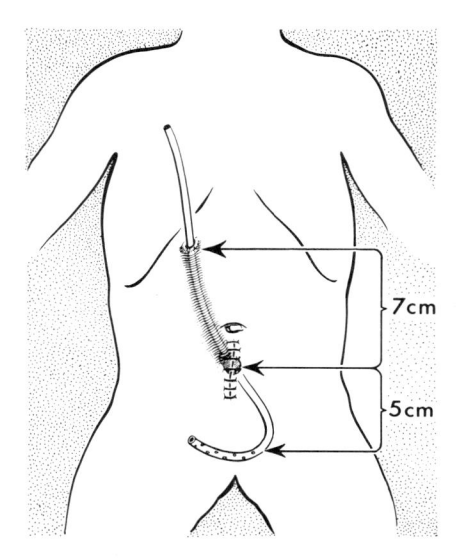

Figure 1. A chronic silastic peritoneal catheter in an infant. The single cuff is positioned at the peritoneal entrance site (the middle arrow). Note a vertical tunnel is preferred for infants.

peritoneal catheters. Some of our catheters have been tailor-made with two Dacron cuffs positioned at each end of a subcutaneous tunnel and two flat Silastic discs in the distal intra-abdominal part of the Silastic catheter (Oreopoulos-Zellerman catheter).[5] Currently, we are using the standard pediatric Tenckhoff catheter. The fixed cuff is removed and the mobile cuff is fixed in place using Silastic glue with a distance of 5 cm between the cuff and the first drainage hole. This seems to be the ideal length to prevent complications of faulty pelvic position because of excessive catheter length or leakage of fluid back along the catheter tunnel observed when the catheter is too short.

Patients are given prophylactic antibiotic 1 hour before operation (tobramycin 1.5 mg/kg; cephalothin 20 mg/kg intravenously). A general anesthetic is necessary with children. A 2–3-cm midline incision is made below the umbilicus (Fig. 1). The peritoneum is opened and the catheter tip is directed toward the pelvis, at times using a Fogarty catheter inserted into the Tenckhoff catheter as an aid to positioning. Correct catheter placement is ascertained by x-ray film; the fenestrated end and particularly the tip must lie in the pelvis. Frequently the catheter needs to be repositioned. Once this is achieved, the wound is closed with the single cuff buried between the peritoneum and the sheath of the rectus abdominis muscle. A long subcutaneous tunnel (5–7 cm), placed vertically and just lateral to the umbilicus, leads the catheter from the peritoneum to the skin exit site. The catheter is irrigated with a reasonable volume of dialysis fluid and then drained by gravity to prove good function. Once catheter placement and function have been verified, the patient is removed from the operating room. The vertical and midline position of the catheter facilitates dressing changes and prevents kinking of the catheter.

Thereafter a precise catheter break-in schedule is followed as shown in Table 3. The dialysis fluid used can be 0.5% or 1.5% dextrose concentration with additives (heparin, 500 units/liter; cephalathin, 50 mg/liter). Approximately one-half the predicted volume (1500 ml/m^2 of body surface or 50 ml/kg body weight) of dialysis fluid is used to prevent stretching the wound and thus causing a leak. The volume of fluid is gradually increased over a number of days until the comfortably accommodated volume is reached. A week of intermittent peritoneal dialysis is recommended to achieve metabolic stability, ensure catheter function, and familiarize the child with dialysis and the nurses. Currently, small-volume bags are not available and thus in our

TABLE 3.

Technique for CAPD

1. Insert peritoneal catheter.
2. Intermittent peritoneal dialysis with no dwell time for 8-12 hours.
3. Intermittent peritoneal dialysis with 5-10 minutes dwell time for 20 hours.
4. Stabilization period. Daily intermittent peritoneal dialysis for 4-6 hours for 7 days.
5. Start CAPD training—about 2 weeks.

pharmacy the prescribed volume for CAPD is aliquoted under a laminar flow hood into transfer packs (Fenwall Laboratories, Division of Travenol Laboratories). We accept a shelf life of 30 days under refrigeration.

The CAPD training per se takes about 2 weeks. One nurse is assigned to the patient and/or the parent. The first week is directed to teaching the principles of sterile technique, how to change a dialysis bag, and how to change the dressing, which is done twice weekly or more if necessary. The second week is devoted to teaching the physiology of dialysis, taking blood pressure, deciding on the required dialysis fluid–dextrose concentrations, the importance of diet, and the complications of CAPD, especially the signs and symptoms of peritonitis. Early home treatment of probable peritonitis is taught, which includes obtaining a sample for culture and adding antibiotics to the fluid prior to traveling to the hospital.

RESULTS

Six of the 15 patients were treated by CAPD for 6 months or more. They attained a linear growth rate of 0.43 ± 0.21 cm/month on dialysis. Three patients gained and three patients lost weight, one of these had psychological eating problems and one was sick from hypertension, eventually requiring nephrectomies (Table 4).

The blood urea nitrogen (BUN) fell in 13 of the 15 treated patients by an average of 34 ± 28 mg/dl and plasma creatinine fell in 13 by an average of

TABLE 4.
Height and Weight Changes in Patients on CAPD

Patient Number	Time on CAPD (months)	Height (cm) S[a]	Height (cm) L[b]	Weight (kg) S	Weight (kg) L
1	14.5	151	158.8	38.6	45
2	12	134	137.5	30.9	29.5
3	10.5	151	152	45.8	45
4	1	98.1	100	19.3	20.9
5	14	95	103	13.2	13.3
6	4	144	144.5	38.4	42.4
7	4	79.5	79.5	8.0	8.2
8	4	79	81	8.5	8.3
9	6	111	115	15.9	18
10	3	61.5	62.3	4.8	5.3
11	1	83	83	9.3	9.8
12	6	118	120.5	20.7	20.4
13	1.5	75	75	8.9	9.1
14	2	68	71	7.8	7.7
15	2	109	110	16.0	17.0

[a] S = start of CAPD.
[b] L = last recording.

TABLE 5.
Blood Results

Patient Number	Blood Urea Nitrogen (mg/dl) S[a]	Blood Urea Nitrogen (mg/dl) L[b]	Creatinine (mg/dl) S	Creatinine (mg/dl) L	Hemoglobin (g/dl) S	Hemoglobin (g/dl) L	Total Protein (g/dl) S	Total Protein (g/dl) L	Albumin (g/dl) S	Albumin (g/dl) L
1	84	66	10.1	9.3	7.2	9.4	6.3	7.2	3.7	4.9
2	76	83	12.0	10.3	6.9	5.6	6.7	6.1	4.4	3.3
3	89	82	16.6	11.0	3.8	6.0	5.6	6.0	3.5	3.7
4	48	36	9.4	7.0	4.9	4.9	6.0	4.8	2.9	3.8
5	112	74	4.0	4.5	7.1	9.5	5.9	6.3	2.9	3.8
6	24	52	6.5	9.6	7.4	7.4	5.5	7.5	1.9	3.8
7	96	44	8.5	5.8	5.4	5.5	6.7	7.5	4.1	4.6
8	72	34	7.8	6.9	6.3	6.1	7.4	6.2	4.3	3.4
9	63	56	11.6	10.1	3.6	6.6	8.1	8.2	3.9	4.5
10	38	14	6.2	3.7	6.5	7.6	6.5	4.6	4.3	2.7
11	55	48	2.6	1.3	6.6	7.8	6.7	7.9	4.1	4.5
12	155	55	5.1	2.9	5.4	8.5	6.6	6.7	3.7	3.9
13	136	67	10.7	5.3	5.4	7.5	7.3	8.1	4.6	4.5
14	48	24	4.2	3.6	6.4	7.2	6.9	7.0	4.5	3.9
15	78	46	5.3	3.8	6.6	7.6	8.1	7.3	4.4	4.1
Mean ± S.D.[c]	78 ± 36	52 ± 20	8.0 ± 4.8	6.3 ± 3.1	6.0 ± 1.2	7.1 ± 1.4	6.7 ± 0.8	6.8 ± 1.1	3.8 ± 0.8	4.0 ± 0.6

[a] S = at start of CAPD.
[b] L = last recording.
[c] S.D. ± standard deviation.

2.2 ± 1.6 mg/dl (Table 5). The last mean value for BUN and plasma creatinine were 52 ± 20 mg/dl and 6.3 ± 3.1 mg/dl, respectively. The hemoglobin (Hb) increased in 11 of the 15 patients. The mean Hb at the start of CAPD was 6.0 ± 1.2 g/dl and increased to 7.1 ± 1.4 g/dl after dialytic therapy. The mean increase in Hb in the six patients treated for longer than 6 months was 2.2 ± 1.1 g/dl and their last mean Hb value was 7.6 ± 1.7 g/dl.

The total plasma protein increased in 11 of the 15 patients and fell in four of the patients; however, changes in either direction were not great, that is, the mean increase was 0.6 ± 0.6 g/dl and the mean decrease was 0.9 ± 0.3 g/dl. Two of the patients were hypoproteinemic and patient 10 had consequent edema. A similar trend was observed for plasma albumin with only one patient with obvious hypoalbuminemia of 2.7 g/dl, the mean for the 15 patients being 4.0 ± 0.6 g/dl.

Peritoneal fluid protein loss is shown on Table 6. The average daily protein loss for nine patients was 0.24 ± 0.09 g/kg body weight. In the four older patients (> 6 years) the mean daily protein loss was 0.16 ± 0.02 g/kg body weight, whereas the younger children experienced greater protein loss, 0.30 ± 0.06 g/kg body weight. The average intake, loss, and absorption of dextrose via the peritoneal route for nine patients is shown on Table 6. The mean dextrose absorption was 2.32 ± 1.05 g/kg body weight. In this small group of patients it appears the younger children absorb on a per unit weight basis a greater amount of dextrose; 2.74 ± 1.06 g/kg/day versus 1.79 ± 0.87 g/kg/day. In spite of the considerable peritoneal dextrose intake no hyperglycemia was observed.

COMPLICATIONS

There were eight episodes of peritonitis, which occurred in six patients during the study period of 80 patient-months (Table 7). Two patients had peritonitis twice. This corresponds to a peritonitis incidence of 40% of the patients, or one episode every 10.7 patient-months. Three teenagers and two small patients managed by their mother or baby-sitter developed peritonitis during the first 3 months of CAPD. The causal organisms were *Streptococcus viridans* in two, *Staphylococcus epidermidis* in two, *Staphylococcus aureus* in two, and α-hemolytic *Streptococcus* in one. In a number of these episodes a break in sterile technique was felt to be responsible for the peritonitis. All patients responded quickly to peritoneal lavage with dialysis fluid containing antibiotic.

Three patients developed hernias (two ventral, one inguinal), two requiring surgery. Three infants were difficult feeders; patient 10 has required nasogastric tube feeding for the past 3 months and for 1 month her dialysis fluid has contained amino acid (1.5 Dianeal, 1% Travasol) to prevent peritoneal amino acid loss.

RENAL TRANSPLANTATION RESULTS

Six patients have received renal transplants, all with the kidney placed retroperitoneally. The catheter has been removed either at the time of surgery

TABLE 6.
Exchanges of Dextrose and Protein in Dialysate

Patient Number	Total Protein (g/kg/day)	Dextrose Input (g/day)	Dextrose Output (g/day)	Absorption (g/kg/day)
1[a]	0.18	45	10.1	0.78
3[a]	0.16	150	19.5	2.90
6[a]	0.14	87.5	17.4	1.65
8	0.35	13.5	1.2	1.48
10	0.30	27	4.2	4.30
11	0.31	22.5	1.5	2.17
13	0.35	30	1.7	3.11
14	0.20	22.5	2.1	2.65
15[a]	0.14	37.5	6.7	1.81
Mean ± S.D.	0.24 ± 0.09			2.32 ± 1.05

[a] Older than 6 years.

TABLE 7.
Complications in Patients on CAPD

Patient Number	Complications
1	Peritonitis twice (*Streptococcus viridans, Staphylococcus epidermidis*) Scrotal swelling
2	Poor appetite
3	Peritonitis once (*Staphylococcus aureus*)
4	Catheter site infection
5	—
6	Peritonitis once (*Streptococcus viridans*)
7	—
8	Peritonitis once (*Staphylococcus epidermidis*) Ventral incisional hernia
9	—
10	Poor appetite, ventral hernia Peritonitis once (α-hemolytic *Streptococcus*)
11	Cloudy sterile fluid once (eosinophils)
12	Severe hypertension, required nephrectomy
13	Poor appetite, inguinal hernia; peritonitis once (*Staphylococcus aureus*)
14	Poor appetite
15	Cloudy fluid once

or within 1 week of surgery. The only complication was sanguineous ascites in one patient, which subsided with removal of the catheter.

DISCUSSION

To date we have been encouraged by our experience with CAPD in children and infants. There are no other published experiences with CAPD in children. However, Brouhard et al.[6] reported their experience with home intermittent peritoneal dialysis in 19 patients, showing it to be an acceptable form of chronic dialytic therapy. The major indication for CAPD at the onset of our program was for children who had no alternative. All vascular access sites for hemodialysis had been used and the likelihood of an early renal transplant was remote because they had rejected previous allografts and had a high titer of cytotoxic antibodies. These were usually older children and they accepted CAPD well. They were able to perform bag changes and were pleased with their new-found freedom because of fewer trips to the hospital and no major dietary restrictions. However, we found they usually needed some help with bag changes, especially if they required four exchanges per day.

Our indications for CAPD appears to be changing. Seven of the last 10 patients have been younger than 5 years of age. The reason for selecting CAPD was because they were small patients and therefore creation and maintenance of a shunt or fistula would have been difficult. We have a number of small children who have severe renal insufficiency. We know that such children usually do not grow and eventually develop significant renal osteodystrophy. It is now possible to maintain CAPD on even a very small infant. Consequently, CAPD permits the pediatric nephrologist to start dialysis earlier on these small children and hopefully enhance growth and prevent osteodystrophy. Our small patients have invariably been picky eaters and it may be necessary to modify the dialysis fluid. Since we showed that the younger patient tended to lose a greater amount of protein in the dialysate, it was not surprising that one of our young patients developed nutritional hypoproteinemia and edema. Consequently, we added amino acid to the dialysis fluid and have been impressed with her improved health and correction of the hypoproteinemia. This was instituted primarily to prevent amino acid loss, but it may in fact be that the peritoneum can be used as an alternative route for parenteral nutrition.

Hemodialysis in the small child is usually feasible only in a highly skilled pediatric dialysis center. Thus, children who require chronic hemodialysis are required to live near such a center until a transplant is found. This is obviously a major disruption to the family, causing psychological and financial strain. CAPD permits such children to live at home and be managed entirely by the parent and the family doctor and only to return to the transplant center when an allograft becomes available. We are unable to answer the important question of how well small children do on CAPD because of too few patients and the short time on CAPD. If we can show that a 5-kg patient on CAPD will grow to a size suitable for renal transplantation, that is, 10 kg, and have healthy bones, then the clinical picture of dialysis and transplantation in young children will change markedly for the better.

ACKNOWLEDGMENT

This work was partly supported by the National Institutes of Health (Contract No. NO1-AM-8-2213).

References

1. Popovich, R. P., Moncrief, J. W., Nolph, K. D., Ghods, A. J., Twardowski, A. J., and Pyle, W. K.: Continuous ambulatory peritoneal dialysis. *Ann Intern Med* **88**: 449, 1978.
2. Oreopoulos, D. G.: The coming of age of continuous ambulatory peritoneal dialysis (CAPD). *Dial Transplant* **8**: 460, 1979.
3. Oreopoulos, D. G., Robson, M., Izatt, S., Clayton, S., and de Veber, G. A.: A simple and safe technique for CAPD. *Trans Am Soc Artif Intern Organs* **24**: 484, 1978.
4. Oreopoulos, D. G., Katirtzoglou, A., Arbus, G., and Cordy, P. E.: Dialysis and transplantation in young children. (Letter to the Editor.) *Br Med J* **1**: 1628, 1979.
5. Oreopoulos, D. G., Izatt, S., Zellerman, G., Karanicolas, S., and Mathews, R. E.: A prospective study of the effectiveness of three permanent peritoneal catheters. *Proc Dial Transplant Forum* **6**: 96, 1976.
6. Brouhard, B. H., Berger, M., Cunningham, R. J., Petrusick, T., Allen, W., Lyndh, R. E., and Travis, L. B.: Home peritoneal dialysis in children. *Trans Am Soc Artif Intern Organs* **24**: 90, 1979.

CHAPTER TWENTY-NINE

Ultrafiltration in the Young Patient on CAPD

E. C. KOHAUT,* M.D.

S. R. ALEXANDER,† M.D.

CONTINUOUS AMBULATORY PERITONEAL DIALYSIS (CAPD) has been evaluated as an alternate form of therapy for children with end-stage renal failure in our institution over the past year. Since its development by Popovich et al.,[1] we have viewed this form of dialysis with great interest. Dialysis therapy for the pediatric population has always been less than ideal. One particular problem has been the maintenance of salt and water balance in patients in whom restriction of salt and water is not always met with 100% compliance. Many children on both hemodialysis and intermittent peritoneal dialysis are not under adequate control of blood pressure.[2,3]

One attractive feature of CAPD is the purported ability to remove relatively large amounts of salt and water,[1,4] therefore allowing greater intake of these substances. This paper addresses that hypothesis as it applies to the young patient.

METHODS

A total of seven children have been placed on CAPD at the University of Alabama in Birmingham. Additional data have also been collected from six patients who have been maintained on CAPD at the University of Oregon in Portland.

All solutions used were commercially available dialysis solutions containing standard concentration of electrolytes, calcium, and magnesium. Before each study period several rapid in and out exchanges were done to try to minimize error created by dead space. Varying volumes of solutions were

---

*The Departments of Pediatrics, University of Alabama in Birmingham, Birmingham, Alabama, and †University of Oregon in Portland, Portland, Oregon

222   CAPD Update

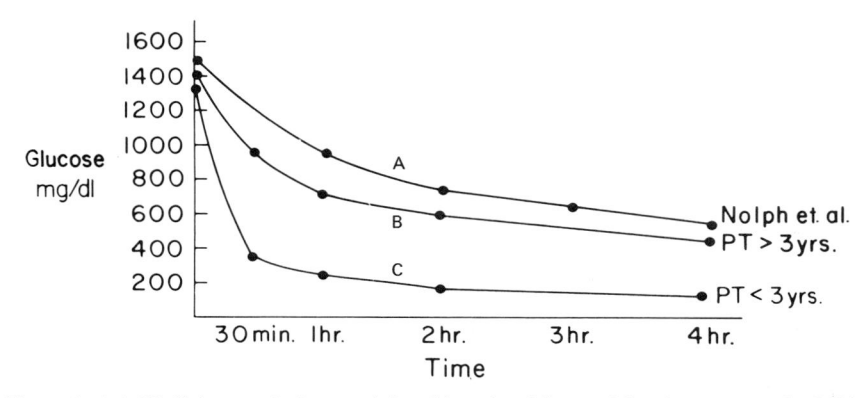

Figure 1. A 1.5% dialysate solution was infused into the abdomen. Line A represents the fall in glucose concentration related to time in a group of adult patients studied by Nolph *et al*. Line B demonstrates that glucose concentration fell slightly faster in children >3 years of age and even faster (line C) in children <3 years of age.

used in different sized patients; however, these volumes always were between 20 and 30 ml/kg. The solutions were then placed in the abdomen and left in the abdominal cavity for varying periods of time. At the end of the time period, the solutions were drained by gravity. All studies were done on patients whose catheters were working well and drainage was accomplished within less than 10 minutes. Before another study was done, in and out exchanges were again done to minimize any error introduced by undrained fluid. Blood studies were done at midpoint of each study period. Data were

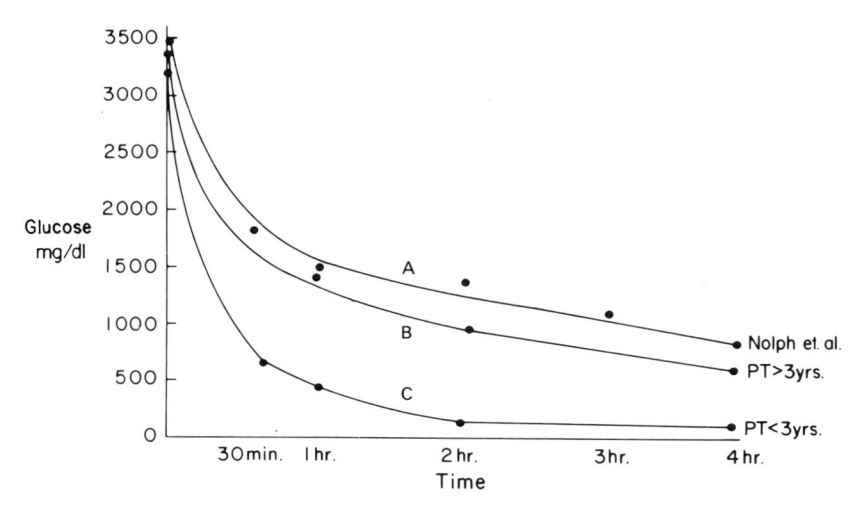

Figure 2. A 4.25% dialysate solution was infused into the abdomen. Line A represents the fall in glucose concentration related to time in a group of adult patients studied by Nolph *et al*. Line B demonstrates that glucose concentration fell slightly faster in children >3 years of age and even faster (line C) in children <3 years of age.

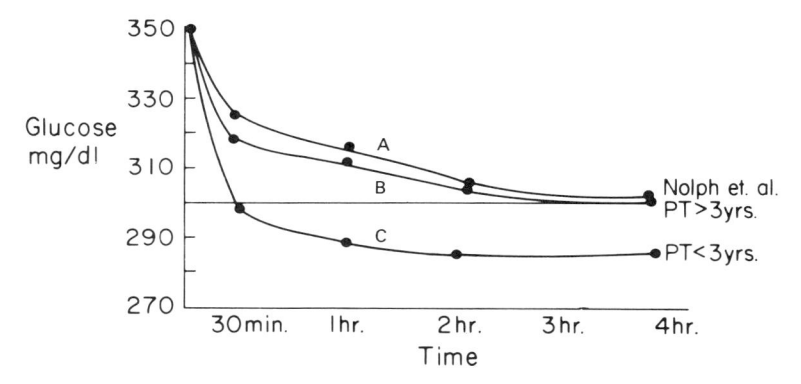

Figure 3. A 1.5% dialysate solution was infused into the abdomen. Dialysate OSM is plotted against time. Dialysate OSM fell slightly faster in children >3 years of age (line B) than adults studied by Nolph *et al.* (line A) and much faster in children <3 years of age (line C).

also collected concerning the dialysis schedule and sugar concentrations required by 13 patients to keep them in balance. Average fluid balance is also presented.

RESULTS

Figure 1 demonstrates the drop in dialysate glucose as a function of time after a 1.5% dialysate was infused. This is compared to previously published adult data.[5] As is seen, the patients who were older than 3 years of age had a curve below but similar to the adult patients; however the patients younger than 3

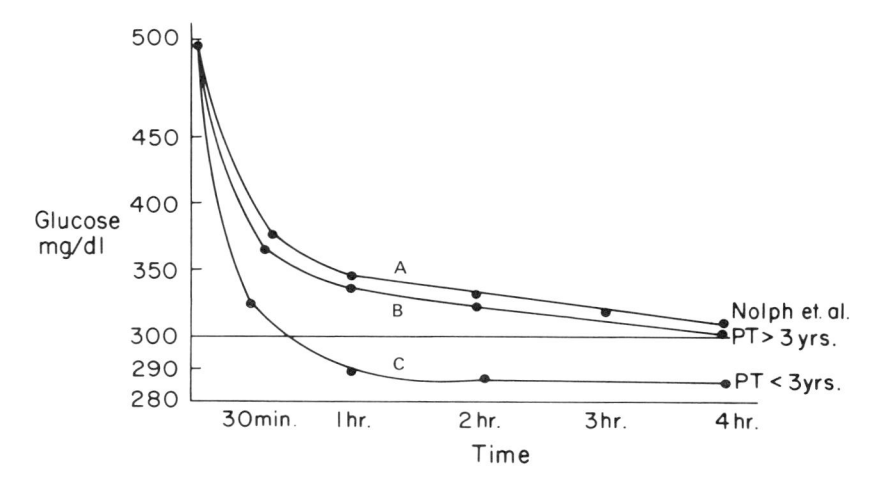

Figure 4. A 4.25% dialysate solution was infused into the abdomen. Dialysate OSM was plotted against time. Dialysate OSM fell slightly faster in children >3 years of age (line B) than adults studied by Nolph *et al.* (line A) and much faster in children <3 years of age (line C).

had a more rapid drop in dialysate glucose. Figure 2 demonstrates similar findings when a 4.25% dialysate solution was infused, although the patients older than 3 years of age reduced dialysate sugar concentration more rapidly than the adult patients, the difference being small. Of the patients younger than 3, dialysate glucose fell much faster. Figures 3 and 4 demonstrate the change in dialysate osmolality as a function of time, after infusion of 1.5% dialysate and 4.25% dialysate. In both instances the patients older than 3 years of age had a more rapid drop in osmolality than the adult patient population, but the difference was small. The patients younger than 3 had dropped dialysate osmolality dramatically, in some cases dialysate osmolality fell below serum osmolality. Table 1 demonstrates the effect that this had on volume. As can be seen in the newborn patients and the 1.5-year-old patient studied, ultrafiltration was not achieved with either a 1.5% or a 4.25% dialysate. Table 2 presents data both from the patients in Birmingham and Portland. This table is meant to demonstrate the various clinical maneuvers undertaken to attempt to dialyze these patients effectively. It can be seen that use of 4.25% dialysate was widespread. Some patients required a few rapid passes during the day to enhance fluid removal. Ultrafiltration was never successful in the two neonates studied in anything resembling a routine CAPD protocol. There were two patients in the 18-month age range. One patient followed by Alexander in Portland is effectively controlled with a dialysate with 2.3% glucose concentration in all passes. In the other 18-month-old from Birmingham, we were never able to produce ultrafiltration; however this patient had a good urine output and we never really had to remove fluid aggressively. Another young patient, a 31-month-old, also from Portland, is effectively controlled with a negative balance of 636 cc/m^2. He requires a constant dialysate sugar of 2.5%. The older patients are also

TABLE 1.
Effect of Osmolality on Volume

	Volume Infused	Volume Drained
1.5% Dialysate—4-Hour Pass		
Newborn	50	39
Newborn	80	58
1.5 years	210	180
5.5 years	500	550
15 years	1,000	950
15 years	1,200	1,250
18 years	2,000	1,830
4.25% Dialysate—4-Hour Pass		
Newborn	50	37
Newborn	80	66
1.5 years	210	190
5.5 years	500	605
15 years	1,000	1,150
15 years	1,200	1,356
18 years	2,000	2,300

TABLE 2.

The effects of the rapid drop in osmolality are noted. Many of the very young patients maintained positive dialysate balances and were unable to continue CAPD

Age	Pass Volume	Sugar Concentration	Fast Passes	Dialysis Balance/M^2	Urine Output/M^2	Comment
Newborn	50	8—4.25% 1—1.5%	Yes	+333	0	Unable to dialyze
Newborn	80	8—4.25% 1—1.5%	Yes	+280	0	Unable to dialyze
19 months	200	5—2.3%	No	−289	0	Stable
18 months	180	2—4.25% 3—1.5%	Yes	+146	936	Unable to continue CAPD
1.5 years	325	5—2.5%	No	−636	0	Stable
6 years	700	2—4.25% 3—1.5%	Yes	−1,501	0	Stable
6 years	300	4—2.5%	Yes	+590	1,454	Unstable
7 years	350	5—1.5%	No	+466	926	Stable
15 years	1,000	2—4.25 3—1.5	Yes	−1,050	0	Stable
15 years	1,500	3—4.25% 2—1.5%	Yes	−1,707	0	Stable
16 years	1,000	3—4.5% 2—1.5%	No	−700	0	Stable
18 years	2,000	2—4.25% 3—1.5%	No	−850	0	Stable

requiring multiple passes with 4.25%, some of them requiring short 4.25% passes to maintain fluid balance. However, as one can see from the amount of ultrafiltration being produced, this is not due to any serious problem in ability to ultrafiltrate these patients; rather it is to compensate for a large water and salt intake.

DISCUSSION

We feel the data presented suggest that children do transport sugar across the peritoneal membrane at a greater rate than adults. Nolph et al.,[6] in a study of 13 uremic patients undergoing peritoneal dialysis, have demonstrated that there is a significant variability in peritoneal glucose transport. Since the number of patients studied is small, it is possible that we are just dealing with a selected population, and the increased rate of glucose transfer seen has nothing to do with age. More patients need be studied before this conclusion can be made. The data are also lacking in that glucose transfer rates were not calculated because we felt the possibility may exist that volumes were inaccurate due to inadequate drainage. However, we do feel the drop in glucose concentration and osmolality is a valid determination since wash outs were done prior to each study period.

The rapid drop in glucose concentration reduced the osmolality of the dialysate, thus reducing the period of time when an adequate osmolar gradient existed to promote fluid transfer. In the children older than 3 years of age, since the concentration of glucose did not fall much more rapidly than it did in the adult group studied by Nolph et al.,[5] this did not cause a significant problem. Adequate ultrafiltration was obtained by using high glucose concentrations and at times one or two rapid passes per day. However, in the very young child and the neonates studied, the drop in glucose concentration and the subsequent drop in osmolality made it impossible to ultrafiltrate these patients by anything close to a normal CAPD schedule.

The changes we did make in the normal CAPD protocol enabled us to ultrafiltrate large amounts of salt and water in the older patient group. This enabled us to put them on unrestricted salt and water intake, which we feel is beneficial to them in terms of their attitudes concerning dialysis and may also be beneficial in improving caloric intake, which is probably the most important determinant of growth.

References

1. Popovich, R. P., Moncrief, J. W., Nolph, K. D., Ghods, A. J., Twardowski, Z. J., and Pyle, W. K.: Continuous ambulatory peritoneal dialysis. *Ann Intern Med* **88**: 449–456, 1978.
2. Counts, S., Hickman, R., Garbaccio, A., and Tenckhoff, H.: Chronic home peritoneal dialysis in children. *Trans Am Soc Artif Intern Organs* **19**: 157, 1973.
3. Jones, J. M. B., Cameron, J. S., Bewick, M., Ogg, C. S., Meadow, S. R., and Ellis, F. G.: Treatment of terminal renal failure in children by home dialysis and transplant. *Arch Dis Child* **46**: 457, 1971.
4. Oreopoulos, P. G.: The coming of age of continuous ambulatory peritoneal dialysis. *Dial Transplant* **8**: 460, 1979.
5. Nolph, K. D., Twardowski, Z. J., Popovich, R. P., and Rubin, J.: Equilibration of peritoneal dialysis solutions during longdwell exchanges. *J Lab Clin Med* **93**: 246–256, 1979.
6. Nolph, K. D., Rosenfeld, P. S., Powell, J. T., and Danforth, E.: Peritoneal glucose transport and hyperglycemia during peritoneal dialysis. *Am J Med Sci* **259**: 272–280, 1970.

CHAPTER THIRTY

Kinetics of Peritoneal Dialysis in Children

ROBERT P. POPOVICH, Ph.D.

W. KEITH PYLE, Ph.D.

DAVID A. ROSENTHAL, B.S.

STEVEN R. ALEXANDER, M.D.*

J. WILLIAM BALFE, M.D., F.R.C.P. (C)†

JACK W. MONCRIEF, M.D.‡

INTRODUCTION

CONTINUOUS AMBULATORY PERITONEAL DIALYSIS (CAPD) is a new treatment modality for treatment of patients with end-stage renal disease.[1-3] In the past several years CAPD has been applied to thousands of adult patients, encompassing virtually every country, with viable dialysis programs. The clinical results demonstrate that CAPD exhibits certain advantages over hemodialysis.[4-6] These include elimination of the need for routine blood access, greatly reduced dietary restrictions, simplicity of operation, patient mobility, and continuous biochemical and fluid control. These advantages indicate that CAPD may be an attractive alternative to hemodialysis or even classical intermittent peritoneal dialysis (IPD) in the treatment of infants and children.

The infusion schedule required to maintain an adult at satisfactory blood urea nitrogen (BUN) and plasma creatinine levels has been presented by Popovich et al.[7-9] These results are based upon knowledge of metabolite generation rates and the transport characteristics of the peritoneum. However, only minimal corresponding transport data are available on metabolite kinetics for infants and children.[10] These mainly involve clearance studies concomitant with short residence time IPD schedules.

The purpose of this research is to determine the mass transfer characteristics of the peritoneum in children. Based upon these clinical results, a

---

Biomedical Engineering Program, Department of Chemical Engineering, University of Texas, Austin, Texas
*Department of Pediatrics, University of Oregon Health Science Center, Portland, Oregon.
†Division of Nephrology, Hospital for Sick Children, Toronto, Ontario, Canada.
‡Acorn Research Laboratory, Austin Diagnostic Clinic, Austin, Texas.

preliminary computer analysis of the child-peritoneal dialysis system is presented to predict infusion volumes required to maintain adequate biochemical control on a four exchange per day CAPD schedule.

METHODS

Patients are placed on CAPD clinical schedules as outlined in detail elsewhere.[11,12] Prior to dialysate infusion, 0.5 μC of iodine-131 as radioiodinated human serum albumin (RISA) per 100 ml of dialysate is aseptically added to standard Dianeal® (1.5% or 4.25% dextrose) and mixed via repeated inversion of the bag. Drainage of the previous infusion is prolonged in order to remove as much dialysate as possible, and the tagged dialysate is infused. Immediately following infusion, an initial dialysate sample is obtained. This is accomplished by allowing approximately 10% of the infused dialysate to flow rapidly into a 100-ml Volutrol® that has been placed in-line. The sample is removed and the remaining dialysate is rapidly reinfused. Total sample time was less than 60 seconds in all cases. Additional dialysate samples are obtained at 15, 30, 60, 90, 120, 240, 360, and 480 minutes following infusion. Blood samples are obtained immediately prior to dialysate infusion, at 180 and 240 minutes of dwell time, and immediately after initiation of drainage.

All samples were analyzed for BUN, creatinine, and uric acid utilizing a Technicon SMAC® analyzer. Glucose concentration was measured using a Beckman Analyzer II®. RISA samples were counted using a Camberra Single Channel Analyzer Model 1772® with counter timer and amplifier connected to a 2-in. well crystal detector from Nuclear Chicago Corporation.

The volume of dialysate fluid present in the peritoneal cavity was computed using the degree of dilution of the RISA.[13,14] The data were corrected for the small amount of RISA mass transfer, which occurred during the exchange. Mass transfer-area coefficients were computed for each solute from analysis

TABLE 1.
Mass Transfer-Area Coefficients[a]

Solute	Patient 1 (7.0 kg)		Patient 2 (8.2 kg)	Patient 3 (11.7 kg)		Patient 4 (14.7 kg)	
Dextrose (%)	1.5	4.25	4.25	1.5	4.25	1.5	4.25
Urea	2.59	2.78	6.14	7.50	—	5.02	10.40
Creatinine	1.49	—	1.51	4.27	2.45	4.74	3.55
Uric acid	0.88	0.88	2.59	4.39	4.29	5.38	3.41
Glucose	1.26	2.07	3.35	3.07	5.22	4.41	2.63

[a] Values given in ml/minute.

TABLE 2.
Mean Mass Transfer-Area Coefficients[a]

Solute	1 (7.0 kg)	2 (8.2 kg)	3 (11.7 kg)	4 (14.7 kg)	Adult Reference
Urea	2.69	6.14	7.50	7.71	33.6
Creatinine	1.49	1.51	3.36	4.15	23.5
Uric acid	0.88	2.59	4.34	4.40	19.5
Glucose	1.67	3.35	4.15	3.52	18.1

[a] Values given in ml/minute.

of the concentration versus time profiles and the known ultrafiltration rates. The details of the various computations are presented elsewhere.[15]

RESULTS

Peritoneal mass transfer characteristics were measured in seven studies on four children at the University of Oregon Health Science Center with an age

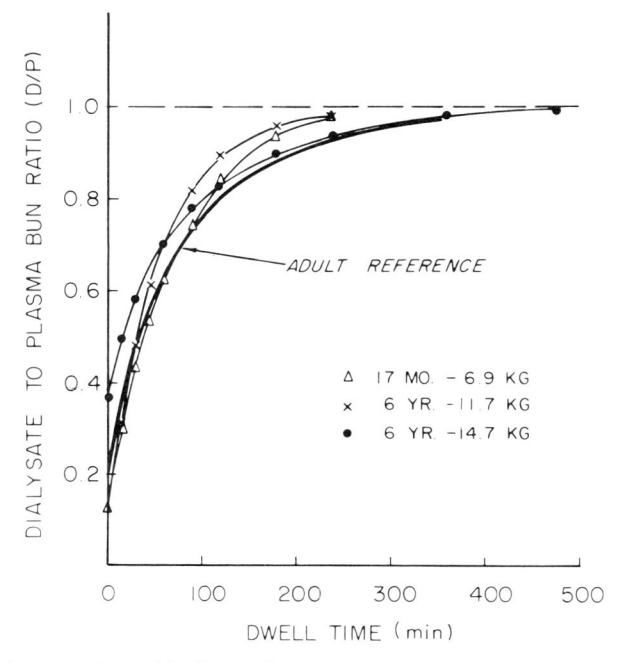

Figure 1. Dialysate to plasma blood urea nitrogen concentration ratio versus dwell time for 1.5% dextrose dialysate in three patients.

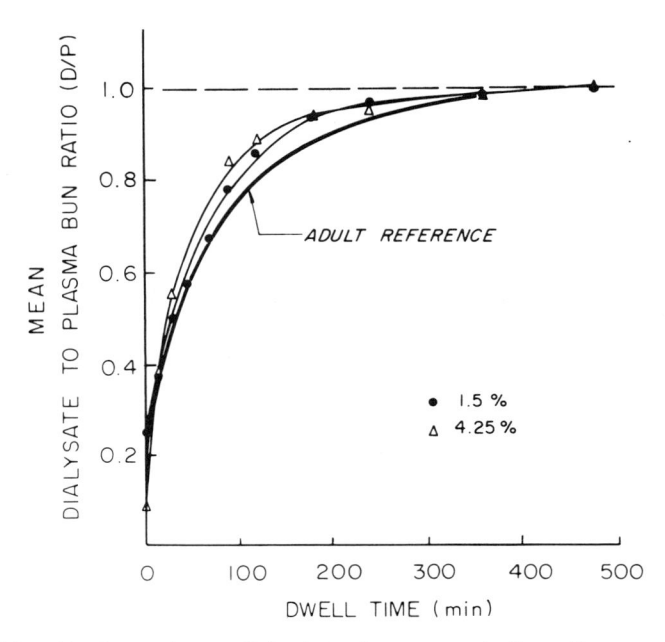

Figure 2. Mean blood urea nitrogen dialysate to plasma concentration ratios versus dwell time for 1.5% and 4.25% dextrose dialysate.

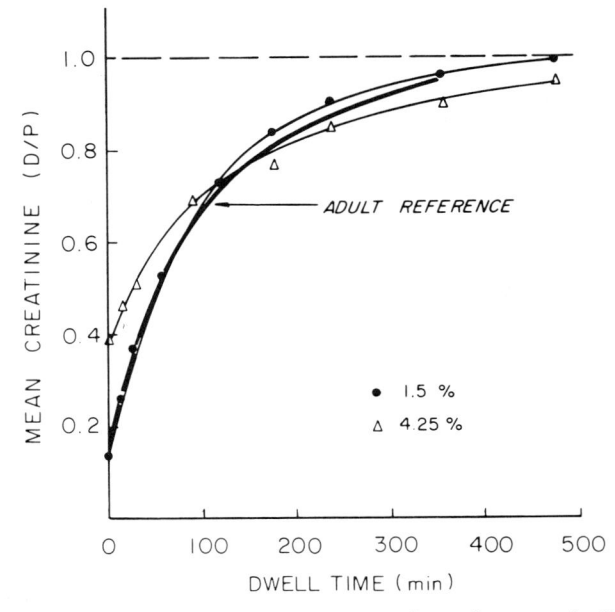

Figure 3. Mean creatinine dialysate to plasma concentration ratios versus dwell time for 1.5% and 4.25% dextrose dialysate.

range of 17 months to 6 years. Three concomitant RISA studies were performed on dialysate volume versus time.

The mass transfer-area coefficients (KA) computed for the individual concentration versus time profiles are presented in Table 1. Multiple studies were obtained in some instances. Averaged results for each child are presented in Table 2.

Representative individual BUN concentration versus time profiles expressed as a dialysate to plasma concentration ratio are presented in Figure 1 for 1.5% dextrose dialysate. Corresponding mean values for adults are also presented for reference. The mean (the average for all children) BUN concentration versus time values for 1.5% and 4.25% solutions are presented in Figure 2. Similar results for creatinine, uric acid, and glucose are presented in Figures 3–5. In all cases mean adult values for a 4.25% dextrose are presented for reference.

The actual dialysate volume in the peritoneal cavity as a function of dwell time following completion of infusion for 1.5% and 4.25% dextrose dialysate for patient 4 is presented in Figure 6. Similar results for patient 2 with 4.25% dextrose are presented in Figure 7.

DISCUSSION

The mass transfer-area coefficients computed from the individual solute concentration versus time profiles are presented in Table 1. Although some

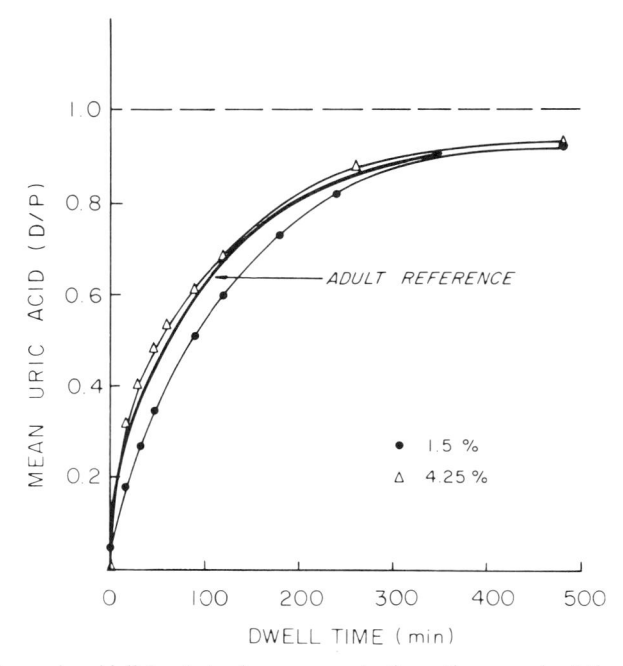

Figure 4. Mean uric acid dialysate to plasma concentration ratio versus dwell time for 1.5% and 4.25% dextrose dialysate.

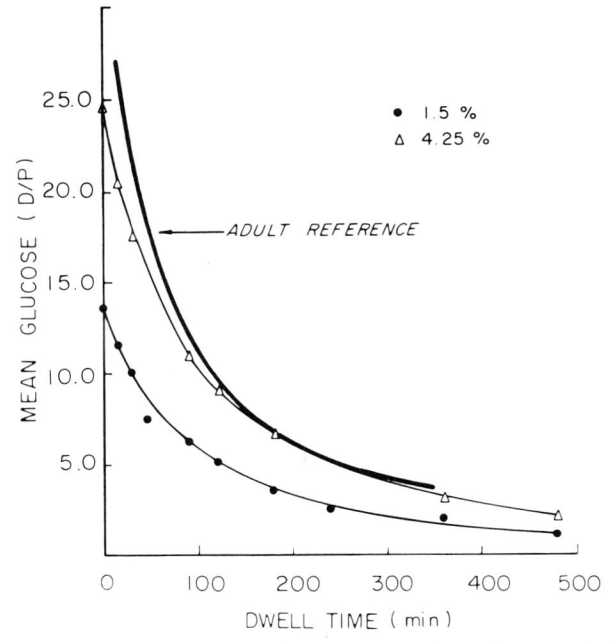

Figure 5. Mean glucose dialysate to plasma concentration ratio versus dwell time.

data scatter is obtained (a characteristic of these parameters), an effect of the size or weight of the child is evident. No consistent differences are noted between the 1.5% and 4.25% dialysate. As described elsewhere,[15] the effects of ultrafiltration are separately accounted for in evaluating the mass transfer-area coefficient. The mean mass transfer-area coefficient is presented in Table 2 with an adult reference value obtained from the mass transfer correlation of Popovich et al.[9] Table 2 further illustrates that the value of the mass transfer-area coefficient decreases with decreasing child weight.

The mass transfer-area coefficient is a measure of the rate of mass transfer, which would occur if the dialysate metabolite concentration level was somehow maintained at zero at all times (the maximum possible dialysis rate). It is also equal to the area available for mass transport divided by the sum of all resistances the metabolite encounters as it diffuses from the blood capillaries into the dialysate fluid. If the anatomical and physiological characteristics of the peritoneum in the child per unit area are similar to that in adults, the sum of the resistances would be similar. Under these circumstances, the results suggest a decrease in transport area with decreasing size. This also suggests that the mass transfer coefficients might be correlated to the adult values by some scaling factor related to size. Table 3 presents the value of the BUN mass transfer-area coefficients scaled to adult values (70 kg with 1.73 m² surface area) by body surface area and by weight. Scaling by body surface area results in coefficients consistently less than the adult

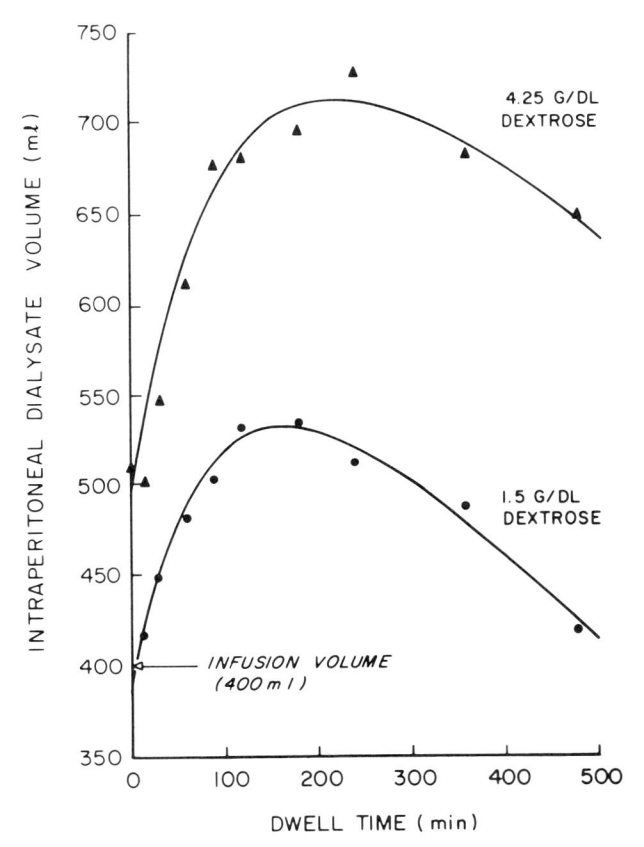

Kinetics of Peritoneal Dialysis in Children   233

Figure 6. Intraperitoneal dialysate volume versus dwell time for patient 4.

TABLE 3.
Mean Blood Urea Nitrogen Mass Transfer-Area Coefficients Scaled by Body Surface Area and Weight

Patient	KA[a] (ml/minute)	Surface Area (m^2)	Wt (kg)	KA Scaled by Surface Area	KA Scaled by Weight	Adult Reference
1	2.69	0.34	7.0	13.7	26.9	33.6
2	6.14	0.38	8.2	28.0	52.4	33.6
3	7.50	0.51	11.7	25.4	44.9	33.6
4	7.71	0.65	14.7	20.5	36.7	33.6
Mean				21.9 ± 5.4	40.2 ± 9.5	33.6

[a] KA is mass transfer-area coefficients.

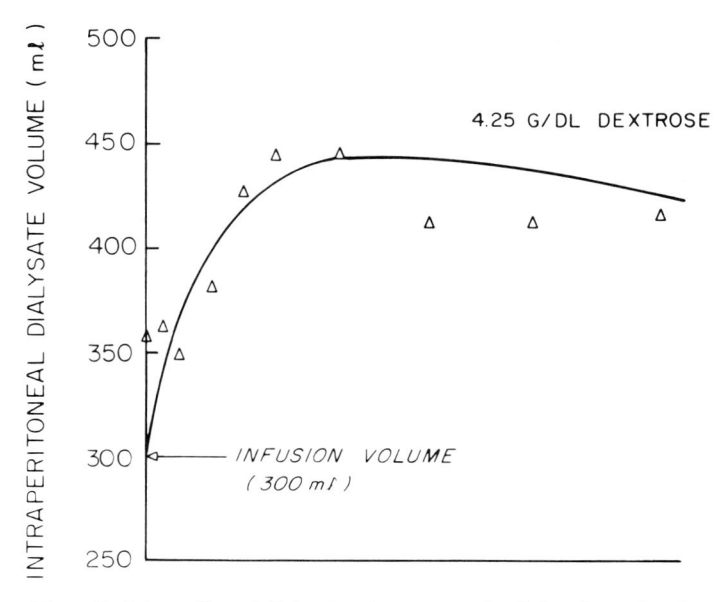

Figure 7. Intraperitoneal dialysate volume versus dwell time for patient 2.

reference values. Scaling by weight appears to yield significantly better correlation with the scaled values scattering around the reference point. The mean scaled value by surface area is greater than two standard deviations from the reference value.

Table 4 presents mean scaled mass transfer-area coefficients for all solutes scaled by body surface area and weight. In all cases, coefficients scaled by body surface area fell significantly below the adult reference values ($p < 0.05$). The mean coefficients scaled by weight scatter around their respective adult values. Consequently, the limited experimental data suggest that the mass transfer-area coefficient is directly proportional to body weight. Additional confirmation of this important relationship will be required, since only four children were involved in this preliminary investigation.

The actual volume of dialysate present in the peritoneal cavity as a function of dwell time for 1.5% and 4.25% solutions in patient 4 is presented in Figure

TABLE 4.

Mean Solute Mass Transfer-Area Coefficients Scaled by Body Surface Area and Weight

Solute	Mean Scaled by Surface Area	Mean Scaled by Weight	Adult Reference
Urea	21.9 ± 5.4	40.2 ± 9.5	33.6
Creatinine	9.2 ± 2.0	16.9 ± 3.1	23.5
Uric acid	10.7 ± 3.7	19.5 ± 6.4	19.5
Glucose	11.8 ± 2.9	21.7 ± 5.1	18.1

6. A rapid increase in dialysate volume above that infused is obtained in the early portion of the residence phase. This occurs under the influence of a high osmotic driving force due to substantial glucose concentration gradients across the peritoneum. Dialysate volume reaches a maximum when the glucose has been substantially dialyzed. Following this, the dialysate fluid is reabsorbed at a nearly constant rate of approximately -0.45 ml/minute.* The 4.25% dialysate results in more net ultrafiltered fluid and has a fluid volume peak that occurs at a later dwell time than that for the 1.5% solution. The maximum ultrafiltered fluid above the 400-ml infused volumes were approximately 330 and 140 ml, respectively. Dwell times corresponding to maximum ultrafiltration were approximately 4 and 3 hours, respectively.

Only a single dialysate volume curve with a 4.25% solution was obtained for patient 2. A maximum net ultrafiltration of approximately 140 ml above the 300 ml infused was obtained after a dwell period of about 3 hours.

The magnitude of ultrafiltration measured in the children was sufficient to maintain good fluid balance control using the two dextrose solutions. These results are quite similar in their general characteristics to those obtained with 2.0-liter infusions in adults.[16]

Instantaneous ultrafiltration rates can be obtained from the slope of the dialysate volume versus dwell time curve. Performing this differentiation yields the ultrafiltration rate curves presented in Figure 8. Maximum rates of ultrafiltration are significantly below those of adults[15] (2.5–3.0 ml/minute compared to 11.7–16.6 ml/minute, respectively). The reduced maximum ultrafiltration rates could be caused by a smaller area for transport, as already outlined.

The maximum ultrafiltration rates were scaled to adult values by body surface area and by weight. The mean results are presented in Table 5. Again, reasonable correlation is obtained if the maximum ultrafiltration rate is assumed to be directly proportional to body weight for the limited data available. Mean glucose concentration versus time curves for the children are presented in Figure 5. Similar results are obtained compared to adults,[17] implying similar osmotic driving forces. This supports the hypothesis that the reduced mass transfer-area coefficients in children are caused by a smaller effective transport area roughly in proportion to body weight.

TABLE 5.
Maximum Ultrafiltration Rates Scaled by Body Surface Area and Weight

Dextrose (%)	Mean Ultrafiltration Rate Scaled by Surface Area	Mean Ultrafiltration Rate Scaled by Weight	Adult Reference
1.5[a]	5.3	9.5	11.7
4.25	9.6 ± 1.7	17.8 ± 3.5	16.6

[a] Single measurement.

*Negative ultrafiltration rates indicate net fluid transfer from dialysate into the blood; positive rates indicate transfer from blood to dialysate.

236   CAPD Update

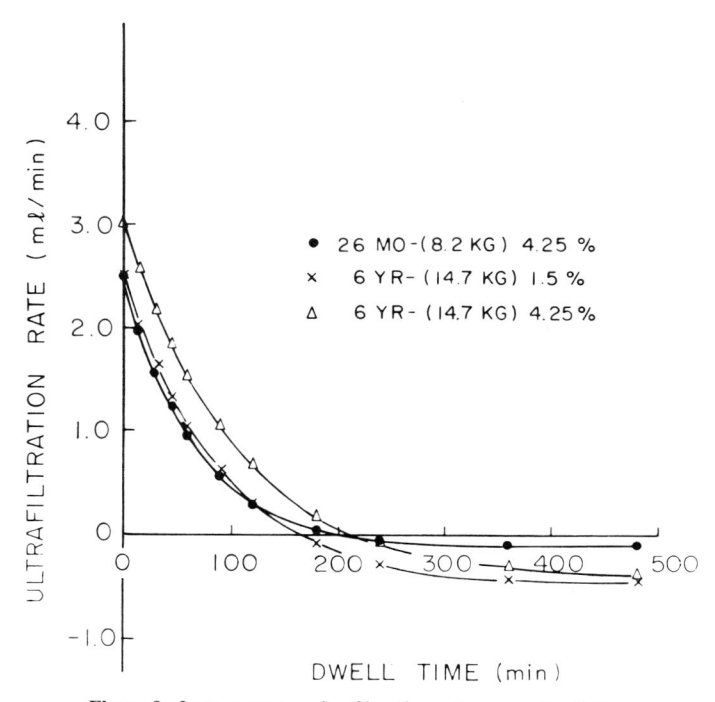

Figure 8. Instantaneous ultrafiltration rate versus dwell time.

A BUN dialysate to plasma concentration ratio versus dwell time for 1.5% dialysate in the three patients studied are presented in Figure 1. Note that similar results are obtained despite the fact that different volumes were infused with different sized children. The results are also quite similar to that obtained for adults. This is interesting in view of the fact, previously outlined, that the mass transfer-area coefficients are so small for these children relative to adults. Figures 2–5 demonstrate that this is also generally true for creatinine, uric acid, and glucose. An explanation for this similarity lies in an analysis of underlying transport theory.

The basic mass transport equations describing the change in the dialysate concentration as a function of dwell time is[15]

$$\frac{d(V_D C_D)}{dt} = KA(C_p - C_D) + (1 - \sigma)Q_u \overline{C}_p, \tag{1}$$

where V_D is the dialysate volume, C_D is the dialysate metabolite concentration, C_p is the plasma metabolite concentration, KA is the mass transfer-area coefficient, σ is the metabolite reflection coefficient, $\overline{C}_p$ is the function defining a mean concentration gradient across the peritoneum, and Q_u is the ultrafiltration rate.

Expansion of the accumulation term yields

$$V_D \frac{dC_D}{dt} + C_D \frac{dV_D}{dt} = KA(C_p - C_D) + (1 - \sigma)Q_u \overline{C_p}. \qquad (2)$$

Since $dV_D/dt = Q_u$, Equation (2) can be rearranged to the form

$$\frac{dC_D}{dt} = \frac{KA}{V_D}(C_p - C_D) + \frac{Q_u}{V_D}[(1 - \sigma)\overline{C_p} - C_D]. \qquad (3)$$

It has been demonstrated that the mass transfer-area coefficient, KA, varies in direct proportion to body weight. The same appears to be valid for the ultrafiltration rate, Q_u. Therefore if the infused dialysate volume, V_D, is also decreased proportionally to decreasing weight, then the terms KA/V_D and Q_u/V_D will be constant regardless of any patient size.

The actual infused volumes for the four patients are presented in Table 6. Also presented are the infused volumes predicted by taking a weight ratio based upon 2,000 ml for a 70-kg adult. The actual volumes infused closely correspond to those predicted by the weight ratio. For these circumstances, KA/V_D and Q_u/V_D will be nearly constant for any sized child or adult resulting in nearly identical solutions for C_D/C_p curves. In other words, even though the rate of metabolite transport is reduced in proportion to weight, the capacity of the infused dialysate to absorb toxins has also been proportionally reduced by weight to yield similar D/p curves.

The results of this investigation suggest that the effective peritoneal surface area for mass transfer varies in direct proportion to body weight. Esperanza and Collins[10] measured the peritoneal surface area in infants and adults. Their anatomical results show a gross peritoneal surface area in infants approximately twice that of adults relative to body weight. One possible explanation for this difference is a comparison of the size of the infants involved. The smallest infant investigated in our study was 7.0 kg. The average weight of the infants studied by Esperanza and Collins was 2.7 kg. It may be possible that a signficant change in the peritoneal surface area to body weight relationship might exist between these different sized infants. Also, we measured the mass transfer-area coefficient, not the over-all peritoneal surface area. The percentage of effective mass transfer area relative to the gross anatomical peritoneal surface area could vary between these different sized infants concomitant with growth and maturation. Addi-

TABLE 6.
Infused Dialysate Volumes in Proportion to Body Weight

Patient	Weight (kg)	Actual Infused Volume (ml)	Infused Volume by Weight Proportion (ml)
1	7.0	200	200
2	8.2	300	240
3	11.7	400	340
4	14.7	400	420

tional mass transfer-area coefficient measurements will be required to confirm and elucidate this apparent difference.

Esperanza and Collins[10] also measured BUN clearances in a 2.95-kg infant. They concluded that "peritoneal dialysis in a newborn infant was twice as efficient as it usually is in adults," based upon scaling their measured clearances to adult values by weight. One reason they obtained such large relative clearances when scaled to adult values is because of the very large infused volumes they used. The infusion volume predicted on a strictly weight basis is 2.95 kg/70 kg times 2,000 ml or about 85 ml. They infused 250 ml per exchange. Infusion of this large quantity of dialysate results in the dialysis becoming essentially mass transfer limited (the concentration of BUN in the dialysate never approaches equilibrium with the plasma). An elevated mass transfer rate and clearance is obtained. Scaling this clearance by weight levels yields clearance values about normal. Popovich and Moncrief[8] have shown that adult peritoneal dialysis clearances with dwell times on the order of 45 minutes also exhibit dialysate flow rate limitations. Thus, the comparison is not being made in equal terms; they would have to compare their clearance to those obtained in adults with infusion of volumes in the range of 5–6 liters per exchange. A better comparison of relative efficiency is to utilize the mass transfer-area coefficient, since these are at least theoretically independent of infused volumes or dwell times used. Clearance measurements can be strongly dependent on both parameters, and comparisons can be difficult to interpret.

COMPUTER SIMULATIONS

A computer program has been devised at the University of Texas at Austin which predicts dialysate concentration versus dwell time profiles and drained volumes from fundamental mass transfer parameters.[18] By coupling these results to known metabolite generation rates, one can predict daily infusion volumes necessary to obtain a specified plasma metabolite concentration level for any given set of conditions.

An analysis of this type was performed for creatinine. The mass transfer-area coefficients and ultrafiltration rates were assumed to scale by weight. Residual renal clearance was assumed to be negligible as a worst case basis. Creatinine generation rates for children and adults were obtained from an analysis of the literature.[19-21] This analysis plus the other details of this simulation are beyond the scope of this paper and will be published elsewhere.

The results of this preliminary analysis are presented in Figures 9 and 10. Estimated infusion volumes required to maintain a plasma creatinine concentration ranging from 6 to 14 mg/dl are presented as a function of patient weight. Two separate curves are presented to facilitate greater ease of interpretation at the lower end of the weight range.

Data points corresponding to actual infused volumes and weights of the four children being treated at the Oregon Health Science Center are presented in Figure 9 for comparison. The mean plasma creatinine level of these patients is approximately 7.0 mg/dl. The mean corresponding value

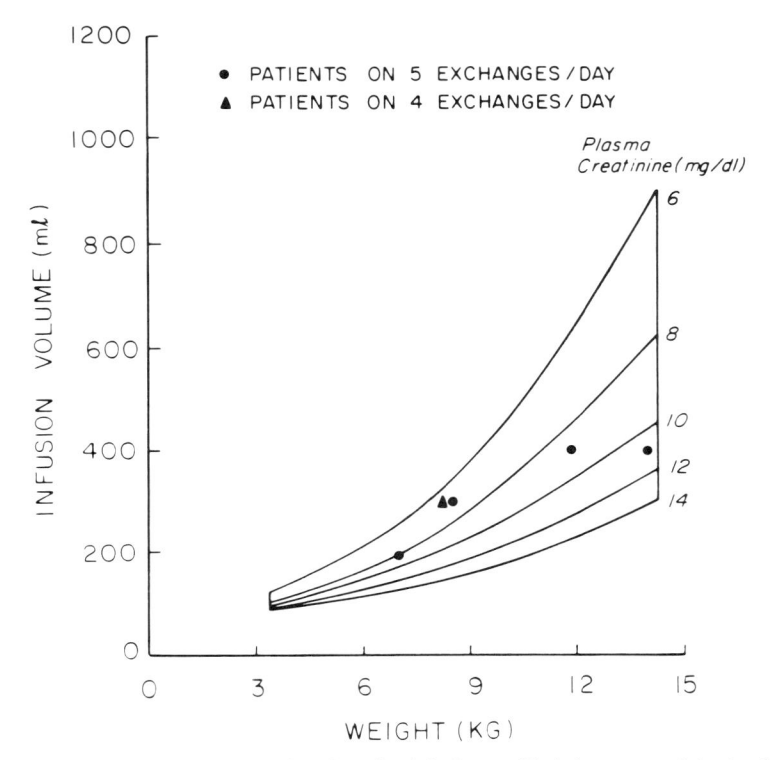

Figure 9. Infusion volumes as a function of weight for specified plasma creatinine levels.

obtained from Figure 9 (for the corresponding weights and volumes) is 8.6 mg/dl. Figure 9 predicts higher resulting creatinine levels because it is based upon a CAPD schedule of four exchanges per day. The children just noted are all on five exchanges per day. Scaling the 7.0 mg/dl clinical results from five to four exchanges per day in direct proportion to the number of exchanges yields a predicted clinical value of about 8.7 mg/dl for the four children. This is in good agreement with the mean value of 8.6 mg/dl predicted in Figure 9.

Figures 9 and 10 also illustrate clinical data from the Toronto Hospital for Sick Children. All these children have negligible renal function and are on four exchanges per day. A predicted mean value of 9.4 mg/dl for the conditions noted compare reasonably well with the clinical mean of 8.7 mg/dl. Finally, the predicted creatinine value for a 70-kg patient on four exchanges per day with 2.0-liter infusions is approximately 13.3 mg/dl. This is also in good agreement with a mean value of 12.8 mg/dl for adult patients with small to zero residual renal clearance at the Austin Diagnostic Clinic.[22]

In summary, Figures 9 and 10 can be utilized to obtain an estimate of the infusion volume required to maintain a child at the desired creatinine level. These curves are based on averaged data and should only be utilized to obtain an initial estimate. Considerable individual variations in peritoneal transport

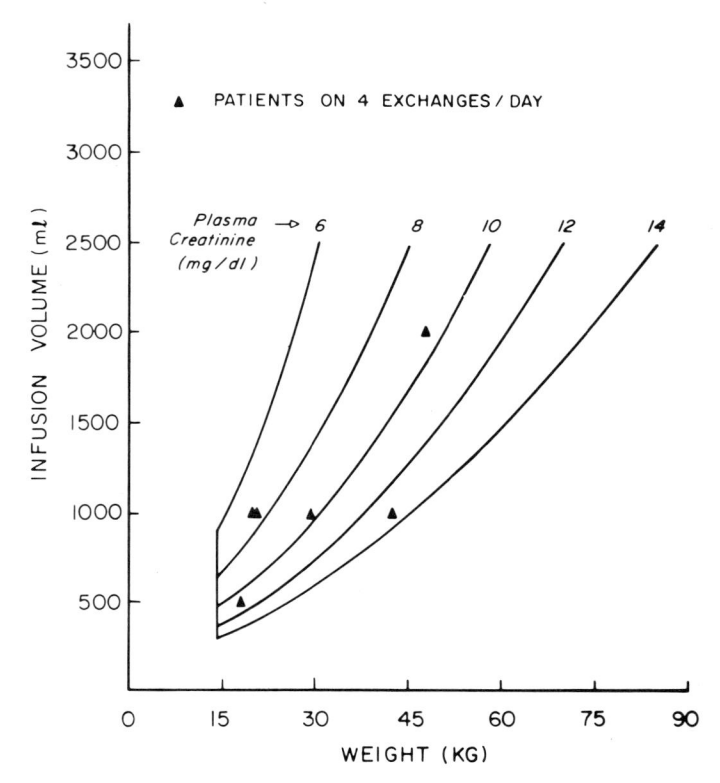

Figure 10. Infusion volumes as a function of weight for specified plasma creatinine levels.

characteristics are common. Also, steady-state creatinine levels are based on drained volumes, not infused volumes. The pediatric nephrologist will have to adjust the ratio of 1.5% and 4.25% solutions to obtain a proper fluid balance. The ratio selected will affect the drained volumes and, thus, the creatinine level. Generation rates can also vary.

CONCLUSIONS

Detailed peritoneal transport characteristics have been clinically measured in four children with a weight range of 7.0–14.7 kg. The mean mass transfer-area coefficients for BUN, creatinine, uric acid, and glucose and the maximum ultrafiltration rate were found to be directly proportional to body weight. Based upon these clinical results, a computer analysis of the child-peritoneal dialysis system was performed resulting in an estimate of the infusion volume as a function of child weight required to maintain a desired creatinine plasma level. These should form the basis for a first estimate of infusion volume, which can be adjusted depending on the particular circumstances involved.

It is the hope of the authors that this preliminary analysis will assist the pediatric nephrologist and stimulate further research into this important new scientific area.

References

1. Popovich, R. P., Moncrief, J. W., Decherd, J. F., Bomar, J. B., and Pyle, W. K.: The definition of a portable/wearable equilibrium peritoneal dialysis technique. *Abstr Am Soc Artif Inter Organs* **5**: 64, 1976.
2. Popovich, R. P., Moncrief, J. W., Nolph, K. D., Ghods, A. J., Twardowski, Z. J., and Pyle, W. K.: Continuous ambulatory peritoneal dialysis. *Ann Intern Med* **88**: 449, 1978.
3. Oreopoulos, D. G., Robson, M., Izatt, S., et al.: A simple and safe technique for continuous ambulatory peritoneal dialysis. *Trans Am Soc Artif Intern Organs* **24**: 484, 1978.
4. Moncrief, J. W., Popovich, R. P., et al.: Clinical experience with continuous ambulatory peritoneal dialysis. *J Am Soc Artif Intern Organs* **2**(3): 114, 1979.
5. Moncrief, J. W., and Popovich, R. P.: Peritoneal dialysis for a greater number of patients. *Controversies in Nephrology,* Schreiner, G. E., Ed. Georgetown University Press, Washington, D.C., 1979.
6. Moncrief, J. W., and Popovich, R. P.: Continuous ambulatory peritoneal dialysis. In *Today's Art in Peritoneal Dialysis,* Trevino, A., Ed. S. Karger, New York, 1979.
7. Popovich, R. P., Pyle, W. K., et al.: Preliminary verification of the low dialysis clearance hypothesis via a novel equilibrium peritoneal dialysis technique. *Trans Aust Conf Heat Mass Transfer* **2**: 217, 1977.
8. Popovich, R. P., and Moncrief, J. W.: Kinetic modeling of peritoneal transport. In *Today's Art in Peritoneal Dialysis,* Trevino, A., Ed. S. Karger, New York, 1979.
9. Popovich, R. P., Pyle, W. K., Bomar, J. B., and Moncrief, J. W.: Chronic replacement of kidney function. *AIChE Symp Series, Peritoneal Dialysis* **75**(187): 31, 1979.
10. Esperanza, M. J., and Collins, D. L.: Peritoneal dialysis efficiency in relation to body weight. *J Pediatr Surg* **1**: 162, 1966.
11. Alexander, S., Tseng, C. H., Maksym, K. A., Campbell, R. A., Talwalkan, Y. B., and Kohaut, E. C.: Clinical parameters in continuous ambulatory peritoneal dialysis for infants and children. This volume.
12. Balfe, J. W., Irwin, M.-A., and Orepoulos, D. G.: An assessment of continuous ambulatory peritoneal dialysis (CAPD) in children. This volume.
13. Bauer, F. K.: Radioisotope dilution methods: Measurement of body composition. In *Nuclear Medicine,* W. H. Blaud, Ed. McGraw-Hill Book Co., New York, 1971, pp. 574–592.
14. Alpert, S. N.: Blood volume, In *Nuclear Medicine,* W. H. Blaud, Ed. McGraw-Hill Book Co., New York, 1971, pp. 593–619.
15. Pyle W. K., Moncrief, J. W., and Popovich, R. P.: Peritoneal transport evaluation in CAPD. This volume.
16. Rubin, J., Nolph, K. D., Popovich, R. P., Moncrief, J. W., and Prowant, B.: Drainage volumes for continuous ambulatory peritoneal dialysis. *J Am Soc Artif Intern Organs* **2**(2): 54, 1979.
17. Nolph, K. D., Popovich, R. P., et al.: Equilibration of peritoneal dialysis solutions during long dwell exchanges. *J Lab Clin Med* **93**: 246, 1978.
18. Popovich, R. P., Moncrief, J. W., Nolph, K. D., Pyle, W. K., and Sawyer, J. W.: Physiological transport parameters in peritoneal and hemodialysis. Third Annual Report No. N01-AM-3-2205 to Artificial Kidney—Chronic Uremia Program, National Institutes of Health, 1977.
19. Arant, B. S., Edelman, C. M., and Spitzer, A.: The congruence of creatinine and inulin clearances in children—Use of the Technicon auto analyzer. *J Pediatr* **81**(3): 509, 1972.
20. Clark, L. C., Thompson, H. L., Beek, E. I., and Jacobson, W.: Excretion of creatine and creatinine by children. *Am J Dis Child* **81**: 774, 1951.
21. Shull, B. C., Haugley D., Koup, J. R., Baliah, T., and Li, P. K.: A useful model for predicting creatinine clearance in children. *Clin Chem* **24**(7): 1167, 1978.
22. Moncrief, J. W.: Personal communication, April 23, 1980.

CHAPTER THIRTY-ONE

Renal Osteodystrophy in Patients on Continuous Ambulatory Peritoneal Dialysis (CAPD): A Biochemical and Radiological Study

V. CALDERARO, M.D.

D. G. OREOPOULOS, M.D., Ph.D., F.R.C.P.(C)

E. H. MEEMA, M.D., F.R.C.P.(C)

R. KHANNA, M.D.

C. QUINTON, R.N.

D. CARMICHAEL, M.Sc.

RECENTLY, AN INCREASING NUMBER OF patients with end-stage renal disease are maintained on continuous ambulatory peritoneal dialysis (CAPD). To date, there has not been any report on the evolution of renal osteodystrophy in patients undergoing this treatment. In this chapter we will present the results of our biochemical and radiological studies in 28 patients who have been on CAPD from 6 to 23 months.

PATIENTS AND METHODS

Twenty-eight patients (10 men and 18 women) with ages ranging from 22 to 74 (average 51.3) years have had one or more follow-up examinations during CAPD treatment. They all underwent CAPD using the Toronto Western Hospital technique.[1]

In addition to CAPD, the patients were treated with 50,000 units of vitamin D_3 once a week and phosphate binders. During the last part of the study, five patients received 1,25 dihydroxyvitamin D_3, the doses being adjusted to maintain their serum calcium at the upper limits of normal.

Routine biochemical investigations included measurement of serum calci-

---

Departments of Medicine and Radiology, Toronto Western Hospital, Toronto, Ontario, Canada and University of Toronto, Toronto, Ontario, Canada

um, phosphorus, and CO_2 content at monthly intervals. Serum 25-hydroxyvitamin D_3 and plasma immunoreactive parathyroid hormone concentrations were measured every 6 months.

Radiological investigations were performed every 6 months and included measurement of bone mineral mass, density, and cortical thickness in the proximal radius and a skeletal survey.[2]

Finally, we measured the peritoneal calcium balance in 21 samples from seven patients who were admitted to a Metabolic Ward.

RESULTS

Biochemical investigations

Table 1 shows the changes in plasma calcium, phosphorus, calcium times phosphorus product, 25-hydroxyvitamin D_3, and parathyroid hormone in relationship to the duration of CAPD. There were no significant changes in serum calcium, whereas mean serum inorganic phosphorus decreased from an initial value of 5.7 mg/dl to 4.9 mg/dl during the first 6 months and remained unchanged thereafter. Serum alkaline phosphatase increased significantly from an initial mean value of 131 units/ml to 187 units/ml at 12 months and remained unchanged at 24 months.

Due to the decrease in serum phosphorus, the calcium times phosphorus product also decreased and remained within normal limits.

Plasma levels of 25-hydroxyvitamin D_3 remained within normal range,

TABLE 1.

Changes in Serum Calcium, Phosphorus, Alkaline Phosphatase, Carbon Dioxide Content and Calcium Times Phosphorus Product with Time on CAPD

	\multicolumn{4}{c}{Duration of CAPD (Months) ($\bar{x} \pm$ S.D.)}			
	0	6	12	12-24
Serum Calcium (mg/dl)	9.6 ± 1.0	9.8 ± 0.6	9.7 ± 0.5	9.8 ± 0.7
Serum phosphorus (mg/dl)	5.7 ± 2.1	4.9 ± 1.3[b]	4.8 ± 0.9[b]	5.0 ± 0.9[b]
Serum alkaline phosphatase (iu/ml)	131 ± 90	155 ± 64	187 ± 92[b]	164 ± 48
Serum Carbon dioxide content	20.9 ± 3.9	21.9 ± 2.1	22.3 ± 2.0	22.4 ± 1.0
Calcium times phosphorus product	53.6 ± 20	46.9 ± 12	46.4 ± 8	47.7 ± 10
25-hydroxyvitamin D_3 (ng/ml)[a]	—	24 ± 11.5	29 ± 8.5	34 ± 18
Immunoreactive parathyroid hormone (ng/ml)[a]	—	0.38 ± 0.2	0.46 ± 0.3	0.47 ± 0.3

[a] Normal range for 25-hydroxyvitamin D_3, >10 ng/ml and for immunoreactive parathyroid hormone, 0-0.25 ng/ml.
[b] Indicates significant change.

whereas plasma immunoreactive parathyroid hormone was increased initially and remained elevated throughout the study.

Radiological investigations

Table 2 shows the changes in bone mineral mass, density, and cortical thickness. Although the mean values showed decreasing trends, this was statistically significant only for the combined cortical thickness ($p < 0.05$).

Subperiosteal resorption increased in 28% of the patients. An additional 10 patients (36%) in whom subperiosteal resorption was increased to start with, remained abnormal throughout the study. Only in three patients (10%) did subperiosteal resorption improve. Intracortical resorption remained unchanged in nine patients, became worse in 13, and improved only in two.

Fractures

New fractures developed in three patients (two pathological and one traumatic); they all healed. In addition, in two patients who had pathological fractures (and histologically proved osteomalacia) when started on CAPD the fractures healed with marked callus formation during the CAPD treatment. It should be stressed that they were all receiving vitamin D_3.

Arterial calcifications remained unchanged, and no new calcifications developed while on CAPD.

The mean peritoneal calcium balance was found to be negative at 50 ± 36 mg/day ($\bar{x} \pm$ S.D.).

DISCUSSION

The fact that serum calcium remained unchanged despite the continuous negative peritoneal calcium balance indicates the effectiveness of some compensatory mechanisms: either an increase in calcium absorption from the gut or an increase in calcium release from the bone. Increased bone resorption is indicated by the increase in parathyroid hormone levels as well as by the

TABLE 2.

Changes in Bone Mineral Mass and Density and Cortical Thickness with Time on CAPD

	Duration of CAPD (Months) ($\bar{x} \pm$ S.D.)			
	0	6	12	12–24
Bone mineral mass (mg/cm^2)	531 ± 135	515 ± 114	537 ± 127	497 ± 107
Bone mineral density (mg/cm^3)	940 ± 100	900 ± 160	960 ± 160	930 ± 160
Cortical thickness (mm)	5.59 ± 0.9	5.58 ± 0.8	5.48 ± 0.8	5.20 ± 0.86

maintenance or even deterioration of bone resorption in a significant number of patients.

CAPD seems to be superior to intermittent peritoneal dialysis in controlling serum phosphorus and as a result, the serum calcium times phosphorus product was normal in most patients.

The increased serum alkaline phosphatase probably reflects the persistence of hyperparathyroid bone disease, since liver function tests were normal (unpublished data).

Persistence or even progression of radiologically diagnosed subperiosteal resorption was found in these patients despite treatment with vitamin D_3 or 1,25-dihydroxyvitamin D_3. In contrast, osteomalacia seemed to respond to treatment with CAPD, since callus formation occurred both in pathological and traumatic fractures. Previous experience[3] has shown that treatment with vitamin D_3 or even with 1,25 dihydroxyvitamin D_3 usually fails to heal osteomalacic fractures. It now appears that this treatment may be more effective in patients undergoing CAPD. CAPD may be enhancing calcification of bone collagen. A calcifying defect in patients with renal osteomalacia has been ascribed to either immaturity of the bone collagen[4] or to the presence of circulating inhibitors of calcification.[5] In the past we have shown that intermittent peritoneal dialysis is effective in removing circulating inhibitors of calcification[6] and it is possible that CAPD may be superior to intermittent peritoneal dialysis in this respect. Similarly, it is possible that CAPD may contribute to the maturation of collagen and thus facilitate calcification by removing unidentified toxins,[7] which may be responsible for the immaturity of the collagen.

Arterial calcification did not progress, probably because most of these patients had normal calcium times phosphorus products. This is in contrast to progression of arterial calcification in patients treated with intermittent peritoneal dialysis who usually have increased calcium times phosphorus product.

In conclusion, whereas the osteitis fibrosa element of renal osteodystrophy progresses in patients maintained on CAPD, osteomalacia seems to improve. Perhaps a higher dialysate calcium and a more vigorous use of vitamin D_3 or its analogues could arrest the progression of osteitis fibrosa in these patients.

ACKNOWLEDGMENT

This work was supported by the United States National Institutes of Health, Chronic Uremia and Artificial Kidney Program (Contract No. NO1 AM8 2213), and Medical Research Council of Canada (Grant MA-3889).

References

1. Oreopoulos, D. G., Robson, M., Izatt, S., Clayton, S., and deVeber, G. A.: A new method for a simpler and safer CAPD. *Trans Am Soc Artif Intern Organs* **24:** 484, 1978.
2. Meema, H. E., Harris, C. K., and Porrett, R. E.: A method for determination of bone salt content or cortical bone. *Radiology* **82:** 986, 1964.

3. Velentzas, C., Oreopoulos, D. G., Pierratos, A., Meema, H. E., Rabinovich, S., Meindok, H., Husdan, H., Murray, T. M., Ogilvie, R., and Katirtzoglou, A.: 1,25-Dihydroxyvitamin D_3 in the treatment of renal osteodystrophy. *Can Med Assoc J* (in press).
4. Russel, J. E., Termine, J. D., and Avioli, L. V.: Abnormal bone mineral materation in the chronic uremic state. *J Clin Invest* **52**: 2848, 1973.
5. Yendt, E. R., Connor, T. B., and Howard, J. E.: In vitro calcification in rachitic rat cartilage in normal and pathological sera with some observations on the pathogenesis of renal rickets. *Bull Johns Hopkins Hosp* **96**: 1, 1955.
6. Oreopoulos, D. G., Pitel, S., and Husdan, H.: Contrasting effects of hemodialysis and peritoneal dialysis on the inhibition of in vitro calcification by uremic serum. *Can Med Assoc J* **110**: 43, 1974.
7. Oreopoulos, D. G., and Funck-Brentano, J. L.: Continuous ambulatory peritoneal dialysis. *Ann Intern Med* **89**: 1009, 1978.

CHAPTER THIRTY-TWO

Histological Renal Bone Disease in Patients on Continuous Ambulatory Peritoneal Dialysis

R. GOKAL, M.D., M.R.C.P.

H. A. ELLIS, F.R.C.PATH.

M. K. WARD, M.R.C.P.

D. N. S. KERR, F.R.C.P.

INTRODUCTION

RENAL OSTEODYSTROPHY INFLUENCES the quality of life and contributes to the morbidity of patients with end-stage renal failure.[1] It comprises osteitis fibrosa (OF), due to secondary hyperparathyroidism, and sometimes, in addition, there is osteomalacia (OM).[2] Potent stimulators of parathormone (PTH) hypersecretion in chronic renal failure are hyperphosphatemia and hypocalcemia (the latter due to acquired vitamin D resistance and decreased intestinal calcium absorption).[3]

Continuous ambulatory peritoneal dialysis (CAPD) is rapidly gaining world-wide acceptance as a mode of therapy for renal failure.[4] We and others have previously reported better calcium and phosphate control in CAPD than in hemodialysis[5,6] and better management of renal osteodystrophy may well be anticipated in these patients. To date there have been no reports on renal osteodystrophy as assessed by bone histology in CAPD.

In this study we summarize briefly our preliminary experiences of renal bone disease in CAPD patients using paired bone histology.

Departments of Medicine and Pathology, University of Newcastle upon Tyne, Newcastle upon Tyne, England, Royal Victoria Infirmary, Newcastle upon Tyne, England

PATIENTS AND METHODS

CAPD as a definitive mode of therapy was introduced in Newcastle in January 1979.[7] In the first 17 months 48 patients were managed by the CAPD technique.

This report is concerned with paired bone histological studies in eight patients, four male and four female (Table 1). A transiliac bone biopsy specimen using a Bordier trephine[8] was obtained from each patient at the start of CAPD and then annually or if the patients left the CAPD program.

Six patients had biopsies at 1 year and the other two at 5 and 6 months, respectively. One had clinical bone disease. Six were on calcium carbonate, 500 mg three times a day, and four were on 1 α-hydroxycholecalciferol, 1 μg daily. Histological OF was graded on a scale of increasing severity (0–5).[9] The presence of OM was sought in plastic embedded undecalcified sections. A diagnosis of OM is based on the presence of an excess of osteoid with wide seams and a reduced mineralization front.[9] Serum ionized calcium and PTH levels were measured by previously reported methods.[5] Biochemical analysis of serum was performed monthly and skeletal radiology was undertaken initially and at the time of the second biopsy.

All patients underwent four exchanges a day of Travenol peritoneal dialysis fluid containing 1.75 mmol/liter calcium and 35 mmol/liter lactate.

RESULTS

With the exception of patient 3, all showed a distinct improvement or no change in the bone histological status over the study period. Patient 6 had previously been managed on maintenance hemodialysis therapy for 5 years and had severe symptomatic bone disease at the onset of CAPD, which necessitated parathyroidectomy four months later. Patient 3 had developed OF grade 1 (from 0) a year later but had low ionized calcium levels.

In four patients (Numbered 2, 5, 7, and 8) there was improvement in histological OF, and two of these were receiving vitamin D therapy. None of the patients had OM initially and none developed it. Radiological renal osteodystrophy was evident in three patients, all of whom had severe histological OF. However, in one patient with severe histological OF the skeletal radiography was normal. Serum alkaline phosphatase levels were normal in all but two patients.

DISCUSSION

Over the short period of study, there has been no deterioration in the bone histology of the patients and some improvement in five. In one this was related to parathyroidectomy and in two partly to vitamin D therapy. These early results are encouraging, suggesting that control of renal osteodystrophy may be achieved by CAPD.

Noninvasive methods for studying renal osteodystrophy have their draw-

TABLE 1.
Details of Bone Histology in Relationship to Biochemistry, Skeletal Radiology, and Duration of CAPD[a]

Patients	Bone Histology Grades At Start of CAPD OF	OM	2nd Biopsy OF	OM	Duration of CAPD	Treatment with 1α OHCC	Serum Ionized Calcium (mmol/liter) (1.15–1.3)	Serum Phosphate (mmol/liter) (0.8–1.5)	Parathormone (u/liter) (1.5)	Serum Alkaline Phosphatase	Skeletal Radiology
1	0	0	0	0	1 Year	—	N	1.8–1.9	2–3.4	N	N
2	1.5	0	0	0	1 Year	—	N	1.5–2.0	1.6–4	N	N
3	0	0	1	0	1 Year	—	L	1.5–1.9	1.1–2.5	N	N
4	1	0	0	0	1 Year	+	L	1.5–2.0	1–2.2	N	N
5	2.5	0	1.5	0	1 Year	+	N	1.3–1.7	4–8	H	RO
6	4	0	0	0	1 Year	+	N	2.0–2.7	6–8	H	RO
7	4	0	2.5	0	6 Months	+	N	1.7–2.0	4–6	N	RO
8	3	0	2	0	5 Months	—	N	1.2–1.6	2.4–5	N	N

[a] The normal range for the biochemical parameters is given in parentheses. The values for serum phosphate and parathormone were available on a monthly basis, the highest and lowest figures are given. Patient 6 had parathyroidectomy 4 months after starting CAPD. OF: osteitis fibrosa (graded 0–5, see text); OM: osteomalacia; N: within normal range; L: below normal range; H: above normal range; RO: renal osteodystrophy.

backs and we have always laid great stress on histological evidence for renal osteodystrophy. Even in this limited study, no correlation of histological grading and clinical features, alkaline phosphatase or skeletal radiology was found; this is in keeping with our previous experience.[10] The patients in Newcastle receive calcium carbonate, 500 mg three times a day if the ionized calcium is low or in the low to mid normal range.[5] This not only helps to promote calcium levels but by its phosphate binding action helps in controlling the phosphate and may also help in the control of acidosis. The role of regular vitamin D replacement has not been established but 25-hydroxycholecalciferol levels may be low.

It would appear that this form of therapy may allow better control of renal osteodystrophy. However, long-term studies are needed with detailed quantitative histological studies of serial bone biopsies before any final conclusions can be reached regarding the effectiveness of CAPD in alleviating or preventing bone disease in patients with end-stage renal failure.

References

1. Avioli, L. V., and Teitelbaum, S. L.: The renal osteodystrophies. In *The Kidney,* Brenner, B. M. and Rector, F. C., Eds. W. B. Saunders, Philadelphia, 1976, pp. 1542–1594.
2. Ellis, H. A., Pierides, A. M., Feest, T. G., Ward, M. K., and Kerr, D. N. S.: Histopathology of renal osteodystrophy with particular reference to the effects of 1αhydroxy vitamin D_2 in patients treated by long-term haemodialysis. *Clin Endocrinol* 7 (Suppl): 31s–38s, 1977.
3. Fournier, A., Sebert, J. L., Coevoet, B., *et al.:* Current status of the management of renal osteodystrophy. *Proc Euro Dial Transplant Assoc* 15: 547–568, 1978.
4. Oreopoulos, D. C.: The coming of age of continuous ambulatory peritoneal dialysis (CAPD). *Dial Transplant* 8: 460–462, 1979.
5. Gokal, R., Fryer, R., *et al.:* Calcium and phosphate control in CAPD patients. In *CAPD: Proceedings of an International Symposium,* Legrain, M., Ed. Excerpta Medica, Amsterdam, 1980, pp. 283–291.
6. Oreopoulos, D. G., Robson, M., Faller, B., *et al.:* Continuous ambulatory peritoneal dialysis: A new era in the treatment of chronic renal failure. *Clin Nephrol* 11: 125–128, 1979.
7. Gokal, R., McHugh, M., Fryer, R., *et al.:* CAPD, one year's experience in a U.K. Dialysis unit. *Br Med J* 281: 474–477, 1980.
8. Bordier, P., Matratt, H., Miravet, L., *et al.:* Mesure histologique de la masse et de la resorption des travres osseuses. *Pathol Biol* 12: 1238–1243, 1964.
9. Ellis, H. A., and Peart, K. M.: Azotaemic renal osteodystrophy: A quantitative study on iliac bone. *J Clin Pathol* 26: 83–101, 1973.
10. Alvarez-Ude, F., Feest, T. G., Ward, M. K., *et al.:* Haemodialysis bone disease: Correlation between clinical, histologic and other findings. *Kidney Int* 14: 68–73, 1978.

CHAPTER THIRTY-THREE

Treatment of *Candida* Peritonitis with Peritoneal Lavage

MICHAEL J. BLUMENKRANTZ, M.D.

PERITONITIS CAUSED BY *Candida albicans* or *Candida tropicalis* accounts for only 2–4% of episodes of peritonitis in a maintenance peritoneal dialysis program. Although the incidence of *Candida* peritonitis is relatively low, the illness is generally so severe that its occurrence represents a major medical care problem. This chapter will present an approach to the diagnosis and treatment of *Candida* peritonitis, which has resulted from personal experiences over the past 9 years and a review of published reports.[1-6]

There are a number of factors that may predispose to the development of candida peritonitis: 1) the use of an "open" peritoneal dialysis system using the manual exchange of 2-liter containers of dialysate, 2) a debilitated host, especially a diabetic, and 3) the prior use of antibiotics.

With the exception of unusual cases, peritonitis represents a breakdown of the sterile techniques used in performing peritoneal dialysis. Since *Candida* peritonitis often occurs in patients who have been undergoing antibiotic therapy for bacterial peritonitis, its occurrence reflects a serious breakdown of sterile procedures. The use of automated equipment for peritoneal dialysis reduces the likelihood of such accidents because it reduces the number of times that human error can result in contamination. When peritoneal dialysis is performed by manual exchanges of dialysate, the potential for infection is high.

Candida peritonitis should be suspected, especially in the debilitated patient, the diabetic patient, and the patient who has undergone recurrent frequent episodes of peritonitis. The likelihood of *Candida* peritonitis is increased in patients with persistent peritonitis despite antibiotic therapy and when bacterial cultures of the peritoneal fluid are negative. Cultures of peritoneal fluid for *Candida* species may take several days to demonstrate the

---

Medical and Research Services, Veterans Administration Wadsworth Medical Center, Los Angeles, California

organism. Gram's stain of a concentrated dialysate specimen may reveal hyphae or spores. The patient is often toxic in appearance, persistently febrile with a persistent peripheral leukocytosis; abdominal tenderness with rebound may be severe. Abdominal pain during dialysate inflow is frequent. Dialysate effluent is not only cloudy but often contains large amounts of fibrin material and clumps of hyphae.

Two approaches to the treatment of *Candida* peritonitis have been advocated. One involves the removal of the permanent Tenckhoff catheter and treatment with intravenous amphotericin B. This approach has the advantages of decreased peritoneal protein loss, a possible reduction in patient morbidity, and the removal of a foreign body that can be colonized by fungi. It has the disadvantage of possibly resulting in the development of multiple/ massive peritoneal adhesions and recurrent episodes of peritoneal abscess. Resumption of peritoneal dialysis is often impossible because of the loss of peritoneal space. This necessitates the permanent transfer of the patient to maintenance hemodialysis. Unfortunately, it is often obligatory for the patient to remain on peritoneal dialysis for medical or social reasons.

The alternative form of treatment for *Candida* peritonitis (Table 1) is to leave the peritoneal catheter in place but to use it to effect not only dialysis, but also peritoneal lavage. Peritoneal lavage may provide several advantages for the treatment of peritonitis occurring in patients undergoing maintenance peritoneal dialysis. High intraperitoneal antibiotic concentrations can be attained and sustained; there is control over serum levels. Continuous peritoneal lavage may also prevent intraperitoneal loculation and adhesion formation and preserve peritoneal dialysis potential. To prevent obstruction of the catheter, lavage should be uninterrupted; dialysate should be pumped in at a high rate, 400–500 ml/minute. Dwell time and outflow should be short. Heparin added to the dialysate often reduces the amount of fibrin debris and may prevent catheter obstruction.

Amphotericin B is the antibiotic of choice. It is a polyene antibiotic consisting of a macrolide ring containing 38 carbon atoms.[7] It binds avidly to ergosterol, the principal sterol in fungal membranes, resulting in leakage or lysis of the fungal cell. It is either fungistatic or fungicidal, depending on dosage. In addition to its antifungal effects, amphotericin B has immunoadjuvant properties. Amphotericin B is marketed as Fungizone, which is a bile salt

TABLE 1.

A Suggested Treatment Regimen Using Peritoneal Lavage for the Treatment of Candida Peritonitis

1. Dialysate pumped into peritoneal cavity (400-500 ml/minute). Short dwell time (2-4 minutes), do not interrupt lavage
2. Amphotericin B to dialysate (1-2 mg/liter) via dextrose pump (50-100 mg/500 ml D_5W at setting of 10 ml/liter of dialysate)
3. 5-Fluorocytosine to dialysate concentrate (50 mg/liter dialysate or 2 g/2 liter concentrate), plus 20,000 u of heparin/2 liter concentrate
4. 5-Fluorocytosine and amphotericin B intravenously (see text)
5. Oral and parenteral nutrition (see text and Table 2)

complex. It forms a colloidal suspension when hydrated. In the presence of electrolytes or at low pH the antibiotic will form visible aggregates and come out of solution. It is this latter property that precludes adding the antibiotic to the dialysate concentrate used with some of the automated dialysate delivery systems. Most *Candida* infections can be treated with a dialysate level of 1 to 2 µg/ml. To accomplish this when using reverse osmosis equipment, 50–100 mg of amphotericin can be added to 500 ml of D_5W or $D_{50}W$; this solution should be added to the dilute dialysate at the rate of 10 ml/liter of dialysate via the dextrose pump on the machine. Neutralization of the dialysate pH by the addition of either sodium bicarbonate or sodium hydroxide may reduce abdominal pain.

With severe infections, amphotericin should be administered intravenously as well, since transperitoneal absorption is probably low and adequate blood levels may not be obtained. An accelerated dosage schedule should be used; a 1-mg test dose followed immediately by 0.25 mg/kg of body weight; following this a daily dose of 0.5 mg/kg of body weight should be given.[7] Amphotericin blood levels should be monitored.

Because of the difficulty in treating systemic candidiasis with amphotericin alone, the use of a combination of flucytosine and amphotericin has been advocated by many.[7] They are synergistic and their use concomitantly will prevent emergence of resistant strains. The use of flucytosine may also permit a decrease in the dose of amphotericin B, thereby reducing the toxicity from the latter antibiotic.

Flucytosine (5-fluorocytosine) is a fluorinated pyrimidine. Its antifungal properties result from its conversion to the antimetabolite 5-fluorouracil. Entry into the fungal cell is via cytosine permease, an enzyme not present in mammalian cells. Like amphotericin, it is either fungistatic or fungicidal, depending on dose. It has considerably fewer side effects than amphotericin. However, resistance develops commonly and therefore it should be administered concomitantly with amphotericin B. The peritoneal clearance of flucytosine is similar to that of creatinine.[2] For patients with *Candida* peritonitis a loading dose of 20–30 mg/kg of body weight should be administered intravenously. Dialysate levels of 50 µg/ml (50 mg/liter of dialysate or 2 g/2-liter bottle of concentrate) will generally result in adequate blood levels.[2-4] The blood level of flucytosine should be monitored.[8]

It is important that considerable attention be paid to maintaining an adequate nutritional intake in these patients in order to minimize tissue breakdown. Protein losses may be very large and intravenous nutrition may be necessary. A suggested regimen for nutrition by peripheral vein is shown in Table 2. A solution containing 4.25 or 5% amino acids (both essential and nonessential) with low concentrations of dextrose (7.5 to 10%) is used. Two or 2.5 liters are infused daily into a peripheral vein. Water soluble vitamins and trace elements are added. Insulin may be added not only to control hyperglycemia but also for its anabolic effect. Since the patient is undergoing dialysis, the addition of electrolytes to the parenteral solution is generally not required. If the patient becomes phosphate depleted, dibasic potassium phosphate or dibasic sodium phosphate may be added to the intravenous solution. Five hundred milliliters of a 20% lipid emulsion may be infused daily through a

TABLE 2.

A Regimen for Parenteral Nutrition by Peripheral Vein in
Patients Undergoing Peritoneal Dialysis

Intravenous Infusion	Quantity of Nutrients (g)	Energy[a] (kcal)	Volume (liters)
Crystalline amino acids (4.25 or 5%)	100-128	350-435	2.0-2.5[b]
Glucose (7.5-10%)	150-250	555-925	
Lipid emulsion (20%)	100	1,100	0.5

Dialysis Schedule:
Intermittent peritoneal dialysis: 5-7 liter/hour, utilize dialysate with 2.5-4.25% dextrose concentration for ultrafiltration

Monitor:
Serum glucose, sodium, potassium, bicarbonate, and phosphate

[a] Additional calories derived from glucose absorbed from dialysate.
[b] Add insulin, trace elements, vitamins.

Y-infusion set concurrently with the amino acids and glucose. High concentrations of dialysate dextrose are generally needed to remove the fluid infused. Glucose absorbed across the peritoneum provides additional energy.

During intravenous nutritional therapy, it is important to monitor serum glucose, sodium, potassium, bicarbonate, and phosphate levels and to check the serum for lipemia. Studies remain to be done to assess the efficacy of this method of nutritional support. If sufficient nutrients cannot be administered by peripheral vein or if prolonged nutritional therapy is required, total parenteral nutrition by central vein should be used.[9]

ACKNOWLEDGMENT

Supported in part by USPHS Contract AM-5-2218, USPHS CRC Grant RR 865 and VA Research Funds.

References

1. Bayer, A. S., Blumenkrantz, M. J., Montgomerie, J. Z., Galpin, J. E., Coburn, J. W., and Guze, L. B.: Candida peritonitis: Report of 22 cases and review of the English literature. *Am J Med* **61:** 832–840, 1976.
2. Holdsworth, S. R., Atkins, R. C., Scott, D. F., and Jackson, R.: Management of candida peritonitis by prolonged peritoneal lavage containing 5-fluorocytosin. *Clin Nephrol* **4:** 157–159, 1975.
3. Barnes, R., Brown, D., Silva, J., et al.: Candida peritonitis complicating peritoneal dialysis. *Abstr Am Soc Nephrol* 1975, p. 27.
4. Andersen, K. E., and Olsen, H.: Case report: Candida peritonitis in a patient receiving chronic intermittent peritoneal dialysis. *Scan J Infect Dis* **10:** 92–93, 1978.
5. Mandell, I. N., Ahern, M. J., Kliger, A. S., and Andriole, V. T.: Candida peritonitis

complicating peritoneal dialysis: successful treatment with low dose amphotericin B therapy. *Clin Nephrol* **6**: 492–496, 1976.
6. Arfania, D., Everett, E. D., Nolph, K. D., and Rubin, J.: Unusual causes of peritonitis in patients on peritoneal dialysis. *Arch Intern Med* (in press).
7. Medoff, G., and Kobayashi, G. S.: Strategies in the treatment of systemic fungal infections. *N Engl J Med* **302**: 145–155, 1980.
8. Kaspar, R. L., and Drutz, D. J.: Rapid, simple bioassay for 5-fluorocytosine in the presence of amphotericin B. *Antimicrob Agents Chemother* **7**: 462–465, 1975.
9. Kopple, J. D., and Blumenkrantz, M. J.: Total parenteral nutrition. In *Clinical Disorders of Fluid and Electrolyte Metabolism,* 3rd ed., C. R. Kleeman and M. H. Maxwell, Eds. McGraw-Hill, New York, 1979, pp. 413–458.

CHAPTER THIRTY-FOUR

Treatment of Peritonitis (in Patients on CAPD)

D. G. OREOPOULOS, M.D., Ph.D., F.R.C.P. (C), F.A.C.P.

S. VAS, M.D., Ph.D., F.R.C.P. (C)

R. KHANNA, M.D.

BEFORE A PHYSICIAN TREATS A PATIENT on continuous ambulatory peritoneal dialysis (CAPD) for peritonitis, he should have the results of several important procedures, namely, 1) examination of the patient, 2) Gram's stain of the effluent, 3) white cell count and differential of the effluent, and 4) culture of the dialysate.

Examination of the patient

Patients on CAPD should be seen as soon as the symptoms of peritonitis develop. They should be asked if, in the days preceding the appearance of the symptoms, they noticed any technical failures, because in our experience 2–4 days elapse after an external contamination before signs and symptoms of clinical peritonitis develop. Any alteration in bowel habits, especially constipation, should be noted because constipation, accentuated by the intake of phosphorus binders, may lead to peritonitis. In extreme cases, the formation of fecaliths may lead to impaction and subsequent bowel perforation. Radiographs of the abdomen (three views and a flat plate) can give useful information in patients with fecal impaction. The main presenting symptoms in this condition are cloudy fluid and abdominal pain. The patient with these symptoms should be examined for evidence of rebound tenderness and the presence and character of bowel sounds, fever, nausea, vomiting, or diarrhea. The examiner should pay particular attention to the skin exit site and the condition of the subcutaneous tunnel.

The appearance of the patient at the time of the examination has consider-

---

Department of Medicine, Toronto Western Hospital, Toronto, Ontario, Canada and University of Toronto, Toronto, Ontario, Canada

TABLE 1.
Clinical Presentation in 35 Episodes of Peritonitis

Symptoms and Signs	Patient's Appearance	
	Ill (%)	Well (%)
Cloudy effluent	100	100
Cramps—abdominal pain, gas pain	92	50
Rebound tenderness	85	36
Nausea or vomiting	77	9
Fever (38°C.)	23	9
Diarrhea	23	0
Decreased bowel sounds	31	0
Total patients	37 (13)	63 (22)

able prognostic importance. In our unit, during the last year, 37% of the patients who presented with peritonitis looked ill in contrast to the 63% who said they were feeling well despite the presence of intra-abdominal infection (Table 1). In addition, this table shows the frequency of other symptoms and signs of peritonitis in these two groups.

Gram's stain

Done by an experienced technologist, this stain will identify the offending organisms in up to 40–50% of cases and enable the attending physician to begin the proper antibiotics immediately. In addition the Gram's stain can identify the presence of fungi and, if it shows the presence of multiple organisms, may provide the first indication of fecal peritonitis. The presence of gram-positive rods with negative aerobic cultures also suggests the presence of anaerobic organisms and thus fecal peritonitis.

White cell count and differential of the effluent

This test may differentiate those cases in which the turbid effluent is due to fibrin or eosinophils from those in which the cloudiness is due to infection. Finally, white blood cell count (WBC) may assist in the follow-up of treatment, especially when the patient continues on CAPD. Figure 1 shows the relationship of the number of white blood cells in the effluent to its appearance. Clear fluid contains from 2×10^3 to 10×10^4 WBC/ml.

Culture of the dialysate

In all cases, a concentrated sample of effluent at least 10 ml should be cultured for aerobic organisms (using agar plate and meat broth) and for anaerobic organisms, using a technique previously described.[1]

Our experience to date suggests that blood cultures make no contribution to the investigation because they are always negative. This experience indicates that peritonitis in CAPD patients is different from surgical peritonitis.

TREATMENT OF PERITONITIS

Management at the Toronto Western Hospital depends on our estimate of the severity in each case. We will describe these approaches under three headings.

Lavage with antibiotics

This procedure is indicated principally for the severe infections but can also be applied for a short period (1 or 2 days) in mild cases.

Usually we lavage the peritoneal cavity using Dianeal solution that contains antibiotics and heparin, the latter to prevent fibrin clot and adhesion formation. The first-line antibiotics are cephalothin (100 mg/liter) for the gram-positive organisms and tobramycin (10 mg/liter) for the gram-negative ones. If the Gram's stain shows no organisms, we administer both antibiotics until the results of culture are obtained. If for various reasons these antibiotics cannot be used, we use one of the second-line antibiotics (Table 2). The lavage (no dwell time) is continued until we obtain three negative daily cultures, at which time the patient is converted to CAPD with the same antibiotic for an additional 7 days.

Some other important points in the management of peritonitis are the following: 1) If the patient is vomiting or has paralytic ileus, he should be kept in a fasting state and may require a nasogastric tube. Otherwise, the patient is allowed to eat. 2) Aluminum hydroxide should be discontinued and special attention should be paid to maintain good bowel movements with oral laxatives or enemas. Occasionally, abdominal pain, which may persist after the infection has cleared, may be due to severe constipation. 3) To offset depletion during prolonged dialysis, potassium (3 or 4 mEq/liter) should be added to the dialysate. 4) Finally, to compensate for the increased protein losses during the peritonitis, we recommend the intravenous administration of 50 g of albumin daily.

Removal of the permanent catheter

This becomes necessary when the peritonitis persists and does not respond to treatment. Usually the peritonitis should respond to treatment within 24 or 48 hours; if it does not, the cultures of the effluent will remain positive, the effluent remains cloudy, and the abdominal pain persists. In these exceptional cases, some abnormality, such as a contaminated catheter, tunnel abscess, intraperitoneal abscess, or bowel perforation, may be maintaining the infection, which usually is characterized by the presence in the effluent of anaerobes or mixed organisms. Detection of an intra-abdominal abscess may require the use of ultrasound, computerized axial tomography, or a combination of liver and lung scans. Screening of the diaphragmatic movements under

Appearance of the Effluent

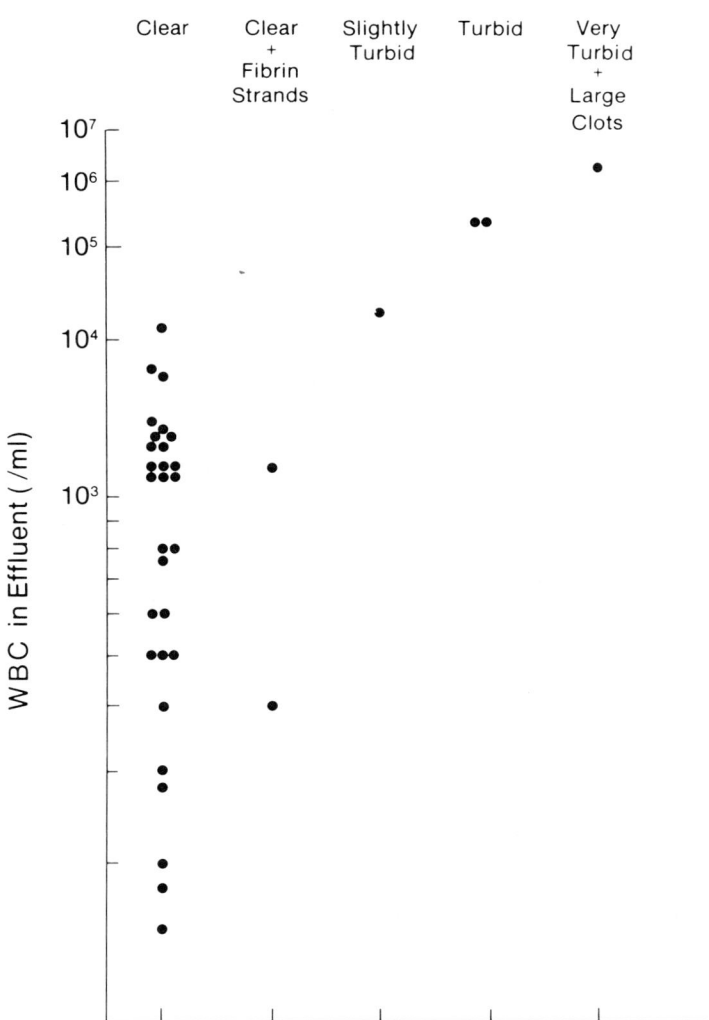

Figure 1. WBC count is related to the appearance of the effluent.

fluoroscopy may prove helpful but in our experience gallium scanning has not proved useful.

In the absence of anaerobes or mixed organisms in the culture, we usually remove the permanent catheter and maintain the patient on hemodialysis for a period of 2–3 weeks, following which we replace the catheter if the patient is free of symptoms. Some investigators have recommended that a new catheter be implanted immediately as soon as the old one is removed, but we believe

TABLE 2.
Second-line Antibiotics and the Concentration Used in Dialysate for Peritoneal Lavage

Vancomycin	30 mg/liter
Cefoxitin	200 mg/liter
Amikacin	50 mg/liter
Ticarcillin	100 mg/liter
Clindamycin	100 mg/liter
Ampicillin	50 mg/liter
Penicillin	50,000 u/liter
Septra	25/5 mg/liter

that in the presence of infection, the new catheter may also become contaminated.

If there are indications of fecal peritonitis (mixed organisms or anaerobes), we usually recommend exploratory laparotomy in addition to the removal of the catheter. The prognosis in these patients is grave because they tend to form intra-abdominal abscesses. Some centers have carried out lavage with four catheters (two for the inflow implanted under the diaphragm and two for the drain implanted in the lower pelvis) and have reported satisfactory results.

CAPD with antibiotics

In mild cases of peritonitis CAPD is continued with dialysate containing antibiotics for a period of 7–10 days. Usually we admit the patient to the hospital, although a few reliable patients have been allowed to carry out their treatment at home. The protocol we follow is as follows. After effluent samples have been taken for Gram's stain, WBC count, and cultures, we initiate three exchanges without dwell time (in–out). The addition of antibiotics to these exchanges is optional. The next step is the antibiotic loading exchange: 2 liters of dialysate with 1000 mg of cephalothin, 100 mg of tobramycin, and 1,000 units of heparin is left in the abdomen for 6 hours. This exchange is followed by exchanges containing the maintainance dose of antibiotics, (that is, cephalothin, 250 mg/liter, tobramycin, 10 mg/liter, and heparin, 500 u/liter), which are left in the abdomen for 4 to 6 hours. This treatment is continued for 8–10 days as long as the effluent is clearing and the cultures become negative. If there is no response to this regimen, we carry out lavage with antibiotics, as described previously.

OUTCOME

The outcome of 119 episodes of peritonitis in 56 patients treated with these approaches is shown in Table 3. After 104 of the episodes, the patients returned to CAPD; of the remainder, nine were transferred to hemodialysis

TABLE 3.
Outcome of 119 Episodes of Peritonitis in 56 Patients Treated with the technique Described in This Chapter

	Episode		Patient No.
	No.	Percent	
Continued on CAPD	104	87	40
Transferred to IPD	4	3	4
Transferred to HD	9	8	9
Died	3	2	3

and four to intermittent peritoneal dialysis; three of the patients died as a result of the peritonitis.

ACKNOWLEDGMENT

We would like to thank the nurses of the Center and Home Peritoneal Dialysis Units and the technologists of the Microbiology Department of the Toronto Western Hospital for their collaboration and Mrs. Fyzina Razack for her assistance in the preparation of the manuscript.

This work was supported by the U.S. National Institutes of Health, Chronic Uremia and Artificial Kidney Program (Contract No: NO1-AM8-2213).

Reference

1. Vas, S., and Oreopoulos, D. G.: Microbiological diagnostic approach to peritonitis of CAPD patients. In *CAPD: Proceedings of an International Symposium,* M. Legrain, Ed. Excerpta Medica, Amsterdam, 1980.

CHAPTER THIRTY-FIVE

Diagnosis and Treatment of Peritonitis

KARL D. NOLPH, M.D.

MICHAEL I. SORKIN, M.D.

INTRODUCTION

CONTINUOUS AMBULATORY PERITONEAL DIALYSIS (CAPD) was begun at our medical center in January of 1977 using peritoneal dialysis solutions in bottles.[1] As shown in Figure 1, the incidence of peritonitis during this early period exceeded six infections per patient-year.[2] A number of changes have taken place since that initial period, including the switch to peritoneal dialysis solutions in bags, replacement of the connecting tubing only monthly by nurses in clinic, and the use of a screw-type titanium adapter.[3] In association with these changes the infection rate has decreased. Certainly also important is the fact that as a program matures, the percentage of the CAPD population representing skilled, experienced patients increases. Most recently, our incidence appears to be between 1 and 2 infections per patient-year. In recent years, 79% of the peritonitis episodes are treated successfully on an outpatient basis. Our approach depends on early diagnosis and treatment. It will be the purpose of this chapter to summarize our approach and some of our results in greater detail.

DEFINITION AND DIAGNOSIS OF PERITONITIS

Peritonitis implies peritoneal inflammation. The etiology in CAPD patients is usually bacterial. Fungal peritonitis does occur, particularly in patients who have been treated repeatedly with antibiotics.[4] So-called "sterile peritonitis" may simply represent failure to identify any infecting organisms, although chemical irritation is frequently hypothesized.

Table 1 shows those clinical findings that justify the diagnosis of peritoni-

---

Division of Nephrology, Department of Medicine, University of Missouri Medical Center and VA Hospital, Columbia, Missouri

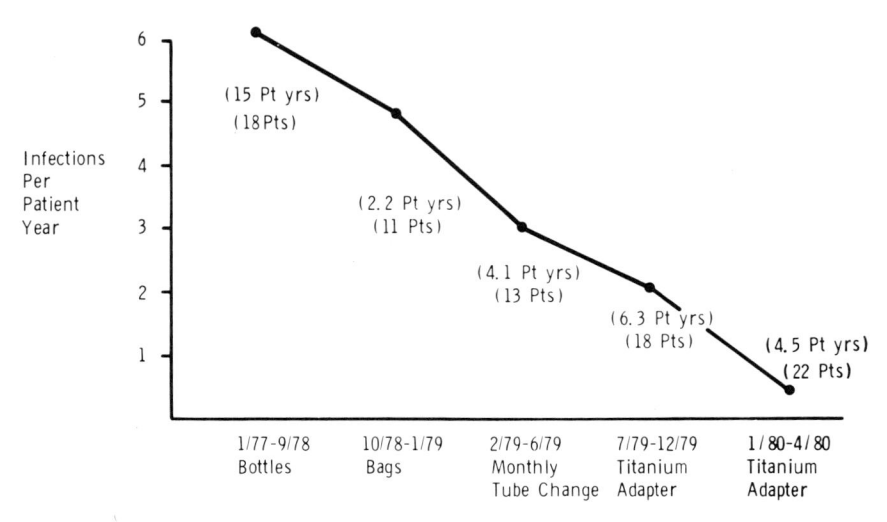

Figure 1. Peritoneal infections per patient-year at the University of Missouri are shown during different periods of the CAPD program. (Reprinted, with permission, from *Am J Nephrol* **1**: 1–10, 1981.)

tis. Peritonitis usually presents with turbid drainage ordinarily associated with abdominal symptoms. Turbid drainage is dialysate that the patient is certain is less clear than usual. The patient should always hold all drainage bags in the light and observe the degree of clarity following completion of the bag exchange procedure. With the first turbid exchange, abdominal symptoms may be mild but are usually present by history or by examination with careful palpation. Increases in dialysate white cell count with peritonitis explain the turbidity. In our experience, turbidity becomes obvious when white cell counts exceed 100–200 cells per mm^3. Patients who are well usually have white cell counts in drainage well below 50 cells per mm^3. With peritonitis, the majority of white cells in dialysate will be neutrophils. In the absence of peritonitis, mononuclear white cells predominate. Cloudy drainage, elevated dialysate white cell count, and an abundance of neutrophils are the three hallmarks of the diagnosis of peritonitis, and, in our experience, these almost always occur together.

TABLE 1.
Diagnosis of Peritonitis

Required	May Be Present, Not Required
Cloudy drainage with abdominal symptoms	Gram's stain positive
Dialysate white cell count, 100/mm^3	Positive culture
Neutrophils >50%	Fever

If the peritonitis is of bacterial or fungal etiology, organisms may be seen on Gram's stain of dialysate. Similarly, with peritonitis of infectious etiology, cultures may be positive. Patients may or may not have fever. The demonstration of organisms in dialysate or fever are not required to make the diagnosis of peritonitis.

Abdominal pain alone without increased turbidity and without an elevated dialysate white cell count should not be considered peritonitis, although dialysate drainage turbidity and white cell count should be followed closely until the cause of abdominal discomfort is established. Turbidity without an elevated white count, pain, or other evidence for peritoneal inflammation occurs rarely in some patients, presumably secondary to leakage of small amounts of lymph into the peritoneal cavity. This is so unusual, however, that turbidity alone should be considered indicative of peritonitis if a dialysate white cell count cannot be obtained. Prior to therapy, if at all possible, dialysate white cell count should be obtained.

ETIOLOGY OF PERITONITIS AT THE UNIVERSITY OF MISSOURI

Because of our high incidence of infection in the early years of CAPD, we have seen many episodes of peritonitis. The distribution of etiologies through our first 25.43 patient-years is shown in Table 2. If one looks at our over-all experience of cultures that were positive, the etiology of peritonitis represents 76% gram-positive organisms, 19% gram-negative organisms, and 5% fungal. The few cases in which we saw no growth on cultures occurred during our earlier experiences. In 35 episodes over the past year in which the filter culture technique was used, the distribution was 63% gram-positive, 23% gram-negative, 14% opportunistic, and 0 no growth.

TABLE 2.

Causative Organisms

	% Frequency[a]
Staphylococcus epidermidis	30
Staphylococcus aureus	13
Streptococci sp.	10
Other gram-positive bacteria	3
Enterobacteriaceae	5
Pseudomonadaceae	5
Acinetobacter sp.	3
Other gram-negative bacteria	3
Candida albicans	2
Nocardia asteroides	1
Aspergillus sp.	1
No growth on cultures	10
Inadequate cultures	14

[a] Represents 131 episodes, 26 patients, 25.43 patient-years.

CULTURE TECHNIQUES

Our patients who live far from the University of Missouri Medical Center are taught to remove dialysate drainage from a bag and place it in a culture bottle without contamination from outside organisms. The dialysate sample is delivered to their community hospital laboratory.

The collection of dialysate is as follows. After washing their hands and masking, the patients place a clamped drainage bag on a work table. Using a sterile needle and syringe, the cap is pulled from a culture bottle and the top cleaned with a Betadine swab. The medication port of the bag is cleaned with Betadine and allowed to dry for a few minutes. The needle is inserted into the bag through the medication port, being careful not to puncture the plastic bag with the needle. Ten milliliters of dialysate drainage are withdrawn from the bag. The needle on the syringe is changed. The fluid is injected into a culture bottle, allowing the vacuum within the bottle to pull about 4–5 ml from the syringe. The syringe is recapped. Both the culture bottle and the syringe go to the laboratory for cultures and sensitivity tests, Gram's stain, and cell count.

In our own laboratory, we inoculate two blood agar plates (0.001 and 0.1 ml). We also inoculate two MacConkey's agar plates (0.001 and 0.1 ml). One milliliter is pipetted into a thioglycolate broth. All are incubated at 37°C in 2–6% CO_2 for at least 48 hours. Anaerobic and fungal cultures are performed if the above are negative.

The filter culture technique is performed as follows: 100 ml of dialysate are obtained in a larger syringe as above. This amount of dialysate is filtered under sterile conditions through a 0.45-μm number 7102 Falcon filter. The filter is removed and placed face down on a blood agar plate. This is also incubated at 37°C in 2–6% CO_2 for at least 48 hours. Even one to two organisms per 100 ml should be trapped on the filter and identified.

THE TREATMENT OF PERITONITIS

Our approach is summarized in Table 3. The development of turbidity should prompt the patient to obtain a dialysate white cell count and culture and contact the training facility. If the white count is greater than 100 cells/mm^3, the patient should be instructed to start therapy immediately. If a white count

TABLE 3.
Treatment of Peritonitis

1. Intraperitoneal cephalosporin (125 mg/liter)
2. Intraperitoneal heparin (500 u/liter)
3. Short exchanges for 6-12 hours
4. Continue 10 days, at least 4 days of intraperitoneal
5. Admission if symptoms remain for more than 12-24 hours
6. If gram-negative organisms on smear or culture, tobramycin or gentamycin 1 mg/kg intraperitoneal or intramuscular, then 5 mg/liter for 10 days

cannot be obtained within 3 hours after a turbid drainage, samples should be collected and therapy should be started without further delay. The technique for obtaining a dialysate sample from a drainage bag at home has been summarized previously.

During the initial training, the patient should be shown how to add antibiotics and heparin to the peritoneal dialysis solution prior to instillation. They should be sent home with arrangements to obtain a supply of cephalosporin and heparin. Cephalosporin, 125 mg/liter of dialysis solution (250 mg/2-liter bag), can then be added by the patient at home if turbidity develops. We have used both cephalothin and cefazolin at this dose. Long trips to the parent center while the patient is ill can usually be avoided. Heparin, 1,000 units/2 liters, should also be added as long as drainage is turbid and contains fibrin-protein particles. Increased numbers of exchanges may be performed with initiation of therapy. A regular schedule should then be resumed, continuing to add antibiotic to all exchanges.

If dialysate turbidity does not decrease and symptoms do not diminish over the next 12–24 hours, the patient should report to the training center. If peritonitis does improve, treatment should be continued for 10 days (at least 4 days of intraperitoneal.) If the patient does not improve, the parent center should repeat the Gram's stain and obtain filter, anaerobic, and fungal cultures. Therapy at this point depends on findings and the results of cultures.

If Gram-negative organisms are found on the initial Gram's stain, we recommend tobramycin or gentamycin (a loading dose intramuscularly or intraperitoneal (1 mg/kg) and then 10 mg per 2 liter exchange (5 mg/liter) for 10 days). If gram-negative organisms only are seen on smear or culture after cephalosporin therapy has been started and if the clinical response has been poor, intraperitoneal cephalosporin should be discontinued and aminoglycoside therapy begun. Do not add both to dialysate solution, since they may be ineffective. If multiple organisms require both aminoglycoside and cephalosporin, cephalexin may be given orally.

For fungal peritonitis, intravenous amphotericin B is recommended. Since there are questions as to the amphotericin levels that can be obtained in the peritoneal cavity and catheter with intravenous therapy alone, and since the fungus is often growing within the catheter, we suggest catheter removal with the initiation of intravenous amphotericin.[4]

EXPECTED CLINICAL RESULTS WITH THERAPY

During the past year, 79% of peritonitis episodes have resolved promptly on an outpatient basis. Those requiring admission are frequently infected by gram-negative organisms or are indicative of underlying complications, such as a ruptured diverticulum.

Figure 2 shows protein concentrations and white cell counts in dialysate during the course of an infection. This patient presented with modestly elevated white cell counts, turbidity, and abdominal discomfort in association with what turned out to be a gram-positive organism. The course was

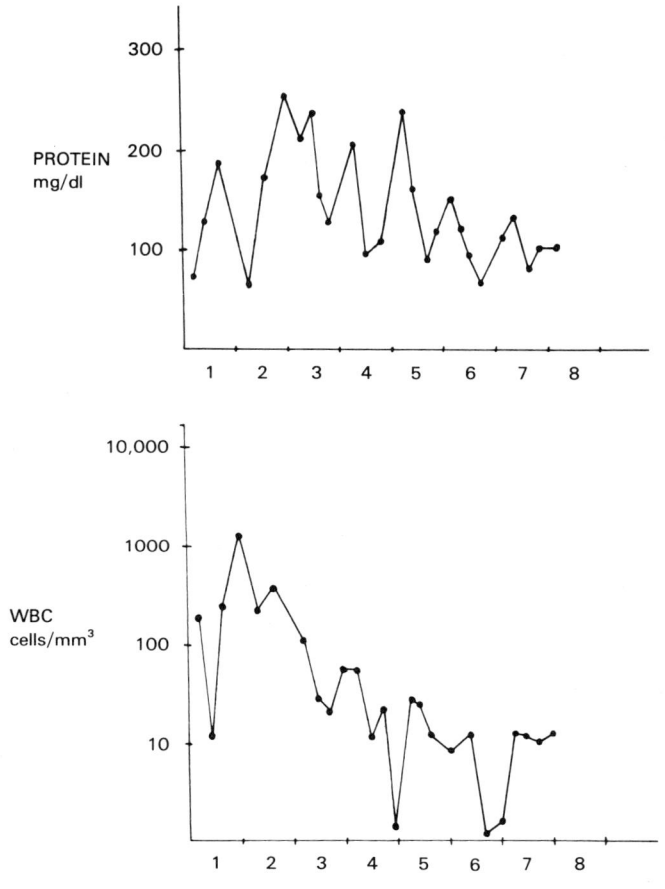

Figure 2. Protein concentrations and dialysate WBC counts were monitored during the course of peritonitis in a patient who contaminated the spike on day 0.

monitored in the Clinical Research Center during intraperitoneal therapy with cephalosporin.

This episode began within 24 hours of a known spike contamination. By the third day, white cell counts were consistently below 100. Protein concentrations in dialysate were also monitored. Note that morning values following an overnight exchange were usually higher and represented by the peaks. There is a progressive fall in the peaks and in the valleys with a return to usual baseline values near 100 mg/dl in about 1 week. This corresponds with our previous reports that peritoneal clearances and peritoneal protein losses are back to baseline within 1 week following prompt therapy of peritonitis.[5]

Table 4 summarizes serial white blood counts during the course of peritonitis in patient A. This patient happened to be seen in clinic when well and presented the next day with peritonitis. Note the prompt rise in white cell

TABLE 4.
Serial WBC Counts/mm³ before and during Peritonitis in Patient A

Date	WBC/mm³	% Neutrophils	% Lymphocytes	% Monocytes
8/14	16	16	38	42
8/15	10,778	83	5	11
8/17	586	75	—	17
8/18	209	85	5	4
8/19	26	48	42	2

count and the striking shift in the differential. Note the prompt fall in white cell count over 4 days with therapy and the return of the usual differential toward normal.

Table 5 shows the median dialysate cell counts and differential with the presentation of peritonitis of different etiology and in the absence of peritonitis. This includes our early episodes of "sterile" peritonitis. The white cell count and differential response appears to be variable from patient to patient, but similar regardless of the etiology of the peritoneal inflammation. We find the responses during gram-negative, gram-positive, and fungal peritonitis, in general, are not distinguishable. Note red cell counts also increased with inflammation.

SUMMARY

Although the incidence of peritonitis appears to be decreasing with increasing experience of CAPD programs and new innovations, it still remains a frequent complication. Until it is eliminated completely, centers must develop means for early diagnosis and treatment. It is our opinion that most can be treated on an outpatient basis with little interruption of the CAPD schedule. If diagnosed early and treated promptly, there is no evidence that peritoneal transport properties are permanently altered.

TABLE 5.
Median Dialysate Cell Counts

Peritonitis	RBC/mm³	WBC/mm³	% Neutrophils
Gram positive ($n = 20$)	309	1,710	74
Gram negative ($n = 20$)	410	5,111	77
Negative culture ($n = 14$)	568	1,217	69
Well patients ($n = 29$)	8	17	18

ACKNOWLEDGMENT

Supported in part by Clinical Research Center grant PHS RR-0028712 and PHS contracts NO1 AM5-2216 and NO1 AM-2217 and NO1 AM9-2208.

References

1. Popovich, R. P., Moncrief, J. W., Nolph, K. D., Ghods, A. J., Twardowski, Z. J., and Pyle, W. K.: Continuous ambulatory peritoneal dialysis. *Ann Intern Med* **88:** 449, 1978.
2. Rubin, J., Rogers, W. A., Taylor, H. M., Everett, E. D., Prowant, B. F., Fruto, L. V., and Nolph, K. D.: Peritonitis during continuous ambulatory peritoneal dialysis. *Ann Intern Med* **92:** 7, 1980.
3. Nolph, K. D., Sorkin, M. D., Arfania, D., Prowant, B., Fruto, L., and Kennedy, J.: Continuous ambulatory peritoneal dialysis—three year experience at a single center. *Ann Intern Med* **92:** 609, 1980.
4. Arfania, D., Everett, E. D., Nolph, K. D., and Rubin, J.: Uncommon causes of peritonitis in patients on peritoneal dialysis. *Arch Intern Med* **141:** 61, 1981.
5. Rubin, J., Nolph, K. D., Arfania, D., and Brown, P.: Follow-up of peritoneal clearances in patients undergoing continuous ambulatory peritoneal dialysis. *Kidney Int* **16:** 619, 1979.

Index

Abdominal pain, 259, 267
Ability to travel, 136
Acetoacetate, 97
Acetobacter, 185
Acid–base control, 95
Acidosis, 95
Adaptation to home dialysis, 172
Adequacy of dialysis, 85
Adolescent patients, 198
Advantages, 135, 227
Advantages of amino acid containing dialysate, 110
Advantages of "cycler," 169
Albumin, changes in, 114
American Society of Nephrology, 27
Amino acids,
    as osmotic agents, 115
    containing dialysate, 109
Amphotericin B, 254, 269
Anatomy of peritoneal transport, 7
Anemia, 21
Angiotensin, 55
Antibiotics, 263, 269
Anxiety, 178
Appetites, 135
Arterialcalcifications, 245
Atherosclerosis, 143
Average fluid transfer results, 41

Bags, 15, 265
Basic Personality Index, 178
Betadine soak, 5-minute, 168
Beta-hydroxybutyrate, 97
Blood pressure, 20, 199
Blood urea nitrogen, 181
Bone mineral mass, 244
Bottles, 265
Bowel perforations, 259, 261
BUN, 181, 183
    changes in, 112

Calcium, 181, 183
Caloric content, 88
    intake, 84, 90
    intake from dialysate glucose, 90

Candida, 184, 253
    allicans, 253
    tropicalis, 253
CAPD exchanges,
    two daily, 122
    three daily, 129
CAPD with antibiotics, 263
Capillary diameters, 70
Carbohydrate metabolisms, 143
Catheter
    adapter, 167
    adapter cracking, 167
    break-in schedule, 214
    contamination, 261
    complications, 139
    cuff erosion, 141
    malfunction, 139
    placement in infants and children, 197, 213
Catheters, lateral placement, 136
    midline incision, 136
Cephalosporin, 269
Change in general health, 135
Changes in
    albumin, 114
    BUN, 112, 114
    skin color and texture, 136
    total protein, 114
    total serum proteins, 110
    weight, 114
Child-peritoneal dialysis system, 228
Children, 10, 198, 211, 227, 238
Cholecystokinin, 56
Chronic intermittent peritoneal dialysis, 181
Chronic metabolic acidosis, 95
CIPD, 181, 183, 184, 185, 186, 187
CIPD patients changing to CAPD, 181
Clearance variation, 75
Cloud fluid, 259
Complications in infants and children, 203
Computer analysis, 228
    simulations, 238
Concentration profiles(s), 41, 44, 45, 46
Concerns, 176
Connection, 168
Connective transport, 36

"Connectology," 8
Contaminated catheter, 261
Contamination risk alleviated by finger guard, 168
Continuous insulin infusion, 160
Convection, 37
Convective protein transfer, 49
  transport, 49
Cortical thickness, 244
Cost, 189
Cost-effectiveness, 171
Co-Trimoxazole, 63
Creatinine, 181, 183
Creatinine generation rate, 76
Culture of the dialysate, 259
Culture techniques, 267
Cultures, 267
"Cycler," 169, 187

Denial, 178
Density, 244
Depression, 178
Dextran, 122
Diabetes mellitus, 143
Diabetics, 10
Dialysate
  bicarbonate, 95
  cell counts, 271
  solution, 148
  volume, 37, 235
  volume curve, 235
  white cell count, 266
Dianeal, Travenol, 195
Dietary
  alternatives, 20
  protein intake, 75
  requirements, 89
  restrictions, 135, 136
  surveys, 88
Differential, 271
  of the effluent, 259, 260
Diffusion, 37
Dilution principle, 38
Dipyridamole, 58
Disconnection, 168
  prevention, 167
Division of Network Administration, 29
D-lactate, 97
Dopamine, 58
Double-locking seal, 167
Dry weight, 199
Dwell time
  prolonged day, 169
  shorter overnight, 169

Economic aspects, 20
Effective transport area, 235
Employment, 174
Employment Adaptation Index, 174
Endogenous urea clearance, 84
Escherichia coli, 185
Evaluation of fluid and solute transport, 38
Exchange, three daily, 129
Exchanges, two daily, 122
Exercise program, 148
Exit site, 259
Exit site infection, 141
Experiments in rabbits, 110
Experience with human beings, 112
Exploratory laparotomy, 263

Family involvement and education, 137
Fecaliths, 259
Fecal peritonitis, 260
Fibrin–protein particles, 269
Filter culture technique, 267, 268
Finger guard, 168
Flucytosine, 255
Fluid
  reabsorption, 40
  transfer, 37, 42, 49
  transport, 36
  volume peak, 235
5-Flourocytosine, 255
Fractures, 245
Funding for research, 2
Fungal peritonitis, 269

Gas diffusion, 68
Gastrointestinal hormones, 56
Gentamycin, 269
Glomerular filtration rate, 85
Glucagon, 56
Glucose
  concentration, 225
  solution, 4.25%, 160
  supply, 9
  transfer rates, 225
Glycoslated hemoglobin, 148
Gram's stain of the effluent, 259, 260
Gripper clamp, 168
Growth of children on CAPD, 196, 215

HCFA, 27, 30
Health Care Financing Administration, 27
Hematocrit, 181, 183
Hemodialysis, 71, 181, 187
Hemoglobin, 181, 183, 217
Heparin, 269

High-density lipoprotein cholesterol, 155
Histamine, 59
HLD, 155
Hollow fiber dialyzer, 68
Home dialyzer, 196
Home training program, 133, 199
Hospital admission rates, 171
Hydrogen ion balance, 95
Hypertriglyceridemia, 143
Hypertriglyceridemia in rabbits on CAPD, 115
Hypervolemia, 20

Independence, 137
Indications for CAPD, 9
  in children, 196, 213
Individualized peritoneal dialysis, 84, 85
Infants, 227
  and children, 198, 227
Infection, 267
  rate, 265
Inflammation, 271
Infusion volume, 238
Insufficient dialysis, 83
Insulin, 148
  absorption, 160
  and ultrafiltration, 154
  infusion, 160
  metabolism, 143
Intercellular channels, 170
Intermittent dialysis, 105
  peritoneal dialysis, 13
Internality–externality, 176
Interstitial resistance, 71
Interstitium, 68
Intracortical resorption, 245
Intraperitoneal abscess, 261
  volume curves, 38, 47
  volume profiles, 45
Introversion, 178
Isoproterenol, 58

Key-grip spike, 168
  crackings, 168
Kinetics, 221
Kinetics of peritoneal transport, 7

L-lactate, 97
Lactate, 97
Laparotomy, exploratory, 263
Lavage with antibiotics, 261
Leakage, 142
Learning modules, 133
Leur-locking system, 167

Libido, increase in, 136
Linear growth rate, 215
Lipid metabolism, 143
Lipoprotein subfractions, 143, 155
Lymph, 267

Maintenance dialysis therapy for infants and small children, 207
Malnutrition, 83
Mannitol, 122
Mass transfer-area coefficient(s), 36, 43, 231, 236
Mass transfer coefficient, 76
Mass transfer parameters, 38
Mathematical model, 36
  modeling, 35
Materials, new, 167
Maximum dialysis, 49
Medicare, 30
Membrane permeability, 85
  transport, 37
Menarchial age range, 136
Menstruation, 136
Mesenteric capillaries, 54
  circulation, 54
Metabolic hydrogen ion generation, 95
Metabolite generation, 75
Metabolite transport, 36, 237
Metarteriole, 54
Milestones, 1
Modeling, 35
MTAC(s), 36, 41, 43, 48, 49, 50

National Institutes of Health, 1
Nitrogen balance, 75, 88, 92
  equilibrium, 92
Nitroprusside, 58
Norepinephrine, 58
Nutrient intake, 83
Nutrition by peripheral vein, 255
Nutritional considerations, 80
Nutritional status, 9, 77, 87
Nutritional therapy, 236

Omentectomy, partial, 199
Organic anion loss, 95
Osmotic agents, 115
Osteitis fibrosa, 246, 249
Osteomalacia, 246, 249
Outflow, total dialysate, 85

Patient acceptability, 189
Patient–peritoneal dialysis model, 36

PDPD, 187
Peclet number, 37
Pediatric CAPD, 196
　population, 189, 221
Peritoneal
　calcium balance, 244
　capillaries, 68
　circulation, 54
　clearances, 270
　fluid protein, 217
　lavage, 254
　permeability, 77
　protein losses, 270
　route, 63
　surface area, 237
　transfer, 65
　transport, 7, 48
　urea clearance(s), 84, 85
　visibility, 80
Peritoneogram, 199
Peritoneum wall, 8
Peritonitis, 8, 13, 21, 59, 63, 183, 184, 185, 186, 187, 203, 217, 253, 259, 265, 267, 269, 270
　definition of, 265
　diagnosis of, 265
　in children, 217
　treatment, 261, 268
Personality inventory, 178
Personnel requirements, 24
Pharmacokinetics, 63
Philosophy of CAPD, 169
Phosphate, 181, 183
Phosphorous binders, 259
Physical well-being of patients, 172
Physiology of peritoneal transport, 7
Placement of peritoneal catheter in infants and children, 197
Plastic bags, 15
Pores, 68
Portal venous pressure, 56
Positive nitrogen balance, 92
Potassium, 59
Prep kit, 168
Prolonged-dwell peritoneal dialysis, 187
Prostaglandins, 57
Protein
　catabolic rate, 76
　concentrations, 269
　intake, 84, 88
　loss, 87, 270
Proteus, 185
Pseudomonas, 185

Psychosocial well-being of patients, 172
Publications, 2

Quality of life, 135, 171

RC(s), 41, 48, 49
Reabsorption rate(s), 42, 47
Recommended dietary allowance, 85
Reflection coefficient(s), 36, 41, 44, 48, 49, 50, 236
Reimbursement, generally, 27–33
　area wage index, 29
　cost, 30
　incentive, 29
　national base rates, 29
　national rate, 28
　self-dialysis, 27
　transition exception, 29
Removal of the permanent catheter, 261
Renal osteodystrophy,
　and CAPD 249–252
　in CAPD, 243–247
Renal transplantation results in children, 217
Renal urea clearance, 85
Research funding, 2
Residual renal function, 83
Rubel, Eugene, 27

Secretin, 56
Self-deprecation, 178
Self-image, 136
Serial clearance data, 80
Serum
　albumin, 181, 183
　calcium, 183
　cholesterol, 157
　metabolites, 21
　proteins, 86
　tryglycerides, 110
　urea nitrogen, 84
Sexual functioning, 176
Sieving coefficients, 48
Sinus tract infection, 141
Skin color and texture, changes in, 136
Skin exit site, 259
Sleeping, improvement of, 135
Small molecules, adequate removal of, 129
Small volume bag technique, 199
Social benefits, 189
Social freedom, 136
Solute
　movement, 7
　transfer, 37
　transport, 38

Index 277

Solution flow, prevention of by gripper clamp, 168
Specifically designed materials, 167
Splanchic blood volume, 55
Stagnant fluid films, 71
 film conditions, 68
Standardized peritoneal dialysis regimen, 83
Staphylococcus, 185
Sterile peritonitis, 9
Streptococcus, 185
Stress, 176
Subperiosteal resporption, 245
Sulfamethoxazole, 63
SUN, 84
Supplies, bulk form, 168
Surgical management of chronic peritoneal catheters, 197
Sympathetic innervation, 56
Symptoms, 105

Taste improvement, 135
Teaching, 133
Teaching aids, 133
Technical aspects, 24
Technique for CAPD, in children, 214
Tenckhoff catheters, 197
Titanium adaptor, 21, 167
Tobramycin, 269
Total daily urea clearance, 85
Total dialysate outflow, 85
Total protein, changes in, 114
Total serum proteins, 181, 183
Toxicity of small and middle molecules, 103
Training, infants and chilren, 199
Training program, 8, 133

Transferrin C_3 and C_4, 89
Transmembrane hydrostatic pressure, 70
Transport resistances, 49
Trimethoprim, 63
Tubing change tray, need for, 168
Tunnel abscess, 261
Turbid drainage, 266

Ultrafiltration, 37, 38, 42, 45, 49, 114, 223, 232
 maximum, 235
 maximum rates, 235
 profile, 40, 41, 42
 rate(s), 40, 54, 71, 117
Unresolved issues, 1
"Up and down" feeling, loss of, 135
Urea clearances, 67, 71, 85
Urea generation rates, 76
Uremic patients, 103
 toxins, 67, 103
 treatments, 11

Very low-density lipoprotein cholesterol, 155
Vitamin B_{12} clearances, 80
VLDL, 155
Volume curve, 40
 profile(s), 47
 selector, 169

Wasting, 83
Weekly clearance, 84
 peritoneal clearances, 71
Weight, changes, in, 144
Well-being of patients, 169, 172
White cell count, 259, 260, 265